Practical Manual of Operative Laparoscopy and Hysteroscopy

Second Edition

Springer
*New York
Berlin
Heidelberg
Barcelona
Budapest
Hong Kong
London
Milan
Paris
Santa Clara
Singapore
Tokyo*

Ricardo Azziz
Professor, Department of
Obstetrics and Gynecology
University of Alabama
School of Medicine
Birmingham, Alabama

Ana Alvarez Murphy
Director, Division of
Reproductive Endocrinology
Department of Obstetrics and Gynecology
Emory University School of Medicine
Atlanta, Georgia

Editors

Practical Manual of Operative Laparoscopy and Hysteroscopy

Second Edition

Illustrated by Rod Powers and Josephine Taylor

With 200 figures in 269 parts

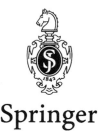

Springer

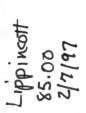

Lippincott
85.00
2/7/97

Ricardo Azziz, M.D., M.P.H.
Professor, Department of Obstetrics
  and Gynecology
University of Alabama School of
  Medicine
618 South 20th St.
Birmingham, AL 35233-7333, USA

Ana Alvarez Murphy, M.D.
Director, Division of Reproductive
  Endocrinology
Department of Obstetrics and Gynecology
Emory University School of Medicine
1639 Pierce Drive
Atlanta, GA 30322, USA

Library of Congress Cataloging in Publication Data
Practical manual of operative laparoscopy and hysteroscopy / [edited
  by] Ricardo Azziz, Ana Alvarez Murphy. — 2nd ed.
        p.   cm.
    Includes bibliographical references and index.
    ISBN 0-387-94696-9 (alk. paper : hrdcvr)
    1. Generative organs, Female—Endoscopic surgery.   I. Azziz,
Ricardo.   II. Murphy, Ana Alvarez.
    [DNLM: 1. Genital Diseases, Female—Surgery.   2.   Laparoscopy—
methods.   3. Hysteroscopy—methods.   WP 660 B895 1996]
RG104.7.P73   1996
618.1'059—dc20
DNLM/DLC   96-21229
for Library of Congress

Printed on acid-free paper.

Production coordinated by Impressions Book and Journal Services, Inc. and managed by Terry Kornak;
  manufacturing supervised by Jeffrey Taub.
Typeset by Impressions Book and Journal Services, Inc., Madison, WI.
Printed and bound by Edwards Brothers, Inc., Ann Arbor, MI.
Printed in the United States of America.

9 8 7 6 5 4 3 2 1

ISBN 0-387-94696-9   Springer-Verlag New York Berlin Heidelberg   SPIN 10524802

To our families for their love and support, and in memoriam of Rod Powers,
a wonderful friend and artist

Foreword to the First Edition

In the past decade, the future of gynecologic endoscopic surgery has been largely unpredictable. Now it is obvious that time has changed gynecology in such a way as to make many of the procedures that were commonly done obsolete. At no other time in the history of gynecologic surgery has such an explosion occurred, thus changing the face of this specialty to such a great degree. But in addition to solving many problems, the past decade has left us with many new and novel dilemmas.

One of the ways in which our field has tremendously evolved is that not only have some procedures become obsolete, but also to some degree gynecologic surgeons have themselves become obsolete. I write this because those not trained in the new techniques have had to go back and learn these surgical procedures in an unconventional way. This "unconventional way" is attending courses, and being supervised and preceptored by members of one's own hospital staff, then finally transmitted into granting of privileges. It is the young who are the leaders and, paradoxically, bringing experience to the field. In many instances, I have seen the resident who is a better endoscopic surgeon than the Senior Attending.

Not only have new techniques and operations been introduced, such as the use of the resectoscope and electrocautery to remove intrauterine myomas, but a new technology has also arisen. Mastery is imperative. One cannot master these techniques by mimicking what other surgeons do, but must understand the principles of the technological advances. Laser physics and properties must be understood and, in addition, optics and television technology are critical to performing excellent endoscopic surgery.

Old timers are playing catch-up ball, but it is the young who are the leaders and pioneers in our field. It is for this reason that this text represents all that is important in endoscopic surgery. It not only is a comprehensive and encyclopedic dissertation on the subject, but it is written by the young leaders in the field. This is a textbook that will go through many editions, passed on from generation to generation of endoscopic surgeons. Not only are the important subjects tackled (i.e., techniques) but also the important principles are covered: adhesion prevention, laser surgery, hemostasis, and instrumentation. Such difficult topics as cost-effectiveness, risk–benefit ratio, and need for randomized clinical studies are attacked with fervor to evaluate results properly.

This is an important text and destined to become a classic. It is comprehensive, principle oriented, and serves a real and tangible need.

I write this foreword with pride as an elder in the field.

Alan H. Decherney, M.D.
Professor and Chair
Department of Obstetrics and Gynecology
UCLA School of Medicine
Los Angeles, California

Acknowledgments

We would like to thank our secretaries, Jo Kirkpatrick and Esther Davidson, for their excellent assistance in the preparation of the manuscripts.

R. Azziz and A. Alvarez Murphy

Contents

Contributors

RICARDO AZZIZ, M.D., M.P.H.
Division of Reproductive Biology and Endocrinology, Department of Obstetrics and Gynecology, The University of Alabama at Birmingham School of Medicine, 619 South 20th Street, Birmingham, Al 35233-7333, USA

RICHARD E. BLACKWELL, PH.D., M.D.
Division of Reproductive Biology and Endocrinology, Department of Obstetrics and Gynecology, The University of Alabama at Birmingham School of Medicine, 619 South 20th Street, Birmingham, Al 35233-7333, USA

ANDREW I. BRILL, M.D.
Department of Obstetrics and Gynecology, The University of Chicago, 820 South Wood Street, Chicago, IL 60612-7313, USA

RICHARD P. BUYALOS, M.D.
Division of Reproductive Endocrinology and Infertility, Department of Obstetrics and Gynecology, University of Kentucky School of Medicine, 800 Rose Street, Lexington, KY 40536-0084, USA

MARIAN D. DAMEWOOD, M.D.
Greater Baltimore Medical Center, Women's Resource Center, 6569 North Charles Street, Suite 406, Baltimore, MD 21117; and Department of Gynecology and Obstetrics, The Johns Hopkins University School of Medicine, 600 North Wolfe Street, Baltimore, MD 21205, USA

JAMES F. DANIELL, M.D.
Women's Health Group, 2222 State Street, Suite A, Nashville, TN 37202, USA

MICHAEL P. DIAMOND, M.D.
Division of Reproductive Endocrinology, Department of Obstetrics and Gynecology, Hutzel Hospital/Wayne State University School of Medicine, 4707 St. Antoine Blvd., Detroit, MI 48201, USA

JACQUELINE N. GUTMANN, M.D.
Department of Obstetrics and Gynecology, Thomas Jefferson University School of
Medicine, 1025 Walnut Street, Philadelphia, PA 19107; and Philadelphia Fertility
Institute, 815 Locust Street, Philadelphia, PA 19107, USA

JOHN S. HESLA, M.D.
The Center for Reproductive Medicine, 799 E. Hampden Avenue, Suite 300, Engle-
wood, CO 80110, USA

WILLIAM W. HURD, M.D.
Division of Reproductive Endocrinology, Department of Obstetrics and Gynecology, Indiana University School of Medicine, 550 University Boulevard, Indianapolis, IN 46202, USA

BRADLEY S. HURST, M.D.
Division of Reproductive Endocrinology, Department of Obstetrics and Gynecol-
ogy, University of Colorado Health Sciences Center, 4200 East 9th Avenue, Box
B198, Denver, CO 80262, USA

JEAN A. HURTEAU, M.D.
Division of Gynecologic Oncology, Department of Obstetrics and Gynecology, Indiana University School of Medicine, 550 University Boulevard, Indianapolis, IN
46202, USA

EUGENE KATZ, M.D.
Greater Baltimore Medical Center, Women's Hospital Fertility Center, 6569 North
Charles Street, Suite 406, Baltimore, MD 21117, USA

ERIC S. KNOCHENHAUER, M.D.
Division of Reproductive Biology and Endocrinology, Department of Obstetrics
and Gynecology, The University of Alabama at Birmingham School of Medicine,
619 South 20th Street, Birmingham, AL 35233-7333, USA

DAN C. MARTIN, M.D.
Department of Obstetrics and Gynecology, University of Tennessee, Memphis, TN
38103; and Reproductive Surgery, 1717 Kirby Parkway, Suite 100, Memphis, TN
38120, USA

ARLENE MORALES, M.D.
Department of Reproductive Medicine, University of California at San Diego, 9500
Gilman Drive, BSB 5046B, La Jolla, CA, 92093-0633, USA

ANA ALVAREZ MURPHY, M.D.
Division of Reproductive Endocrinology, Department of Gynecology and Obstet-
rics, Emory University School of Medicine, 1639 Pierce Drive, Atlanta, GA 30322,
USA

DENISE MURRAY, M.D.
9708 Medical Center Drive, Suite 230, Rockville, MD 20850, USA

CAMRAN NEZHAT, M.D.
Department of Surgery and Department of Gynecology and Obstetrics, Stanford University School of Medicine, 300 Pasteur Drive, Stanford, CA 94305; Center for Special Pelvic Surgery, 5555 Peachtree Dunwoody Road, Suite 276, Atlanta, GA 30342; and 900 Welch Road, Suite 403, Palo Alto, CA 94304, USA

CEANA H. NEZHAT, M.D.
Department of Gynecology and Obstetrics, Stanford University School of Medicine, 300 Pasteur Drive, Stanford, CA 94305; and Center for Special Pelvic Surgery, 5555 Peachtree Dunwoody Road, Suite 276, Atlanta, GA 30342, USA

FARR NEZHAT, M.D.
Department of Gynecology and Obstetrics, Stanford University School of Medicine, 300 Pasteur Drive, Stanford, CA 94305; and Center for Special Pelvic Surgery, 900 Welch Road, Suite 403, Palo Alto, CA 94304, USA

STEVEN F. PALTER, M.D.
Yale Office Laparoscopy Program, Division of Reproductive Endocrinology, Department of Obstetrics and Gynecology, Yale University School of Medicine, 789 Howard Avenue, New Haven, CT 65210, USA

C. PAUL PERRY, M.D.
2006 Brookwood Medical Center Drive, Suite 402, Birmingham, AL 35209, USA

SUJATHA REDDY, M.D.
Division of Reproductive Endocrinology, Department of Gynecology and Obstetrics, Emory University School of Medicine, 875 Johnson Ferry Road NE, Atlanta, GA 30342, USA

HARRY REICH, M.D.
Wyoming Valley GYN/OB Associates, 480 Pierce Drive, Kingston, PA 18704; and Department of Obstetrics and Gynecology, Center for Advanced Laparoscopic Surgery, Columbia University College of Physicians and Surgeons, 622 West 168th Street, New York, NY 10032, USA

JOHN A. ROCK, M.D.
Division of Reproductive Endocrinology, Department of Gynecology and Obstetrics, Emory University School of Medicine, 1639 Pierce Drive, Atlanta, GA 30322, USA

MICHAEL J. SAMMARCO, M.D.
Department of Obstetrics and Gynecology, The University of Chicago, 820 South Wood Street, Chicago, IL 60612-7313, USA

WILLIAM D. SCHLAFF, M.D.
Division of Reproductive Endocrinology, Department of Obstetrics and Gynecology, University of Colorado Health Sciences Center, Campus Box B-198, 4200 East Ninth Avenue, Denver, CO 80262, USA

STEFANIE SCHUPP CHRISTIAN, M.D.
Department of Obstetrics and Gynecology, University of Colorado Health Sciences Center, Campus Box B-198, 4200 East Ninth Avenue, Denver, CO 80262, USA

DANIEL S. SEIDMAN, M.D.
Department of Gynecology and Obstetrics, Stanford University School of Medicine, 300 Pasteur Drive, Stanford, CA 94305, USA

SCOTT M. SLAYDEN, M.D.
Division of Reproductive Biology and Endocrinology, Department of Obstetrics and Gynecology, The University of Alabama at Birmingham School of Medicine, 619 South 20th Street, Birmingham, AL 35233-7333, USA

SAMUEL SMITH, M.D.
Division of Reproductive Endocrinology and Infertility, Department of Obstetrics and Gynecology, Sinai Hospital Baltimore, 2411 W. Belvedere Avenue, Suite 206, Baltimore, MD 21215, USA

YOLANDA R. SMITH, M.D.
Division of Reproductive Endocrinology, Department of Obstetrics and Gynecology, University of Michigan Medical Center, 1500 East Medical Center Drive, Ann Arbor, MI 48109, USA

MICHAEL P. STEINKAMPF, M.D.
Department of Obstetrics and Gynecology, The University of Alabama at Birmingham School of Medicine, 619 South 20th Street, Birmingham, AL 35233-7333, USA

J. BENJAMIN YOUNGER, M.D.
American Society for Reproductive Medicine, 1209 Montgomery Highway, Birmingham, AL 35216-2809, USA

HOWARD A. ZACUR, M.D.
Division of Reproductive Endocrinology and Infertility, Department of Gynecology and Obstetrics, The Johns Hopkins University School of Medicine, 600 N. Wolfe Street, Houck Building, Room 247, Baltimore, MD 21287, USA

Introduction

Peritoneoscopy and culdoscopy were first introduced in the second edition of *TeLinde's Operative Gynecology* in 1953. TeLinde noted, "In many instances we find peritoneoscopy to be a useful procedure. Nevertheless it often left something to be desired." During the subsequent four decades, enormous progress has allowed the expansion of the application of laparoscopy and hysteroscopy throughout gynecology. Thus, it is appropriate and quite useful to have a text devoted solely to this rapidly advancing specialty.

In its second edition, the text *Practical Manual of Operative Laparoscopy and Hysteroscopy* is a complete and honest overview of the field providing the reader with a critical appraisal of the current literature on technique, development, and long-term follow-up. Refreshingly, the authors include not only the American experience but also advances from Europe and Asia.

Ricardo Azziz and Ana Alvarez Murphy have carefully organized the text into general concepts and laparoscopic and hysteroscopic operative techniques. The editors have selected authors of national and international stature to prepare chapters in their areas of expertise. The edited text carefully analyzes the advantages and disadvantages of each operative technique so as to allow readers insight as to the proper place for a particular endoscopic technique in their surgical practices.

Finally, I am particularly pleased and proud to have the opportunity to introduce the second edition. Dr. Azziz and Dr. Murphy were both fellows in reproductive endocrinology and infertility at the Johns Hopkins Hospital and have independently developed an international reputation as authorities in reproductive surgery. I was privileged to have the opportunity to work with both editors and attest to their surgical philosophy of careful study of surgical devices and techniques before their acceptance in clinical practice.

John A. Rock, M.D.
James Robert McCord Professor and Chairman
Department of Gynecology and Obstetrics
Emory University School of Medicine
Atlanta, Georgia

Part I
General Concepts in Operative Endoscopy

1

History of the Development of Gynecologic Endoscopic Surgery

Marian D. Damewood

As early as 500 A.D. a "siphopherot" or tube made of lead and used to bring the internal female genitalia within range of the physician's eye was described (Fig. 1.1).[1] This ancient accomplishment resulted in visualization of the external cervical os through dilatation of the vagina. In the last two decades developments in the techniques of operative laparoscopy and operative hysteroscopy have had a major impact on the specialty of gynecologic surgery. At present, laparoscopy is the most frequently performed gynecologic procedure in the United States. The development of endoscopic surgery has been primarily stimulated by the worldwide need for permanent sterilization methods. Most importantly, improvements in our ability to achieve intraabdominal hemostasis, primarily through the use of electrocoagulation, has made it possible to perform surgical procedures through the laparoscope.

Development of Laparoscopy

The first reported observation of the human peritoneal cavity with an optical instrument was by Jacobaeus in Scandinavia in 1910.[2] However, several developments predated this report. As early as 1805, Bozzani in Germany vi-sualized the urethral orifice with candlelight and a simple tube. This led to Desormeaux's development, in 1843, of the first urethroscope and cystoscope using mirrors to reflect light from a kerosene lamp.[3] After this development Stein, in Germany (1874), developed a photo endoscope. Nitze, also from Germany, added a lens system to the endoscopic tube allowing magnification of the viewed area.[4] The invention of the light bulb in the United States by Thomas Edison had a significant impact on the development of gynecologic endoscopy. Newman in Scotland developed a cystoscope using a small incandescent light bulb at the distal end (1883). Kelling from Germany (1902) first reported peritoneal endoscopy in dogs creating a pneumoperitoneum using a needle and a cystoscope designed by Nitze.[5] Subsequently, Jacobaeus (1910) used a trocar and cannula to induce pneumoperitoneum in women, introducing a Nitze cystoscope through the same cannula to achieve pelviscopy, laparoscopy, or peritoneoscopy.[2]

Several refinements in the technique of peritoneoscopy preceded its application to gynecologic surgery. Orndoff from the United States developed a sharp pyramidal point on the laparoscopic trocar to facilitate puncture.[6] An automatic trocar sheath valve was then intro-

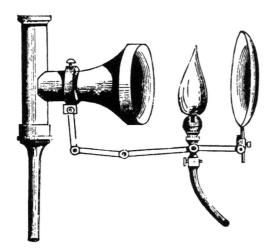

FIGURE 1.1. The "photoendoscope" or sipho-pherot described in the Talmud.[4]

duced to prevent escape of air. Although the first pneumoperitoneum was created using air, Zollikoffer from Switzerland went on to use carbon dioxide (CO_2).[7] A fore-oblique 45° lens system and the use of a second puncture for upper abdominal procedures were introduced by Kalk from Germany (1929).[8] Biopsy instru-

mentation and cauterization of intraabdominal adhesions at laparoscopy was re-reported by Fervers from Germany (1933).[9] This report was followed by the introduction of a single-puncture operating laparoscope by Ruddock in the United States in 1934,[10] and followed almost immediately by Boesch's utilization of a 40° to 50° pelvic elevation during the procedure. In 1937 Hope (United States) used Ruddock's peritoneoscope to diagnose ectopic pregnancies.[11] In the United States, Anderson (1937) and Powers and Barnes (1941) performed endothermal coagulation of the fallopian tube for the purpose of sterilization.[12,13] A laparoscopic uterine suspension was performed in 1942 by Donaldson and colleagues (United States).[14] An alternative approach to peritoneoscopy, the culdoscope, was introduced by Decker in 1944 (Fig. 1.2).

The first gynecologist to use laparoscopy clinically on a wide basis was Palmer in France (1947).[15] He was also responsible for the introduction of the endouterine cannula for uterine manipulation and for the development of chromotubation. Further advancements in our ability to perform surgical procedures at laparoscopy occurred with the introduction of

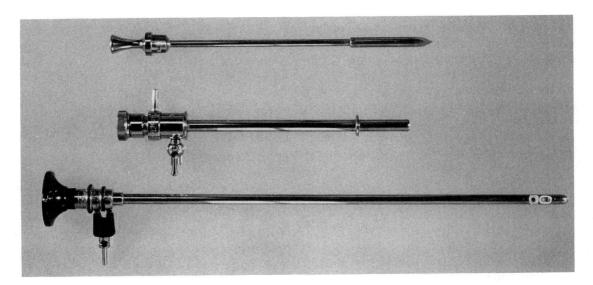

FIGURE 1.2. Decker culdoscope manufactured by American Cystoscope Makers, Inc. Note incandescent distal lamp and 90° viewing angle. From top to bottom: pyramidal trocar, sheath with distal stop, and culdoscope. (Courtesy of Dr. Michael P. Steinkampf.)

TABLE 1.1.   Chronology of the development of laparoscopy.

Investigator	Date	Development
Bozzani	1805	Visualization of urethral orifice with candlelight and simple tube
Desormeaux	1843	Presentation of first urethroscope and cystoscope, using mirrors to reflect kerosene lamplight. First effective endoscope
Stein	1874	Development of photoendoscope
Nitze	1877	Addition of lens system to endoscopic tube, thus allowing magnification of area viewed
Edison	1880	Invention of incandescent lamp bulb
Newman	1883	Development of a cystoscope using a small incandescent light bulb at distal end
Boisseau de Rocher	1889	Separation of ocular part from introducing sheath and use of different telescopes through sheath
Kelling	1901	Creation of air pneumoperitoneum in dogs using a needle, followed by insertion of a Nitze cystoscope
Jacobaeus	1910	Creation of air pneumoperitoneum in humans using a trocar, followed by introduction of a Nitze cystoscope through the trocar. First recorded observation of a human peritoneal cavity with an optical instrument
Orndoff	1920	Development of sharp pyramidal point on the trocar to facilitate puncture and automatic trocar sheath valve to prevent escape of air (peritoneoscopy)
Zollikoffer	1924	Used carbon dioxide instead of air to create pneumoperitoneum
Korbsch	1927	First textbook with an atlas of laparoscopy
Kalk	1929	Developed fore-oblique (45°) lens system. Introduced second puncture for upper abdominal procedures
Fervers	1933	Cauterization of intraabdominal adhesions
Ruddock	1934	Developed single-puncture operating laparoscope. Published results of 900 peritoneoscopies. 100% diagnostic accuracy in 58 cases of ectopic pregnancy
Boesch	1935	Utilization of 40°–50° of pelvic elevation
Anderson	1937	Endothermic coagulation of fallopian tube as a method of sterilization
Powers & Barnes	1941	Sterilization by means of laparoscopy tubal cautery
Decker	1944	Introduction of culdoscopy
Palmer	1947	First gynecologist to use gynecologic laparoscopy clinically. Introduced the endouterine cannula for uterine manipulation and tubal patency testing
Hopkins & Kapany	1952	Introduction of fiberoptics to endoscopy
Palmer	1962	Utilization of electrocoagulation for tubal sterilization by laparoscopy
Frangenheim	1963	Used diathermy for tubal sterilization by laparoscopy
Semm	1963	Automatic insufflation of the pneumoperitoneum and complete pelviscopy instrumentation set
Steptoe	1967	First laparoscopy textbook in the English language
Steptoe & Edwards	1970	Recovery of oocyte with the laparoscope for in vitro fertilization
Clarke	1972	Introduction of instruments for tubal ligation by laparoscopy
Hulka	1972	Introduced clips for tubal sterilization by laparoscopy
Rioux	1973	Development of bipolar cautery for tubal sterilization by laparoscopy
Yoon	1974	Utilization of silastic rings for tubal sterilization by laparoscopy

fiberoptics in 1952 by Hopkins and Kapany. In the early 1960s Harold Hopkins went on to design the rod lens system used in most endoscopes today. Almost concurrently, Frangenheim[16] in Germany (1963) and Palmer in France continued to develop electrocoagulation for tubal sterilization by laparoscopy. The availability of intraabdominal electrocoagulation was a major impetus to the development of pelviscopy, since this type of surgery would not be possible without the ability to achieve intraperitoneal hemostasis. Additional advancements in pelviscopic techniques and instrumentation have been attributed to Kurt Semm of Germany. In 1963, he introduced the use of an automatic insufflator to maintain pneumoperitoneum.[17] Semm is also credited with the introduction of a complete pelviscopy instrumentation set, which has since been updated and modified.

In the 1970s laparoscopy was increasingly used for intraabdominal surgery. Steptoe and Edwards recovered the first oocyte for in vitro fertilization in 1970 using the laparoscope.[18] Until the introduction of transvaginal ultrasound oocyte retrieval in the late 1980s, laparoscopy had formed an integral part of the in vitro fertilization procedure. Laparoscopic tubal sterilization using clips was introduced by Hulka and colleagues in 1972.[19] Rioux (1973) from Canada developed bipolar cautery for laparoscopic tubal sterilization. Yoon of the United States (1974) laparoscopically applied silastic rings, also for tubal sterilization. The chronology of the development of operative laparoscopy is summarized in Table 1.1.

Concurrent with the development in the technology of laparoscopy, a significant body of information was developed. The first textbook with an atlas of laparoscopy was published by Korbsh from Germany in 1927. Ruddock in the United States in the late 1930s published results of 900 laparoscopies.[20] Specific reference in this publication was given to the diagnostic accuracy of laparoscopy with respect to ectopic pregnancy. Two years later Beling, also from the United States, published a review that listed indications for laparoscopy with specific reference to endometriosis, chronic pelvic inflammatory disease, and the diagnosis of ectopic pregnancy. Palmer in 1947 published results of his case series of 250 procedures. The late 1950s and early 1960s saw the introduction of multiple textbooks of gynecologic laparoscopy. A German textbook was published in 1959 by Frangenheim, followed by Thoyer-Rozat[21] with a French version, and Albano and Cittadini[22] with an Italian text on gynecologic endoscopy. The first textbook of laparoscopy published in the English language was by Steptoe from the United Kingdom, in 1967.[23] Cohen and Fear from the United States presented the first American publication of gynecologic laparoscopy, followed by the first American textbook of gynecologic laparoscopy in 1970.[24] Additional large case reports concerning outpatient laparoscopic procedures were reported by Wheeless from the United States in 1970.[25]

Standards for laparoscopic surgery have been set and followed in the United States. In 1972 Phillips founded the American Association of Gynecologic Laparoscopists (AAGL), and during the same year Hulka coordinated the first annual report of Complications Committee of the AAGL.

The impact of diagnostic and operative laparoscopy on gynecologic practice has been significant. Laparoscopy has allowed the gynecologist to establish the diagnosis in a large number of clinical situations and has reduced greatly the need for laparotomy. Additional advances stimulated the laparoscopic treatment of endometriosis, pelvic adhesions, tubal disease, ectopic pregnancies, and ovarian cysts. A significant reduction in cost, postoperative morbidity, and recuperation with respect to laparotomy has also been documented.

Development of Hysteroscopy

Attempts at visualization of the uterine cavity preceded the development of peritoneoscopy. As early as 1000 A.D., Abulkasim used a mirror to reflect light into the vaginal vault. Desormeaux (1853) in France inspected the interior of the uterus with an early endoscope and reported the first "satisfactory" hysteroscopy. In addition, he identified polyps in the uterus of a postmenopausal patient experiencing vaginal bleeding.[26] Aubinais in 1864[27] inspected the uterine cavity with the naked eye and Pantaleoni[28] from Ireland used a cystoscope (Fig. 1.3) initially designed by Desormeaux to identify uterine polyps (1868). Clado (1898) in France described several models of hysteroscopic instrumentation and published material on the technique of hysteroscopy (Fig. 1.4).[29] This accomplishment was followed by the publication of a treatise on hysteroscopy, with specific reference to contact hysteroscopy (Fig. 1.5), by David in 1908.[30]

Further refinements in hysteroscopy were directed at the development of effective distending media and clear visualization of the uterine cavity. Rubin in 1925 combined the cystoscope with CO_2 insufflation of the uterine cavity.[31] In

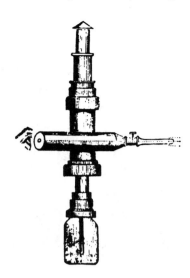

FIGURE 1.3. The first hysteroscope used by Pantaleoni (1868).[29] The alcohol lamp at the bottom provided light for the tapered metal hysteroscope. (Reproduced with permission from Barbot J. History of hysteroscopy. In: Baggish MS, Burbot J, Valle RF, eds. *Diagnostic and Operative Hysteroscopy: A Text and Atlas*, Chicago: Year Book Medical Publishers; 1989.)

1928 Gauss used water to flush blood and distend the uterine cavity.[32] The water source in this case was held 50 cm above the patient. Use of a transparent rubber balloon mounted on the endoscope that was subsequently inflated within the uterine cavity was presented by Silander in 1962.[33] Edstrom and Fernstrom in 1970 introduced high molecular weight dextran as a distension medium.[34] Lindemann in 1970 used CO_2 for uterine distension.[35] These developments increased the clinical utility of hysteroscopy. Developments in hysteroscopy are summarized in Table 1.2.

Since the lens systems of earlier hysteroscopes were inferior, inadequate light and image transmission occurred frequently. At present, most hysteroscopes consist of a lens system surrounded by glass fibers carrying light into the uterine cavity. However, Vulmiere in 1952 used a rigid one-piece mineral glass guide, which when properly treated could not only illuminate but also magnify the image when in direct contact with the object. In 1963 an optical trocar in an italic sheath was used and perfected in 1973 when Barbot introduced it for clinical use in France.[29] In 1979 Baggish reported the first experience with this instrument in the United States.[29] Contact hysteroscopy optics were combined with the principles of modern panoramic hysteroscopy into a single instrument, the microcolpohysteroscope, introduced by Hamou in 1980.[36] As recently as 1987 Baggish introduced a focusing panoramic hysteroscope with a four-channel operating sheath particularly useful for laser procedures.[29]

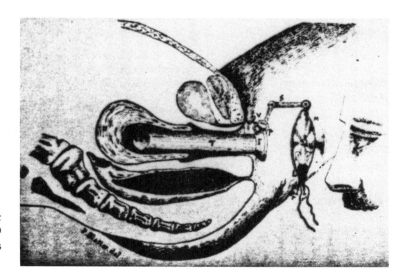

FIGURE 1.4. The hysteroscopic technique of Clado (1898).[29] (Reproduced with permission as in Fig. 1.3.)

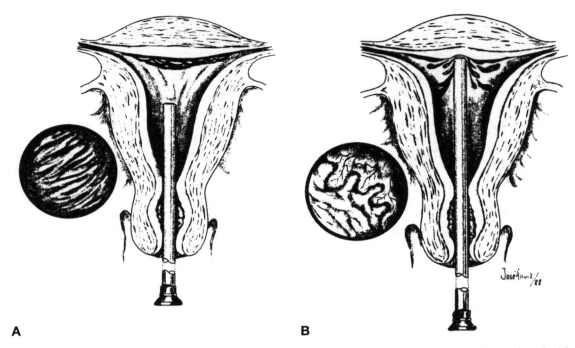

A   **B**

FIGURE 1.5.   Early contact hysteroscope (1907).[29,30] **A:** Before contact. **B:** After contact. (Reproduced with permission as in Figure 1.3.)

TABLE 1.2.   Chronology of the development of hysteroscopy.

Investigator	Date (A.D.)	Development
Abulkasim	1000	Utilization of mirror to reflect light into vaginal vault
Desormeaux	1853	Inspection of interior of uterus with early endoscope, first "satisfactory" endoscope
Aubinais	1864	Inspection of uterine cavity with the naked eye
Pantaleoni	1868	Used cystoscope designed by Desormeaux to identify uterine polyps
Clado	1898	Described several models of hysteroscopic instruments
David	1907	Treatise on hysteroscopy, with specific reference to contact hysteroscopy
Ruben	1925	Combination of a cystoscope with CO_2 insufflation of the uterine cavity
Gauss	1928	Use of water to flush blood and distend uterine cavity. Water source held 50 cm above the patient
Silander	1962	Use of a transparent rubber balloon mounted on the endoscope inflated within the uterine cavity
Edstrom & Fernstrom	1970	Introduction of high molecular weight dextran as a distention medium
Lindemann	1970	Use of CO_2 for uterine distension
Hamou	1980	Introduction of the microcolpohysteroscope
Baggish	1987	Invention of a focusing panoramic hysteroscope and a four-channel operating sheath particularly advantageous for the Nd:YAG laser

References

1. The Talmud.
2. Jacobaeus HC. Uber die Moglichkeit, die Zystoskopie bei Untersuchung seroser Hohlungen anzuwenden. *Munich Med Wochenschr.* 1910; 57: 2090–2092.
3. Gunning JE. History of laparoscopy. In: Phillips JM, ed. *Laparoscopy.* Baltimore: Williams & Wilkins; 1977:6–16.
4. Nitze M. *Uber eine neue Beleuchtungsmethode der Hoblen des menschlichen Korpers.* Wien: Med. Presse; 1879:V20;851–858.
5. Kelling G. Uber Oesophagoskopie, Gastroskopie

und Colioskopie. *Munich Med Wochenschr.* 1902; 49:21–24.

6. Orndoff BH. The peritoneoscope in diagnosis of diseases of the abdomen. *J Radiol.* 1920; 1:307–325.

7. Zollikoffer R. Uber Laparoskopie. *Schweiz Med Wochenschr.* 1924;104:264–272.

8. Kalk H. Erfahrungen mit der Laparoskopie (zugleich mit Beschreibung eines neuen Instrumentes). *Z Klin Med.* 1929;111:303–348.

9. Fervers C. Die Laparoskopie mit dem Cystoskop. Ein Beitrag zur Vereinfachung der Technik und zur endoskopischen Strangdurchtrennung in der Bauchhohle. *Med Klin.* 1933; 29:1042–1045.

10. Ruddock JC. Peritoneoscopy. *West J Surg.* 1934; 42:392–405.

11. Hope RB. The differential diagnosis of ectopic gestation by peritoneoscopy. *Surg Gynecol Obstet.* 1937;64:229–234.

12. Anderson ET. Peritoneoscopy. *Am J Surg.* 1937; 35:36–43.

13. Power FH, Barnes AC. Sterilization by means of peritoneoscopic tubal fulguration. A preliminary report. *Am J Obstet Gynecol.* 1941; 41: 1038–1043.

14. Donaldson JK, Sanderlin JH, jun Harrel WB. Method of suspending uterus without open abdominal incision; use of peritoneoscope and special needle. *Am J Surg.* 1942;55:537–543.

15. Palmer R. Instrumentation et technique de la couldoscopie gynecologique. *Gynecol Obstet.* 1947;46:422–429.

16. Frangenheim H. Tubal sterilization under visualization with the laparoscope. *Geburtsch u Frauenheilk.* 1964;24:470–478.

17. Semm K. Das Pneumoperitoneum mit CO_2. In: Demling L, Ottenjann R, eds. *Endoslopie—Methoden, Ergebnisse. S.* Munchen: Banaschewski; 1967:167–169.

18. Steptoe PC. Laparoscopic studies of the ovaries. *Ned Tijdschr Verloskd Gynaecol* 1970;70:296–300.

19. Hulka JF, Fishburne JI, Mercer JP, et al. Laparoscopic sterilization with a spring clip: a report of the first fifty cases. *Am J Obstet Gynecol.* 1973; 116:751–759.

20. Ruddock JC. Peritoneoscopy. *Surg Gynecol Obstet.* 1937;65:623–639.

21. Thoyer-Rozat J. *La Coelioscopie. Technique-Indications.* Paris: Masson; 1962.

22. Albano VE, Cittadini E. *La celioscopia in ginecologia* (monografia). Palermo: Denaro; 1962:I 420.

23. Steptoe PC. *Laparoscopy in Gynaecology.* Edinburgh, London: Livingstone; 1967.

24. Cohen MR. *Laparoscopy Culdoscopy and Gynecography: Technique and Atlas.* Philadelphia: Saunders; 1970.

25. Wheeless CR Jr. Outpatient sterilization by laparoscopy under local anesthesia in less developed countries. In: Duncan GW, Falb RD, Speidel JJ, eds. *Female Sterilization: Prognosis for Simplified Outpatient Procedures.* New York, London: Academic Press; 1972:125–129.

26. Desormeaux A-J. *L'Endoscopie Uterine, Applications au Diagnostic et au Traitement des Affections de l'Urethre de la Vessie.* Paris: Bailiere; 1865.

27. Aubinais. Union Med. 1864; no. 152.

28. Pantaleoni D. On endoscopic examination of the cavity of the womb. *Med Press Circ.* London 1869;8:26–28.

29. Barbot J. History of hysteroscopy. In: Baggish MS, Burbot J, Valle RF, eds. *Diagnostic and Operative Hysteroscopy: A Text and Atlas.* Chicago: Year Book Medical Publishers; 1986.

30. David CH. *L'Endoscopie Uterine, Applications au Diagnostic et au Traitement des Affections Intrauterines.* Paris: Jacques; 1908.

31. Rubin IC. Uterine endoscopy, endometrioscopy with the aid of uterine insufflation. *Am J Obstet Gynecol.* 1925;10:313–319.

32. Gauss CJ. Hysteroskopie. *Arch Gynaekol.* 1928; 133:18–24.

33. Silander T. Hysteroscopy through a transparent rubber balloon in patients with carcinoma of the uterine endometrium. *Acta Obstet Gynecol Scand.* 1963;42:284–296.

34. Edstrom K, Fernstrom I. The diagnostic possibilities of a modified hysteroscopic technique. *Acta Obstet Gynecol Scand.* 1970;49:327–330.

35. Lindemann J-J. The use of CO_2 in the uterine cavity for hysteroscopy. *Int J Fertil.* 1972; 17: 221–224.

36. Hamou J. Microhysteroscopy: a new procedure and its original applications in gynecology. *J Reprod Med.* 1981;26:375–382.

2

Training, Certification, and Credentialing in Gynecologic Operative Endoscopy

Ricardo Azziz

Introduction

Proper training, certification of competence, and credentialing are important to assure the highest quality of health care, maximizing success and minimizing morbidity. Furthermore, documentation of appropriate skills is essential for the medical-legal protection of the parent institution, the operating room personnel, and the surgeon. While complications are an accepted risk of endoscopic or any surgery, corroboration of a surgeon's training and skill in these techniques will minimize his or her liability in the face of an eventuality.

A common fallacy among practitioners is that the implementation of a uniform and fair credentialing process for operative endoscopy, either in a hospital or outpatient facility, results in an increased risk of litigation. In fact, hospitals and staff members are generally found negligent by the courts if a negative outcome occurs in the face of a failure to institute appropriate and reasonable quality control measures. As has been noted:[1]

"The hospital has the duty to protect its patients from malpractice by members of its medical staff when it knows or should have known that malpractice was likely to be committed upon them. . . . It was negligent in not knowing, because it did not have a system for acquiring knowledge."

Gonzales v. Nork. Superior Court,
Sacrament County, Cal., Nov. 19, 1973

The training and credentialing of endoscopic surgeons has become a pressing and immediate issue in our specialty[2]; pressing, because nonmedical agencies are taking rapid steps to implement credentialing guidelines. For example, the New York State Health Department has issued guidelines specifying "that surgeons must perform at least 15 laparoscopies under supervision" before a hospital may issue privileges permitting them to perform laparoscopic cholecystectomy, laparoscopic hysterectomies, and other advanced endoscopic procedures.[3] Unfortunately, poor or inadequate surgical training and certification has an immediate negative, and potentially fatal, impact on a patient's health. Again as an example, in New York State alone from August 1990 through June 1992, at least 7 patients had died and 185 others suffered serious or life-threatening complications from the performance of laparoscopic cholecystectomies.

Following is outlined the logic behind operative endoscopic training and certification, and a suggested outline for training designed to ensure optimum skill and expertise among gynecologic endoscopic surgeons.[4]

Training, Certification, and Credentialing Schemes

Training refers to the process by which knowledge and skill are acquired; certification refers to the process of documenting the acquired skill or expertise; and credentialing refers to the process by which a hospital governing board recognizes that training and competence of a surgeon and assigns him or her privileges to perform those procedures within the confines of that hospital. Training, certification, and credentialing can be based on a variety of schemes, differing in degree of specificity (Table 2.1). Nonetheless, these three steps form part of the same process and should ideally also follow the same scheme.

Credentials can be assigned on the basis of expertise in gynecologic operative endoscopy as a whole; the surgeon either is skilled or is not skilled in the overall technique. The American College of Obstetricians and Gynecologists (ACOG)[5] and the American Association

TABLE 2.1. Various training, certification, and credentialing schemes.

Most Simple
For operative endoscopy as a whole
For operative laparoscopy and hysteroscopy separately
By skill level, for operative laparoscopy and hysteroscopy separately
By type of procedure
Most Complex

of Gynecologic Laparoscopists (AAGL)[6] currently recommend such a scheme. Second, training and the assignment of privileges may be separated into those for operative laparoscopy and those for operative hysteroscopy. This type of scheme was previously recommended by ACOG.[7,8] A third and more intensive training/certification scheme is that based on specific procedures, documenting separately the skills for performing a laparoscopic-assisted hysterectomy, a presacral neurectomy, a neosalpingostomy, etc. Many hospitals currently utilize this scheme, although it is cumbersome and regressive, particularly in a field as rapidly changing as gynecologic operative endoscopy.

An alternate scheme, of intermediate complexity and that which we prefer, is based on the grouping of laparoscopic or hysteroscopic procedures according to the general skill level needed to complete them[4] (Tables 2.2 and 2.3). We believe that the logic of this scheme is

TABLE 2.2. Suggested skill levels for the training, certification, and credentialing of operative laparoscopy.

Level 1 (Basic operative laparoscopy):
    Ablation/removal of mild to moderate endometriosis, including endometriomas <3 cm in diameter
    Salpingo-ovariolysis of mild to moderate adhesions
    Uterosacral ablation
    Treatment of ectopic pregnancies
Level 2 (Advanced operative laparoscopy):
    Resection of moderate to severe endometriosis
    Resection of ovarian and parovarian cysts, including endometriomas
    Oophorectomy ± salpingectomy
    Neosalpingostomy and fimbrioplasty
    Lysis of moderate to severe peritubal, ovarian, and abdominal adhesions
    Myomectomy
    Appendectomies
Optional Level 3 (Innovative/experimental operative laparoscopy):[a]
    To include the performance of any procedures considered by the institution to be more risky, innovative, or experimental than usual (e.g., presacral neurectomies, nodal sampling, etc.)

[a]This level is not usually used in credentialing; rather, cases designated as level 3 may be reviewed at regular intervals by an appropriate committee (e.g., Quality Assurance) for complications, indications, etc.

TABLE 2.3. Suggested skill levels for the training, certification, and credentialing of operative hysteroscopy.

Level 1 (Basic operative hysteroscopy):
 Removal of polyps, small fibroids, and lost intrauterine devices (IUDs)
 Metroplasties
 Lysis of mild to moderate synechiae
Level 2 (Advanced operative hysteroscopy):
 Lysis of severe synechiae with obliteration of the uterine cavity
 Endometrial ablation
 Resection of larger fibroids

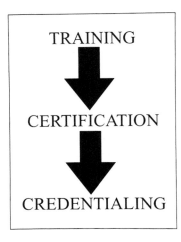

FIGURE 2.1. Surgical training, certification, and credentialing form part of the same process that culminates in the acquisition of the necessary knowledge and skills, documentation of these skills, and the assignment of operative privileges by a hospital or other operating facility. (Reprinted with permission from Azziz R. *Clin Obstet Gynecol.* 1995; 38:313–318.)

optimum because it follows naturally the attainment of surgical skills, it does not require continuous recertification as new applications for gynecologic operative endoscopy are described, and a trainee can realistically obtain sufficient experience in a reasonable amount of time to document competency. A skill level-specific credentialing system is currently recommended by the Society of Obstetricians and Gynaecologists of Canada (SOGC)[9] and the Society for Reproductive Surgeons (SRS) of the American Society for Reproductive Medicine (formerly the American Fertility Society).[10]

Training In Operative Endoscopy

Training refers to the portion of the process by which a practitioner acquires the necessary knowledge and skills to (1) appropriately select patients for surgical treatment, excluding those who would benefit from nonsurgical interventions; (2) select the type of procedure, including approach (e.g., endoscopic vs. laparotomy); (3) counsel and obtain consent from patients; (4) select the necessary instrumentation; (5) perform the procedure; (6) manage and minimize intraoperative complications; (7) manage the postoperative course; and (8) document indications, counseling, procedure, findings, and postoperative course.

Surgical training, certification, and credentialing form part of the same process (Fig. 2.1) culminating in the acquisition of the necessary knowledge and surgical skills, documentation

of these skills, and the assignment of operative privileges by a hospital or other operating facility. Aspiring operative endoscopists must first demonstrate knowledge and appropriate skills in the performance of diagnostic laparoscopy and hysteroscopy. For younger physicians, these techniques may have been incorporated into their residency training. For others these skills are acquired in the midst of an active and independent practice.

Endoscopic surgical training can be divided into three portions, specifically a didactic, an observational, and a tutorial phase (Fig. 2.2).

Didactic/Laboratory

During this portion of their training, the surgeon will review the theoretical aspects of the surgery, including physical principles, patient selection, preoperative evaluation and preparation, surgical technique, alternative treatments, outcome, and morbidity. Generally, attending one or two training courses, complemented by review of an appropriate text, suffices. Unfortunately, there is a tendency among surgeons today to attend a myriad of

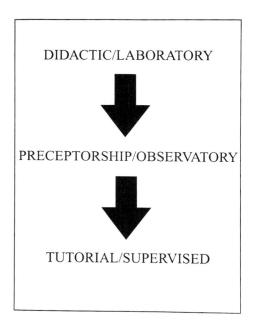

DIDACTIC/LABORATORY

PRECEPTORSHIP/OBSERVATORY

TUTORIAL/SUPERVISED

FIGURE 2.2. Endoscopic surgical training can be sequentially divided into a didactic/laboratory, a preceptorship (observational), and a tutorial (supervised) phase. (Reprinted with permission as in Fig. 2.1.)

such courses without further progression in their training, effectively halting their learning process.

As part of the didactic sessions, the surgeon should develop in the laboratory the skills needed for the performance of operative endoscopy. The laboratory sessions may use inanimate objects (i.e., dry), or use animal parts or live animals (i.e., wet). Generally, the learning objectives for these laboratory sessions should be fairly narrow and specific. Most importantly, surgeons should develop basic spacial orientation and eye–hand coordination skills during these sessions, which often require only a dry lab. Other training objectives that require only a dry lab include learning to suture intraabdominally with a pelvic trainer and developing a familiarity with laser beam characteristics. To learn other techniques, extirpated animal organ models may be used, such as the pig bladder for training in endometrial ablation and other hysteroscopic procedures. However, these models have the disadvantage that intraoperative bleeding does not occur and he-

mostatic skills are not fully tested. Live animal models are often used, although these are rarely required unless the surgeon is developing or learning a particularly high-risk and innovative procedure.

Most operative endoscopy courses today combine didactic teaching with laboratory training. They may also incorporate pretaped videos of surgical procedures (preferably unedited), or even have a small number of televised live cases. However, the surgeon should not assume that 1 or 2 days of laboratory teaching will suffice to develop a specific skill. As noted before, in general the skills acquired in the laboratory are relatively narrow, and complete training requires continued observation of actual surgical procedures and the performance of procedures under supervision (see following). A more detailed discussion of the development of an endoscopic training program is given in Chapter 3.

Observational (Preceptorship)

Having acquired didactic and laboratory training, the surgeon now proceeds to observe live operative endoscopic procedures, generally via a video monitor. Viewing pretaped procedures is not an acceptable substitute, because the trainee must fully appreciate the placement and extraabdominal manipulation of the endoscopic instruments. Although some training courses include live surgery observation, the period of time dedicated to this, by necessity, is relatively limited.

Ideally, the trainee should observe between 10 and 20 cases of the skill level selected (see Tables 2.2 and 2.3). Trainees may complete this portion of their training by spending a week or so observing the procedures of a busy endoscopist or by viewing cases once or twice weekly for approximately 1 to 2 months.

Tutorial (Supervised)

Having observed 10 to 20 live cases of a specific procedure or set of procedures, the physician is now ready to begin performing their own endoscopic surgery, under direct supervision. Physicians should aim to perform at least

5 to 10 supervised cases within the skill level desired. The supervising endoscopist should have proven expertise in the field, *and* should allow the trainee to perform most or all of the surgery. The trainee must be responsible for the preoperative patient selection, preparation, and postoperative management. Unfortunately, this important portion of the training process is the one most frequently not fulfilled. Nonetheless, all organizations currently issuing credentialing guidelines (e.g., ACOG, AAGL, SRS, and SOGC) emphasize that newly trained surgeons should initially perform their surgeries under direct supervision.

Training in operative endoscopy should ideally form part of the obstetric/gynecologic or general surgical residency.[4,11–13] In fact, the Council on Resident Education in Obstetrics and Gynecology (CREOG) of ACOG has developed a program for residency training in operative endoscopy, based on the foregoing scheme.[11] The training of residents is the most effective method for resolving the vast discrepancies in skill levels currently present among practicing gynecologists and general surgeons. Unfortunately, many residency programs have not yet developed this expertise within their curriculum or faculty, resulting in the graduation of many ob/gyn or general surgical residents with little or no training in endoscopic surgery. Training programs should attempt to remedy the deficiency by initially training (or retraining), certifying, and credentialing their faculty. An approach similar to that suggested for initially credentialing staff at a private hospital can be used (see following). Programs may also need to increase participation and involvement by select clinical faculty with expertise in endoscopic surgery.

As pertaining to any rapidly evolving field, new or additional surgical skills should be and often are acquired following the completion of residency training. In this case, practicing surgeons may have to devise their own training program. The entire training/certification process can take as little as 2 to 3 months for each specific skill level being learned. Unfortunately, the popular demand for this type of surgery is increasing exponentially, encouraging many surgeons to perform procedures that they are neither familiar with nor trained to do, often with poor results, increased operative costs, and a rise in patient morbidity and mortality.

Certification and Credentialing

A certificate of competence (documentation of knowledge and skill) must not be issued, for the sake of all involved, until the trainee readily demonstrates, to the supervising surgeon, satisfactory and independent endoscopic skills corresponding to the skill level desired. If endoscopic training was acquired in residency, certification of surgical expertise and skill becomes the domain and responsibility of the program director, and assignment of hospital surgical privileges is per routine. Alternatively, if all or the majority of training was acquired post residency, the certification and credentialing process becomes less well defined.

While a course instructor will be happy to document the trainees' attendance, or tutors will note the cases they supervised, it is unlikely that either one will assume the legal and ethical responsibility of certifying competency. Thus, certification of surgeons acquiring their training post residency is and should be intimately tied to the assignment of privileges (credentialing) by a hospital or other operating facility. The postresidency credentialing process can be based on (a) prior residency training; (b) review of a 12- to 18-month case list; or (c) documented training, including preceptorship and tutorial.

To minimize the possibility of litigious situations, and in view of the increasing demand for operative endoscopic procedures, this author recommends that hospitals and other similar institutions begin their staff credentialing system NOW! The development and implementation of faculty/staff credentialing guidelines should be combined with the development of residency training guidelines, if applicable. The credentialing system should apply to all faculty interested in receiving privileges, without exception, but should be specialty specific (e.g., gynecology, general surgery, plastic surgery). A method that we have found useful for initiating a credentialing process with minimal repercussions has been to use the skill level-specific scheme outlined in Tables 2.2 and 2.3.

Cases are then requested from all surgeons desiring privileges that will illustrate their degree of experience and level of skill. Cases generally cover the preceding 12 to 18 months. We request patient name or number, indications, procedure, pathology, complications, and days of hospitalization. The cases are then reviewed by the standing credentialing committee or an ad hoc subcommittee to determine whether a surgeon has had sufficient experience (i.e., number of cases) for the skill level requested, and whether the complication rate is significantly disparate. Barring any obvious problem, or lack of case numbers, privileges are granted. Faculty or staff who desire more advanced privileges must undertake further training (including a preceptorship and tutorial) either at the same institution, if expertise is available in house, or elsewhere.

The need for devising and implementing a rational and structured training, certification, and credentialing protocol in operative endoscopy has become obvious and unavoidable. Training and credentialing in gynecologic operative endoscopy today depends on the surgeon's and the surgical institution's goodwill and desire for excellence. If we as the concerned practitioners do not rapidly establish such guidelines, other interested parties, namely governments and third-party payers, will and are proceeding to do so unilaterally.

References

1. Furrow BR, Johnson SH, Jost TS, Schwartz RL. *The Law of Health Care Organization and Finance.* St. Paul, MN: West Publishing Co.;1991:25.

2. Azziz R. Operative endoscopy: the pressing need for a structured training and credentialing process. *Fertil Steril.* 1992;58:1100–1102.

3. Altman LK. Surgical injuries lead to new rule. *New York Times.* 1992; June 14, p 1.

4. Azziz R. Training, certification and credentialing in gynecologic operative endoscopy. *Clin Obstet Gynecol.* 1995;38:313–318.

5. The American College of Obstetricians and Gynecologists. Credentialing guidelines for new operative procedures. ACOG Committee Opinion 142, August 1994.

6. American Association of Gynecologic Laparoscopists. Credentialing guidelines for operative endoscopy. September 1992.

7. The American College of Obstetricians and Gynecologists. Credentialing guidelines for operative laparoscopy. ACOG Committee Opinion 106, April 1992.

8. The American College of Obstetricians and Gynecologists. Credentialing guidelines for operative hysteroscopy. ACOG Committee Opinion 107, April 1992.

9. The Society of Obstetricians and Gynaecologists of Canada. Guidelines for training in operative endoscopy in the specialty of obstetrics and gynaecology. SOGC Policy Statement. January 1993.

10. Society for Reproductive Surgeons–American Fertility Society. Guidelines for attaining privileges in gynecologic operative endoscopy. *Fertil Steril.* 1994;62:1118–1119.

11. CREOG Training Guidelines: Advanced Surgical Techniques for Residency Training Programs in Obstetrics and Gynecology, 1994. Available through the Council on Resident Education in Obstetrics and Gynecology, 409 12th Street SW, Washington, DC 20024–2188.

12. Sammarco MJ, Youngblood JP. A resident teaching program in operative endoscopy. *Obstet Gynecol.* 1993;81:463–466.

13. Dent TL. Training, credentialing, and evaluation in laparoscopic surgery. *Surg Clin North Am.* 1992;72:1003–1011.

3

Developing a Training Program in Operative Endoscopy

Michael J. Sammarco

Introduction

Developing skill and competency in any surgical subspecialty requires a combination of innate ability, technical skill, and a thorough understanding of anatomy and instrumentation. In particular, the performance of an operative endoscopic procedure requires a unique blend of surgical skill, technology, and eye-to-monitor coordination, because there is less tactile feedback than with more traditional surgery. Operative endoscopy is not simply an extension of other surgical approaches, and it should not be assumed that a surgeon accomplished in laparotomy will automatically be able to master endoscopic techniques. Traditionally, surgical training has been taught clinically, through observation and tutorial. However, the field of operative endoscopy has advanced rapidly, while the increase in the number of surgeons trained in these techniques during their residency has increased to a lesser degree.

Training programs can be implemented at any level of surgical expertise. Whether the trainees are residents in training or practicing physicians, the basic structure of the training sessions is the same. The following outlines how to organize and prepare for the development of a training program in operative endoscopy.

General Considerations

Regardless of the level of surgical skill present, training sessions should attempt to reproduce actual surgical conditions. This is not to say that the exercises should try to simulate an actual surgical procedure, i.e., hysterectomy, bladder neck suspension, etc., but should attempt to simulate the techniques and situations used to perform those procedures. The type of instruments and equipment used, the positioning of the surgeon and the assistant, the type of suture, and the orientation of the surgical field should be similar to that encountered during actual endoscopic surgery (Fig. 3.1). Furthermore, port location should also be realistic, and placement of unnecessarily large-diameter trocars should be discouraged.

A thorough understanding of the equipment, including its assembly and disassembly, is critical and essential. This includes the ability to "troubleshoot" technical problems as they arise. Endoscopic surgeons should not rely completely on the operating room (OR) staff for technical assistance, but should be prepared to diagnose and repair mechanical problems as they arise. Because not all institutions use the same equipment, the participants should have at least a basic understanding of comparable instruments and their compatibility with other pieces of equipment. A practical example is the compatibility of various light cables with different light sources and laparoscopes. These issues can easily be covered in the didactic portion of the workshops.

The groups of participants should be kept small, no more than three per workstation. This not only creates a more realistic surgical condition but will reduce inefficient use of time and frustration. An "OR attitude" should be encouraged. For example, practicing techniques with instruments that were neither designed nor intended for that use simply promotes the development of bad habits, as does the unrealistic positioning of the trainees around the operative site. Unfortunately, bad habits are easily learned but difficult to change.

The purpose of any training program should be to comprehensively instruct the participants, both didactically and technically. There should be an emphasis on the mastering of basic skills, which will serve as the foundation upon which further skills will develop. Furthermore, it is essential that training include proper patient selection, preoperative preparation and counseling, and realistic expectations. In fact, complications and litigation in operative endoscopy occur more often because of poor patient selection and/or counseling than poor technique.

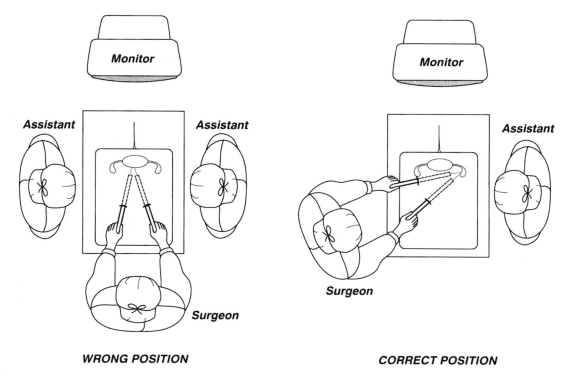

WRONG POSITION   **CORRECT POSITION**

FIGURE 3.1.   Training sessions should attempt to reproduce actual surgical conditions, and the positioning of the practicing surgeon and his/her assistants should be as realistic as possible.

The goal of any training program should be to help the participants develop a level of surgical confidence before entering the operating room, tempered by a realistic assessment of the surgeon's own skill level, the skill level needed to accomplish the procedure, and the need for additional assistance or tutoring. These goals can be accomplished through training sessions that incorporate both didactic and hands-on exercises. These sessions should be carefully planned, with specific objectives outlined, to be completed within a given amount of time. Repetition and review are very effective teaching tools, as is the incorporation of case presentations and review of pretaped surgical procedures. Therefore, it is advantageous to specifically plan exercises in a complementary fashion to emphasize salient points.

The majority of the laparoscopic training exercises can be effectively performed with a pelvic trainer (Fig. 3.2) in conjunction with inanimate or tissue models. Live animals can also be used as teaching models. Nonetheless,

although they very popular with trainees because they add a sense of realism to the exercises, they are more time consuming and more costly than pelvic trainers, while providing little training advantage. While live animals are superior models for demonstrations of dissection and hemostatic techniques, most of the basic skills necessary for the completion of operative endoscopy can be learned from the use of inanimate or tissue models. For example, performing a hysterectomy on a porcine model does not simulate an actual laparoscopic hysterectomy, although the same techniques are used to dissect and ligate major vessels whether in a pig or an actual patient. The training exercises should follow the same basic principles of keeping the groups small and focusing on the application of specific techniques, not on procedures. The focus should always be on the manner and time in which a task is accomplished, not simply on the completion of that task.

Hysteroscopic techniques are better demonstrated on tissue models than in live animals.

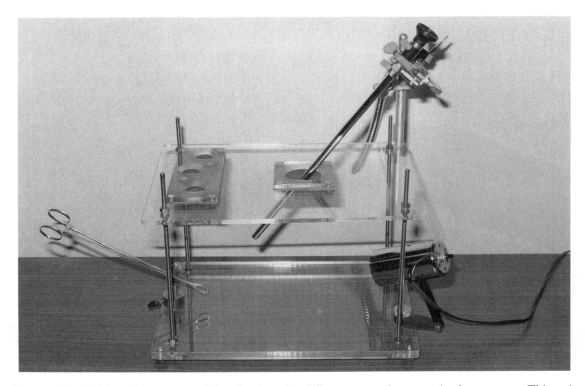

FIGURE 3.2. Pelvic trainers are useful to develop the skills necessary for operative laparoscopy. This unit was constructed in house. (Courtesy of R. Azziz, M.D.)

Familiarity with instrument assembly and disassembly should be strongly emphasized. Because the power settings and the observed tissue effects are markedly dissimilar to those seen at the time of actual surgery, each session should be accompanied by a didactic presentation to emphasize these points. Hysteroscopic workshops generally require less time than laparoscopic sessions.

Laparoscopic Models

To allow operative laparoscopic and hysteroscopic workshops to proceed smoothly, an adequate number of tissue models should be prepared in advance. Models used for laparoscopic training exercises can be constructed from a variety of materials, the type dependent on the objectives of the particular exercise. As the majority of laparoscopic procedures are performed in the pelvis, the models should attempt to maintain a similar spatial relationship. Furthermore, the safety of the participants should not be taken for granted. Because some of the materials or tissues used are potential biohazards, the pelvic trainer and instruments used should always be properly cleaned and disinfected after use. The participants should always wear gloves, not only for their own protection but also to simulate the actual conditions encountered during surgery.

Uterine Models

Sock Uterus

The elastic (ankle) portion of a small tube sock is cut off and stuffed into the toe of the sock. The base is then tied off, and the resulting "uterus" anchored firmly to a piece of wood with either a nail or staple. This model performs well for most exercises, especially for suturing. Adnexal structures, made from tissue or other materials, can be easily attached and replaced.

Silk Pear Uterus

A decorative silk pear is covered with a small sock and anchored top down to a piece of wood. This model can be reused because, when covered with a small sock or a piece of cast stocking, it performs well with any of the adnexal models without becoming soiled.

Placental Uterus

The umbilical cord and membranes are removed from a human placenta. The placenta is then folded over itself into three parts. Each part is sutured to the others to form a flat triangular tube (Fig. 3.3). Although more time consuming and messy to assemble, this model offers some distinctive advantages over the others. The demonstration of knot integrity by ligating the superficial vessels, and the tissue effects of laser or electrosurgical energy, are superior. Unlike the models mentioned earlier, the placental uterus needs to be suspended from the top of the pelvic trainer rather than mounted on a board.

Any of the uterine models can be used with laser or electrosurgical energy sources. Care should always be taken to moisten any flammable materials used and to have the participants wear the appropriate eye protection. If an electrosurgical energy source is to be used, a grounding wire can be attached directly to any of the tissue models or uterine models. The inanimate objects should be covered in conducting gel (Signa Gel, Parker Laboratories, Denver, CO), preferably under the protective sock. Furthermore, the grounding wire should be attached as close as possible to the site where the procedure is to be performed. Higher than normal voltage may be needed.

Tubal Models

Porcine Uteri

The porcine uterus can be used to construct an extremely versatile model for tubal surgery. Preferably, these should be harvested from a nulliparous 150- to 200-lb pig. After removal of the ovaries, the remaining uteri and broad ligaments are sutured/stapled to the uterine model of choice. Such a "tubal" model, attached to a placental uterus, is depicted in Fig. 3.3.

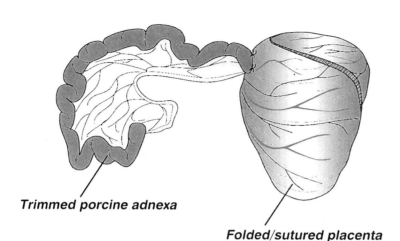

FIGURE 3.3. A tissue model of a uterus and its adnexa can be formed by using a folded and sutured placenta with an attached porcine uteri and broad ligament, representing a tube and mesosalpinx.

Trimmed porcine adnexa

Folded/sutured placenta

Tubal Pregnancy Model

Porcine uteri are stuffed with small pieces of liver or placenta, at 2- to 3-cm intervals throughout the length of the "tube." If fresh liver or placenta is not available, a piece of sponge or a cotton ball can be used. This model is very useful for reviewing laparoscopic linear salpingostomy for an ectopic pregnancy.

Hydrosalpinx Model

The cystic duct is removed from a porcine gallbladder (Fig. 3.4A), and the gallbladder is thoroughly washed and filled with water. The remaining gallbladder is then sutured to the end of the porcine uterus in the "tubal model" (Fig. 3.4B). This model can be used to demonstrate more advanced suturing or tissue-handling techniques, and forces trainees to select the appropriate instruments and port location. This model is generally rather delicate and encourages the participants to use gentle and precise surgical technique. It performs well with laser, electrosurgical, or suturing techniques. If no porcine gallbladders are available, the distal end of the porcine uteri can be splayed to resemble a normal tube (Fig. 3.5).

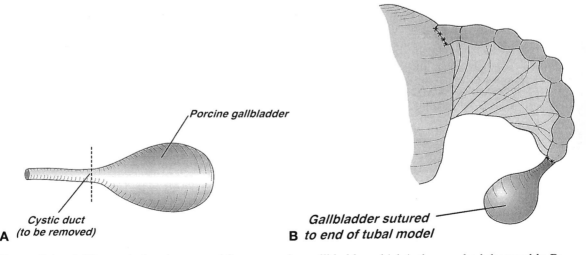

Porcine gallbladder

Cystic duct
A *(to be removed)*

Gallbladder sutured
B *to end of tubal model*

FIGURE 3.4. **A:** The cystic duct is removed from a porcine gallbladder, which is then washed thoroughly. **B:** The gallbladder is then sutured to the end of the porcine uterus (e.g., tubal model; see Fig. 3.3).

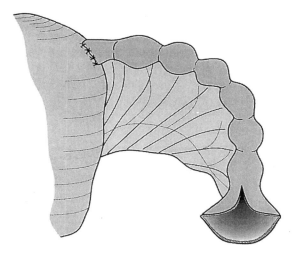

FIGURE 3.5. An open-tube model can be created by splaying the end of the porcine uteri.

Ovarian Models

Nontissue Ovarian Models

If an ovarian model is required to add either additional spatial orientation or for simple procedures, small balloons can be used. A balloon is filled with water and tied, then covered with a second balloon. The inner balloon may be sutured to the "uterus" while the outer balloon is sutured to the "mesosalpinx" (broad ligament of the porcine uterus).

Ovarian Tissue Model

A porcine gallbladder or urinary bladder (after ureters are ligated) is sutured to the uteri broad ligament (i.e., "mesosalpinx"). These models perform well for the demonstration of ovarian cyst aspiration or extirpative procedures. Adhesions can easily be added by attaching a piece of omentum over the "ovary." Endometriosis is added by injecting small amounts of chocolate syrup superficially. Either one of these additions can be used to demonstrate adhesiolysis or vaporization techniques with any energy source.

Attempts have been made to use the porcine ovaries for an ovarian tissue model, but they perform very poorly. Rarely are they very large,

and they tend to be very hard and difficult to suture or incise.

Ovarian Cyst Model

This model best demonstrates the techniques required to perform an ovarian cystectomy. Furthermore, this model does not need to be attached to a uterine or tubal model. A section of porcine liver with the intact gallbladder still attached is used. Dissection should be carried out through the outer capsule of the gallbladder.

Ligature Models

Intra- and extracorporeal knot-tying techniques can easily be incorporated into a number of exercises. Knot-tying tends to be one of the more difficult techniques to master. It is best if sutures are placed through actual tissue so that the tissue will tear if excess force is applied.

Hysteroscopic Models

Operative and diagnostic hysteroscopic techniques can be demonstrated utilizing two different types of models. The *resectoscope box* is best suited to demonstrate the tissue effects of various waveform and energy settings (Fig. 3.6), working within a fluid medium. Pieces of fresh liver or red meat perform well. If tap water is used, inordinately high power settings may be required to produce the desired tissue effect, depending on the mineral content of the water. Often, distilled or sterile water is better.

The *porcine urinary bladder hysteroscopic model* can be used to demonstrate the techniques used for both basic and advanced hysteroscopic surgery. Basic techniques, i.e., directed biopsy, equipment assembly, simple lysis, foreign-body removal, are easily demonstrated by placing sutures or other material through the wall or inside the bladder. The bladder used should only measure $3-4 \times 5$ in. in its resting state, or the cavity will be too large to use. The bladder should be wrapped snugly in aluminum foil to maintain bladder shape, and

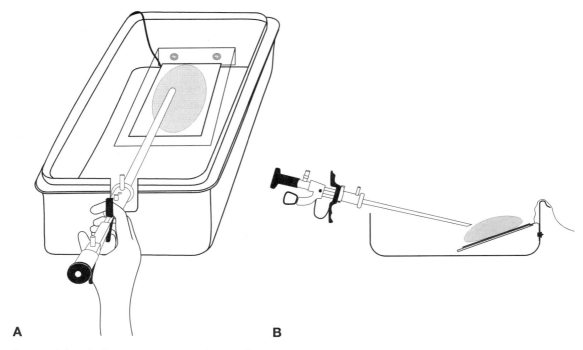

A   **B**

FIGURE 3.6.   **A:** A resectoscopic model can be constructed from a plastic tub, with a notch cut to fit the hysteroscope. **B** A tissue rack can be made from an acrylic picture frame. Holes are drilled into its base and the frame is screwed, with rubber washers, to the tub wall. The rack is covered with a grounding pad or metal sheet and connected to the ground of the electrosurgical generator.

covered with conducting gel (Parker Laboratories) to increase current conductivity. A model that simulates a submucous leiomyoma can be constructed by securely suturing a piece of denuded beef tongue or other fibrous material within the bladder. To do so, a 1-in. cut is made on the bladder wall, the specimen sutured on the inside, and the entry incision repaired.

Both these models perform extremely well and are easily assembled. To perform the exercises, a functioning continuous-flow system must be in place, similar to what is required during surgery. Unfortunately, the tissue effects seen on these models are not similar to those observed during an actual case. Modulated waveforms cause a more obvious effect than unmodulated waveforms when an electrosurgical generator is used. Nd:YAG (neodymium:yttrium aluminum garnet) lasers can also be used, but the wall of the bladder is easily perforated.

These models are only some examples of the type of operative endoscopy teaching tools that can be constructed. It is beyond the scope of this chapter to present all the exercises that can be performed. However, before developing a training program, the specific objectives should be outlined and understood. Not all institutions have the same needs; therefore, not all programs should be formatted the same. A more detailed list of both exercises and learning objectives is available from the Council on Resident Education in Obstetrics and Gynecology (CREOG) of the American College of Obstetricians and Gynecologists.[1]

Reference

1. CREOG Training Guidelines: Advanced Surgical Techniques for Residency Training Programs in Obstetrics and Gynecology, 1994. Available through the Council on Resident Education in Obstetrics and Gynecology, 409 12th Street SW, Washington, DC 20024-2188.

4

Principles of Endoscopic Optics and Lighting

Richard P. Buyalos

Light Sources

Illumination of the peritoneal cavity is essential in laparoscopic and hysteroscopic surgery. There are a variety of light sources with varying spectral emissions and illumination power.[1-3] Light originates from an object when it is heated sufficiently, and the color (wavelength) of the light emitted varies with the temperature of the source. This property of color temperature is measured in degrees Kelvin (K°). Light sources with higher K° contain more high frequency (blue) wavelengths, resulting in a brighter and more accurate image. As light loses heat (lower K°) its spectral emission shifts from blue to red, causing the image to assume a reddish tint.

Until the mid-1960s, endoscopic lighting consisted of the traditional incandescent light bulb. Output was generally between 75 and 250 W, although light sources of less than 150 W were generally avoided in gynecologic en-

doscopy. An incandescent light bulb transforms approximately 97% of electrical energy into heat, while only 2% to 3% is converted into visible light. Ideally, light sources should be equipped with two lamps to facilitate rapid switching should one lamp fail. Preoperatively, both bulbs should be inspected to confirm proper functioning. This is particularly crucial in operative endoscopy where loss of the light source during dissecting or hemostatic procedures would pose a significant risk to the patient.

Some of the light sources employed in gynecologic endoscopy today incorporate 150- to 250-W tungsten/iodine vapor (2800–3200 K°) or halogen-quartz (3200–3400 K°) incandescent lamps. Although these light sources are less expensive, they emit relatively little blue light and are generally insufficient for proper photo documentation (see Chapter 7). A 150- to 300-W mercury halide (5600 K°) or 300-W xenon vapor (6000–6600 K°) arc lamp is preferable as these provide excellent illumination for visualization and photo documentation because of their high content of blue spectral light. The bulb life of mercury halide arc lamps is approximately 250 hr, while the xenon vapor lamp may last up to 1000 hr but is significantly more expensive.

Although the light is extremely hot at its source, most of the heat is dissipated along the length of the light cable. It is for this reason that it is commonly called "cold light." Nonetheless, a significant amount of heat may still be generated at the end of the light cable, which can cause thermal injury to the patient or burn paper drapes or clothing with prolonged direct contact.

The brightness of the image transmitted back into the endoscope depends, to a certain degree, on the reflective quality of the peritoneal surface. Pigmented or blood-covered surfaces will reflect relatively little light in contrast to more reflective structures such as the ovaries. The light intensity decreases by the square of the distance from the endoscope to the image viewed. Doubling the distance between the endoscope and the tissue being examined (e.g., from 3 to 6 cm) increases the light dispersion fourfold (i.e., from 9 to 36). Consequently, far more light is required for panoramic views.

Light Transmission Cables

A dramatic improvement in lighting technology occurred with the development of fiberoptic cables, composed of multiple coaxial quartz fibers. These systems absorb and disperse the heat from the light source with relatively little heat being conducted to the end of the cable, while transmitting light of high illuminosity or "lux." Individual fibers are usually 10 to 25 μm in diameter and consist of an inner core of high refractive index quartz fused to an outer sheath of low index material or cladding (Fig. 4.1). Light transmitted through the fiber is reflected inward by the high index/low index intersurface. Thus, visible light (wavelengths of 400–700 nm) enters the proximal end of the fiber and emerges from the distal end after

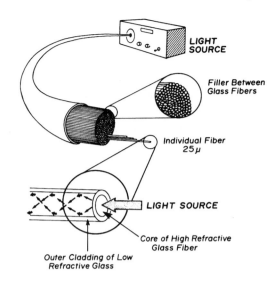

FIGURE 4.1. The structure of fiberoptic cables and individual fibers. Note that at least 30% of the transverse surface of the cable is occupied by low refractory index cladding and nontransmitting interfiber filler cement.

many internal refractions. Between the fibers, cementing them together, is a nontransmitting filler material or cladding.[1,4] Light transmission is enhanced by increasing the number of fibers. The larger the cable diameter, the more fibers can be carried, resulting in improved illumination.

There are two types of fiber bundles (Fig. 4.2). "Incoherent" bundles are produced by packing multiple fibers together in a random arrangement. These systems are usually 1.5 to 2 m in length and transmit light from an external source to the endoscope. In contrast, "coherent" or "oriented" bundles have identical fiber arrangements at both ends of the cable. A "true image" is then transmitted as dots of light through a cable containing as many as 100,000 fibers, each approximately 10 μm in diameter. The image from the distal end of coherent bundles is fused and focused on the ocular of the endoscope. Coherent bundles are significantly more expensive to manufacture, but permit flexion of the endoscope. They are most frequently employed in flexible gastroscopes, colonoscopes, and bronchoscopes. Flexible fiberoptic endoscopes have been de-

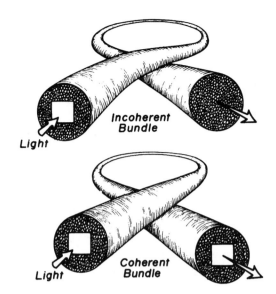

FIGURE 4.2. Types of Fiber Bundles *Top:* Incoherent bundles have their fibers arranged in random order within the fiberoptic cable. *Bottom:* Coherent bundles demonstrate a uniform fiber arrangement from one end of the cable to the other and serve to transmit an image.

veloped for hysteroscopy and laparoscopy but are used less widely in gynecologic endoscopy than endoscopes utilizing glass lenses. Recently, specialized small endoscopes (2 to 3 mm) containing fused fiberoptic bundles rather than glass lenses have been developed (see page 29).

Because of the presence of low refractory index cladding and filler material in the fiberoptic cable, approximately 30% of the light transmitted from the light source to the origin of the cable is lost in the form of heat. A light cable without cladding or interfiber filler has been developed by Karl Storz Endoscopy-America Inc. (Culver City, CA). This "fluid light" cable may improve light transmission by approximately 70% compared to the fiberoptic type.

Care should be exercised when handling fiberoptic cables. Coiling cables too tightly or direct trauma can cause breakage and cracking of the fiber bundles, resulting in loss of their ability to transmit light. Fiberoptic cables should be inspected before each procedure for extensive fiber breakage or central burnout,

which will rapidly reduce light transmission. If more than 30% of the fibers are damaged or if over 2 mm of the central area is burned out, the cable should be replaced. To determine if fiber bundles are damaged, the surgeon can shine the end of the cable on a flat surface at a distance of approximately 10 to 20 cm. Dark spots represent broken fibers and the brown central area indicates oxidation damage. The proximal end of the cable that connects to the light source can burn out with use and high temperatures inevitably turn even glass surfaces and their synthetic packing materials brown from oxidation.

A variety of manufacturers produce light sources and cables. Unfortunately, the specifics of the coupling of fiberoptic cables to either the light source or the endoscope vary widely. Use of available adapters may cause further loss of illuminosity, so it is of paramount importance to minimize ill-fitting or mismatched adapters to maximize light transmission.

Endoscopes

Lens Chains

Endoscopes are composed of an ocular or eyepiece proximally, which is closest to the surgeon's eye or camera, a lens chain or optical relay system, and an objective located at the distal end of the endoscope. The lens system employed in contemporary endoscopes may be divided into three types: classic, Hopkins, and graded index (GRIN) lens systems.[3-6]

In the classic system, the width of the lens is far less than the length of the endoscope and the distance between lenses is relatively large (Fig. 4.3). These endoscopes consisted of a long metal tube containing many thin glass lenses widely spaced within for transmission of a lighted image. The amount of light transmitted by an endoscope is proportional to the square of the index of refraction of the medium interspersed between the lens. Since air has a refractive index of 1.0, the proportional light transmission is also 1.0. When glass is used as the medium, with a refractive index of approximately 1.5, light transmission more

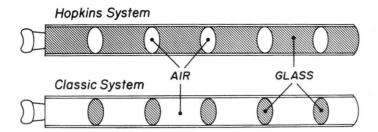

than doubles. Employing these principles, Dr. Harold Hopkins reversed the air/glass spaces within the endoscope, substantially improving light transmission (Fig. 4.3). In the Hopkins lens system, most of the length of the endoscope is occupied by the rod lens. Most laparoscopes and rigid hysteroscopes today employ this lens system.

The GRIN lens system consists of a single rod of glass in which the refractive index decreases gradually from the axis to the periphery (graded). In gynecology this lens system is most often employed in the design of the contact hysteroscope (see Chapter 26).

Types of Endoscopes

Two types of gynecologic endoscopes are available today (Fig. 4.4). "Diagnostic" (straight) endoscopes consist of a central Hopkins lens chain surrounded by fiberoptic bundles projecting light into the peritoneal cavity. In contrast, "operative endoscopes" contain an additional operating channel through which ancillary instruments are placed. The lens chain is angled to bring the eyepiece away from the operating channel. Operating endoscopes contain fewer fiberoptic bundles and therefore transmit less light than straight endoscopes of the same diameter. The exaggerated deflection of the returning light in operative endoscopes reduces the brightness of the image.

Laparoscopes are available in different external diameters,[7-9] but the optical system of operative endoscopes is always smaller than that of straight instruments. For 10- to 12-mm instruments, the diameter of the lens system of an operating versus a straight laparoscope is 2.5 to 3 mm compared to 5 to 6 mm, respec-

tively. Laparoscopes usually have a working focus between 7 and 12 cm, although in most optic systems the true distance for sharp focus is fixed at approximately 5 to 7 cm. The lens in the viewer's eye can compensate for small deviations from this true focus. When the multiple-puncture technique for operative laparoscopy is employed, straight laparoscopes are usually preferred because they provide maximal light transmission with greater image clarity and field of vision.

Hysteroscopes are of smaller diameter than laparoscopes and consequently transmit less light. They also have a greater angle of deflection to maximize their field of vision (see following). Their shorter working distance, approximately 2.5 cm, and the smaller size of the uterine cavity compensate for the decreased illumination.

Viewing Angle, Field of Vision, and Magnification

The distal end of the endoscope has been designed with a variety of viewing angles (Fig. 4.5). Most optics have a direct or 0° deflection system that provides the surgeon with a visual field that is collinear with the true field. This angle of vision was previously denoted as 180°, but the classification has now been standardized to the direction of the view from the optic end of the laparoscope and not toward the viewer. Oblique lens from 5° to 70° are also available. In general, diagnostic or "straight" laparoscopes have a viewing angle of 0°, while operative laparoscopes have a slight deflection of the viewing field of 5° to 10°. As hysteroscopes have less mobility in the uterine cavity, they are available with viewing angles of 0° to

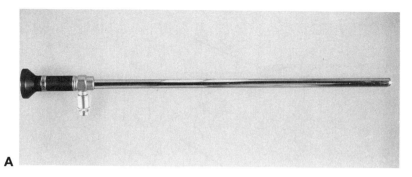

A

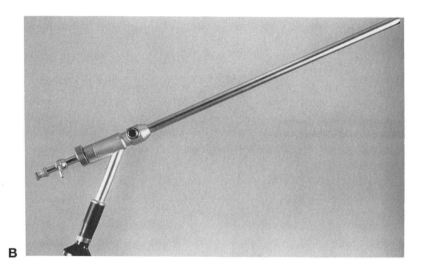

B

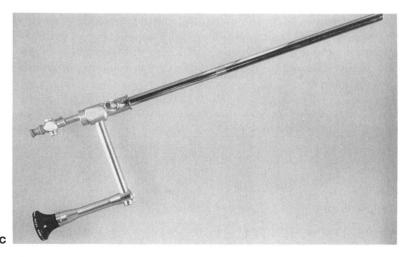

C

FIGURE 4.4. **A:** Diagnostic 0° 10-mm laparoscope (Olympus Corp., Lake Success, NY). **B:** 45° Operating laparoscope with 5-mm operating channel. Stopcock may be removed for placement of CO_2 laser coupler (Olympus Corp., Lake Success, NY). **C:** Right-angle (90°) operating laparoscope with 5-mm operating channel (Richard Wolf Medical Instruments Corp., Rosemont, IL).

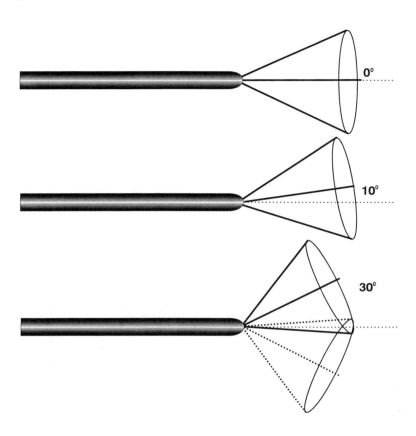

FIGURE 4.5. Representative angle of view for laparoscopes.

70°. It should be noted that the greater the angle of deflection, the greater the loss in illumination.

"Field of vision" refers to the borderlines of the field of view. The wider the viewing angle, the larger the potential viewing borders if the instrument is rotated 180° (Fig. 4.5). However, with an increasing field of vision, there may be some distortion at the periphery. Increased magnification of the field is obtained by moving the laparoscope closer to the desired object. Examples of magnification at different working distances for various makes of operative endoscopes are shown in Table 4.1.

TABLE 4.1. 10-mm Hopkins operating laparoscope with 3-mm operating channel: magnification at different working distances.

Working distance (mm)	Magnification		
	Wolf[a]	Olympus[a]	Storz[a]
3	—	8.2	10
5	—	5.7	6
10	3.19	3.2	3
15	—	2.2	2
20	1.71	1.7	1.5
30	—	1.2	1
50	0.73	0.7	0.6

[a]Personal communication.
Reproduced with permission from Murphy AA. Diagnostic and operative laparoscopy. In: Thompson JD, Rock JA, eds. *Telinde's Operative Gynecology,* 7th ed. Baltimore: Lippincott; 1992:365.

Light Loss

A typical Hopkins endoscope has a dozen or more lens and many air/glass surfaces. The cumulative light loss from these surfaces (4%–7% per interface) can be considerable. Light loss at the air/glass interface is greatly reduced by coating the lens with a thin film of magnesium fluoride, which decreases light reflection to approximately 0.5%. Light intensity is also lost from reflection at light cable–instrument connections. As noted, mismatched, poorly aligned, or loose connections significantly reduce light transmission. Deflection of the viewing angle or of the lens chain (as in operative endoscopes) further reduces light transmission. A typical system may lose at least 75% of the light originating at the source as it emerges from the distal end of the endoscope.[1]

Fogging

The peritoneal cavity has an ambient temperature of 37°C with 100% humidity. When a cold metal instrument such as an endoscope is placed into the abdominal cavity, condensation of water vapor occurs on the glass objective, which results in fogging. This can be prevented by prewarming the endoscope to 40° to 50°C, which can be achieved by simply soaking the instrument for approximately 3 min in hot (50°C) sterile water or saline before insertion into the abdomen. Additionally, a number of manufacturers have designed sterile apparatuses for prewarming endoscopes. Unfortunately, these devices generally require 1 to 2 hr to sufficiently warm the endoscopes because of poor heat conduction in air. The endoscope may also be warmed by placing the objective against the fundus of the uterus or against the large bowel for several seconds. However, this method is generally less satisfactory and may result in some distortion of the field of view from moisture or blood droplet accumulation on the lens surface.

Antifog solutions can be used to minimize fogging by decreasing the surface tension of moisture droplets, causing them to spread out rapidly and almost invisibly over the surface of the lens. However, antifogging solutions can also distort the lens surface sufficiently to compromise the visual image. Fogging that is still present after repeated efforts to clean the lens of the ocular and objective may be evidence of water vapor accumulation within the lens chain. This can be detected by holding the endoscope up to an external light source, such as an operating room light, and looking into either end of the instrument to detect water beads inside the lens chain. If this has happened and additional endoscopes are not available, the endoscope may be utilized temporarily by placing it in a warming oven at approximately 100°C. This converts the water into steam, forcing it to escape from the lens system. After use the endoscope should be returned to the manufacturer for repair to avoid further damage. A laparoscope that incorporates a permanent wash channel designed for distal lens wash and for tissue irrigation is available (Hydro™ laparoscope, Circon ACMI, Santa Barbara, CA). This 10-mm laparoscope is available in both 0° and 30° models.

Specialized Laparoscopes

In addition to the standard laparoscopes that utilize a glass lens, more specialized laparoscopes have been developed. As noted, endoscopes consisting of coherent fiberoptic bundles have been developed, particularly for use as flexible hysteroscopes (see Chapter 26). Microlaparoscopes utilizing fused fiberoptic bundles rather than glass lens are now available (see Chapter 24). Both a 2-mm (Microlap™, Imagyn Medical, Inc., Laguna Niguel, CA) and a 3-mm model (Olympus 3mm Microlaparoscope, Olympus America, Inc., Melville, NY) are available (Fig. 4.6). These "microlaparoscopes" have a complete line of small-diameter (2-mm), handheld instruments designed for microoperative laparoscopy. They are inserted through disposable plastic trocars, which are introduced over a verres needle, and their eyepieces are compatible with standard medical video and camera systems. These microlaparoscopes may facilitate many diagnostic and therapeutic procedures outside the operating room under intravenous sedation or local anesthesia.

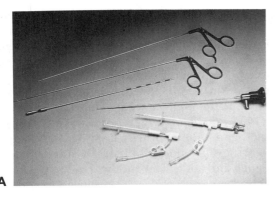

A

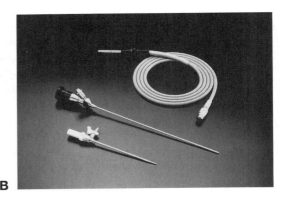

B

FIGURE 4.6. **A:** A 2-mm 0° microlaparoscope, introducer sheaths, and 2-mm operative instruments (Microlap™, Imagyn Medical, Inc., Laguna Niguel, CA). **B:** A 3-mm 0° microlaparoscope (Olympus 3-mm Microlaparoscope), access needle, and light cable (Olympus America, Inc., Melville, NY).

A laparoscope that transmits a video image through a distally placed imaging chip was recently developed (Stereovu™ 3-D Imaging System, Welch Allyn, Skaneateles Fall, NY) (Fig. 4.7). This laparoscope consists of a steel tube that carries the fiberoptic bundle and circuitry for image transmission and is attached via a cable to a combined light source and image processor. A flexible video laparoscope containing a 360° articulating tip is also available (Distalvu™ 360 Video Laparoscope, Welch Allyn).

Instrument Sterilization

In general, endoscopes should be gently cleansed, rinsed thoroughly with water, and then sterilized in metal or glass containers. Disinfecting systems with formalin tablets provide the gentlest method of sterilization but require 24 hr to be completely effective, which may prove impractical in a busy operating room. Disinfection of endoscopes performed at room temperature by soaking in antiseptic solutions such as alkalinized glyceraldehyde (Cydex, Johnson & Johnson Products, New Brunswick, NJ) is effective in 30 to 60 min. Gas autoclaving with ethylene oxide at 50° to 60°C for 2 to 3 hr can safely sterilize endoscopic equipment, but its chief disadvantage is that it requires a 12-hr airing-out period. A rapid sterilization method using peracetic acid at low temperatures (55°C) has been developed (Steri-System I, Karl Storz, Inc.) that safely sterilizes all im-

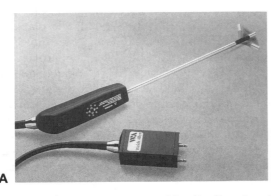

A

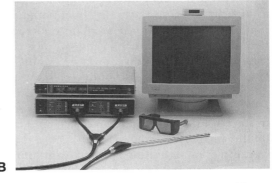

B

FIGURE 4.7. Laparoscopes with distally placed imaging chips. **A:** Flexible tip laparoscope (Distalvu™ 360 Video Laparoscope, Welch Allyn). **B:** Three-dimensional (3-D) imaging system (Stereovu™ 3-D Imaging System, Welch Allyn, Skaneateles Fall, NY).

mersible instruments, including endoscopes and light cables, in 20 to 30 min and requires no airing-out period.

Some manufacturers state that in an emergency sterilization may be accomplished using a gravity displacement steam autoclave at 130°C. However, repeated use of high-temperature autoclaves for this purpose will cause the seals between glass and metal to deteriorate, allowing steam to enter the optic chain, resulting in fogging of the lens system. Furthermore, rapid submersion in cold water following autoclaving, as is done with steel instruments, accelerates the deterioration of these seals. Efforts to improve the seals between glass–metal interfaces or to reduce the difference in the coefficients of expansion between these surfaces have been relatively unsuccessful. Maintenance and sterilization instructions for endoscopic equipment are provided by the manufacturers and should be carefully followed.

References

1. Hulka JF. Biophysics and physiology. In: Hulka J, ed. *Textbook of Laparoscopy*. Orlando: Grune & Stratton; 1985:7–43.
2. Semm K. *Operative Manual for Endoscopic Abdominal Surgery*. Chicago: Year Book Medical Publishers; 1987:46–59.
3. Quint R. Physics of light and image transmission. In: Phillips J, ed. *Laparoscopy*. Baltimore: Williams & Wilkins; 1977:18–23.
4. Hopkins HH. Physics of the fiberoptic endoscope. In: Berci G, ed. *Endoscopy*. New York: Appleton-Century-Crofts; 1976:27–63.
5. Hopkins HH. Optical principles of the endoscope. In: Berci G, ed. *Endoscopy*. New York: Appleton-Century-Crofts; 1976:3–26.
6. Prescott R. Optical principles of endoscopy. *J Med Primatol*. 1976;5:133–147.
7. Soderstrom R. Survey of laparoscopes for ob-gyn use. *Contemp Obstet Gynecol*. 1991;36:115–125.
8. Munro MC. Gynecologic endoscopy. In: Berek JS, Adashi EY, Hillard PA, eds. *Novak's Gynecology*. Baltimore: Williams & Wilkins; 1996:677–725.
9. Murphy AA. Diagnostic and operative laparoscopy. In: Thompson JD, Rock JA, eds. *Telinde's Operative Gynecology*, 7th ed. Baltimore: Lippincott; 1992:361–384.

5

Electrosurgery and Thermocoagulation at Operative Endoscopy

Ricardo Azziz

Introduction

The ability to achieve hemostasis is integral to any laparoscopic procedure and is probably the single most important factor that delayed the evolution and widespread applicability of operative endoscopy. The modalities to achieve hemostasis essentially mirror those of laparotomy surgery. Today there are many hemostatic techniques available including lasers, suturing, clips and staples, and thermocoagulation. Nonetheless, the most widely used and least expensive method of maintaining hemostasis within the pelvis are the electrosurgical modalities. This chapter discusses electrosurgery and briefly reviews the use of thermocoagulation. The use of lasers is discussed in Chapter 6, and sutures, clips, and staples are examined in Chapter 9.

Electrosurgery

American gynecologic laparoscopists use unipolar and bipolar instruments with cutting (undampened) or coagulation (dampened) waveforms more extensively than any other modality to achieve hemostasis. Nonetheless, a thorough understanding of the basic physics of this modality is often lacking. In Fig. 5.1 we see a schematic representation of the various measures of electrical energy.

Tissue Effects

Electric current has the ability to fulgurate, desiccate, coagulate, or cut tissue.

a. *Fulguration* refers to the heating of tissue by sparks of electrical current when the electrode is close to, but not in direct contact with, the tissue. This technique requires relatively high voltages and achieves superficial hemostasis with minimal tissue penetration. It can be used to stop diffuse bleeding such as that occurring after myomectomy.

b. *Coagulation* occurs when the tissue is heated, and protein loses its conformation, subsequently solidifying. Coagulation usually results in tissue blanching and occurs at temperatures of 45° to 60°C.[1]

c. *Desiccation* refers to the evaporation of all liquid until the tissue is completely dry,

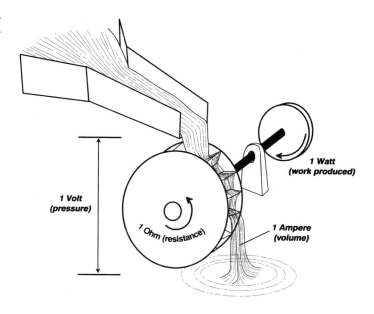

which occurs at higher temperatures than coagulation, 45° to 100°C. The term desiccation, however, is rarely used and coagulation (or electrocoagulation) is used to describe both effects.

d. *Vaporization* occurs at temperatures above 100°C when the intracellular liquid boils, leading to cellular disruption.

During electrosurgery a combination of these tissue effects is usually seen, although generally one type is predominant. Depending on the predominant tissue effect, electrosurgery results in tissue cutting or ablation. The different tissue effects can be achieved by varying the type of current waveform, the power output of the generator, the electric circuit, and the type of electrosurgical instrument tip used.

Electrosurgical Generators and Power Density

Electrosurgery requires generating units that are able to transform the available low-voltage (110 V), low-frequency (60 Hz) alternating electrical current into a high-voltage, high-frequency current. Spark gap circuits and triode vacuum tubes have now been replaced by solid-state units, which are widely employed at laparotomy and laparoscopy.[1,2]

A significant variable determining the type of tissue damage is the waveform of the alternating electrical current. The sine wave may be pure, with continuous regular oscillations (undampened or unmodulated) (Fig. 5.2), or may be released in short bursts (dampened or modulated) (Fig. 5.3). The former is usually referred to as "cutting" and the latter as "coagulation" current. The two may be blended to produce a combination that cuts and coagulates (Fig. 5.4). The undampened waveform vaporizes tissue and is ideal for cutting when applied with an instrument of small surface area such as a needle electrode. If an instrument with a large surface area is used, tissue coagulation is the effect principally seen. Dampened current, on the other hand, has a widespread coagulating effect on the surrounding tissue, including blood vessels, and therefore is useful for hemostasis. Nonetheless, the use of dampened current, by virtue of its extensive coagulation, can produce widespread tissue damage and necrosis.

Additional variations in tissue effects can be achieved with changes in power density, electrosurgical instrument tip, and electric circuit used. Generally, higher power densities

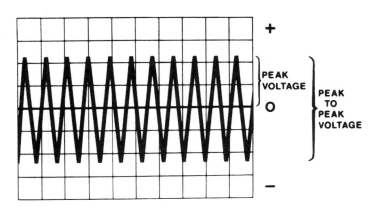

FIGURE 5.2. Undampened (unmodulated) or cutting electric current waveform. (Reprinted with permission from Soderstrom RM. Electrical safety in laparoscopy. In: Phillips J, ed. *Endoscopy in Gynecology.* Downey, CA: American Association of Gynecologic Laparoscopists; 1978: 306–311.)

achieve cutting or ablation, while lower power densities result in tissue coagulation. Power density depends on the power output of the electrosurgical unit and the surface area of the tissue being exposed to this current. The latter can be modified by the size of the electrode tip that comes in contact with the tissue. A small contact surface, such as that seen with a needle electrode, will achieve a higher power density than larger instruments. Hence at the same power output the former may cut or ablate while the latter may coagulate. For instance, the unipolar knife will cut when the energy is applied with the cutting edge of the blade but may coagulate when the instrument is applied on its side.

Types of Electrosurgical Circuits

Two types of electrical circuits, unipolar and bipolar, are employed in electrosurgery, each with its unique advantages and disadvantages, as follows.

Unipolar (Monopolar) Current

In unipolar circuits, the current flows from the generator through the operating electrode,

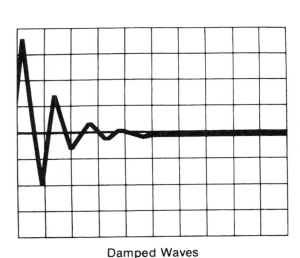

Damped Waves

FIGURE 5.3. Damped (modulated) or coagulating electric current waveform. (Reprinted with permission as in Fig. 5.2.)

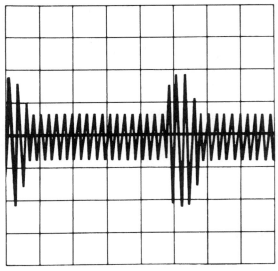

FIGURE 5.4. Blended electric current combines both damped and undamped waveforms. (Reprinted with permission as in Fig. 5.2.)

FIGURE 5.5. Scheme of unipolar (monopolar) electrical circuit.

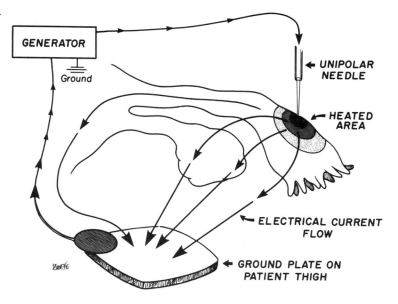

through the patient to the dispersing or "ground" electrode, and finally back to the generator (Fig. 5.5). Any insulated metal instrument can be designed to carry monopolar current (Fig. 5.6). A number of different instruments can be used. For example, the unipolar microtip or needle electrode works well for removal of filmy adhesions and for tissue dissection. Cutting current used is in the range of 20–80 Watts. This minimizes damage to surrounding tissues and is most effective for

lysis of adhesions. The needle electrode is available for use with a cannula (Trident® or Cohen®, Karl Storz, Culver City, CA) that has two ports for irrigation and suction. Additionally, some automatic suction/irrigation devices have a port that allows insertion of the needle electrode. The unipolar knife can be used in much the same way. Scissors can also be obtained with unipolar electrosurgery attachment. These may be used to cut and coagulate simultaneously, as when performing a salpingectomy.

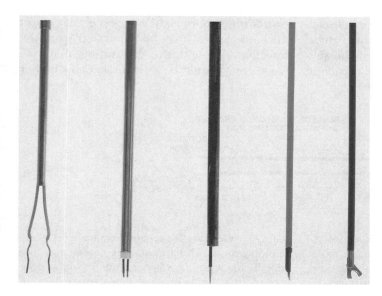

FIGURE 5.6. Electrosurgical laparoscopic instruments (*from right to left*) scissor combined with unipolar capabilities (Richard Wolf Co., Rosemont, IL); knife electrode (Richard Wolf Co., Rosemont, IL); needle point or microtip electrode (Karl Storz, Culver City, CA); Vancaillie microtip bipolar forceps (Karl Storz, Culver City, CA); Bipolar (Kleppinger) paddles (Karl Storz Co., Culver City, CA).

Unipolar electrosurgery was first introduced to laparoscopy as a method of sterilization.[3] However, the method came into disrepute because of the high risk of bowel injury or perforation purportedly resulting from arcing of the high-frequency current. Doubt has since been cast on this theory to explain the complications.[4] Histologic evidence suggests that most bowel perforations thought to result from electrosurgical burns were in actuality secondary to trocar injuries. Nonetheless, thermal injuries may still occur with the use of unipolar electrosurgery. Faulty contact between the ground electrode (in a reference ground system) and the patient may result in the current dispersing through unwanted pathways of lesser resistance and in undesired thermal injury. The bowel, perhaps because of its high concentration of electrolytes and water, seems to be particularly susceptible to this type of injury. To prevent this complication, most electrosurgical units utilize an isolated ground system. These systems have an isolated ground plate, which requires both sides of the plate to be properly applied and an internal circuit in the ground plate to be closed, for the electrosurgical unit to operate.

Another source of complications with the use of monopolar electrosurgical instruments is uncontrolled electrical discharge into the abdomen, after capacitation (charging) of the laparoscope. When a unipolar cautery instrument is placed down the operating channel of a laparoscope (Fig. 5.7), the interfaces between the insulated metal core of the operative instrument (carrying electric current) and the surrounding operative channel act as a capacitor (like a battery), resulting in the accumulation of electrons within the metal of the laparoscope. This accumulated electric current can be discharged in a disperse fashion into the surrounding tissues with little damage. Alternatively, the accumulated electrical energy can be released in a concentrated manner onto bowel or other organs, with subsequent damage.

A number of steps may be used to minimize the risk of organ injury from capacitation. First, monopolar instruments should be placed through the laparoscope only when a metal umbilical trocar is in use, which allows for the accumulated electricity to discharge in dispersed fashion into the surrounding umbilical skin. Second, it is preferable to place these instruments through suprapubic ports, which allow full view of the instrument and sleeve. Third, the use of multiple layers of metal/isolate (e.g., plastic) should be avoided. For example, plastic umbilical retainers should not be used to anchor a metal trocar sleeve through which a laparoscope with an operative channel and a monopolar instrument are placed.

Other monopolar injuries may occur because of breaks, often invisible, in the outer isolating coat of the instrument tip. An injury may occur if the area with the break in the coating comes into direct contact with an organ. Thus, these instruments should be checked regularly for defects, both visually and by placing them when charged near a grounding source (e.g., piece of moist chicken). Sparks may be generated from the defective site and the grounding material. These tests should be done at voltages higher

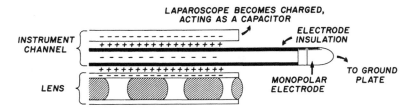

FIGURE 5.7. When an insulated unipolar instrument is used through the operating channel of a laparoscope or via a metal suprapubic puncture, the interfaces may act as a capacitor (i.e., battery), resulting in electric charge building up in the surrounding metal. This accumulated charge may accidentally discharge in a concentrated fashion onto surrounding organs, causing tissue damage.

FIGURE 5.8. Scheme of bipolar electrical circuit.

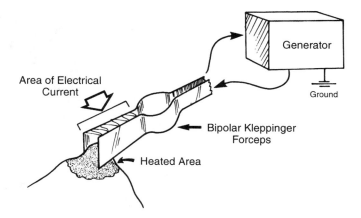

than regularly used clinically to overcome the
resistance of air to electrical current. An isolating sleeve is available that discharges any electrons released through defects in the instrument coating or accumulated capacitance to a
separate ground (Electroshield, Electroscope,
Boulder, CO).

Bipolar Current

In bipolar electrosurgery the circuit is self-
continuing and does not use the patients as
ground. Electrical current flows through two
electrodes so that the current only goes
through the intervening tissue and not the patient's body (Fig. 5.8). Obviously the instrument used to deliver the current must resemble a forcep and be insulated so that the
current returns to the generator through the

second electrode. Bipolar instruments can coagulate and desiccate but, in contrast to
monopolar current, cannot achieve cutting,
because power densities high enough to cause
cell vaporization of tissue cannot be achieved.[1]

Bipolar instruments are best suited for grasping and coagulating vessels or fallopian tubes,
particularly when using large bipolar paddles
(e.g., Kleppinger) (Fig. 5.9). Hemostasis can
best be achieved by first crushing and occluding the open vessel with the bipolar paddles
before coagulation. The microbipolar forceps
(Vancaillie®, Storz, Culver City, CA) are not
truly forceps because there is a fixed distance
between the two electrodes and the tissue to be
coagulated cannot be grasped (Fig. 5.9). This
instrument has a channel for irrigation that is
useful for identifying bleeding areas before coagulation. Bipolar instruments, however, do

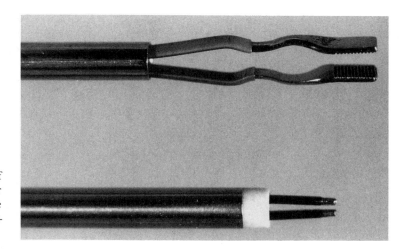

FIGURE 5.9. A close-up view of
the paddles of the Kleppinger
bipolar forceps (*top*) and the
Vancaillie microbipolar unit (*bottom*).

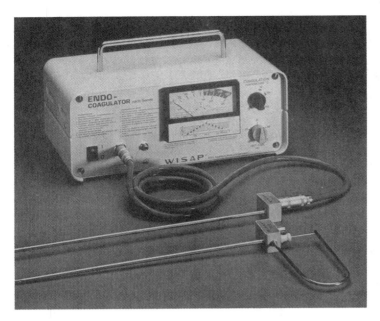

FIGURE 5.10. Thermocoagulator with the point coagulator in the background and the alligator forceps in the foreground. (Reprinted with permission from Garzo VG, Murphy AA. Operative laparoscopic instrumentation. *Semin Reprod Endocrinol.* 1991;9:109–117. Courtesy of WISAP, Saurlach, Germany.)

not work well when placed within a fluid medium. Bipolar forceps can also be used to fulgurate surfaces, with only superficial tissue penetration. This technique may be useful for ablating diffuse superficial endometriosis or for achieving hemostasis in large oozy areas such as the bed of an ovarian cyst or myoma.

Bipolar forceps can use both modulated and unmodulated current to achieve hemostasis, although most often undampened (cutting) current is preferred. As current is applied, tissue resistance increases and the effective power output reduces slowly and then rapidly. The coagulation mode, which has higher peak voltage, will cause desiccation at the surface, which will impede transmission of electrical energy to the endosalpinx through increased surface resistance. Cutting or unmodulated current will achieve slower but more effective heat, deep in the tissue. In fact, fallopian tubes cannot be fully coagulated unless a cutting or unmodulated current is used.[5]

Thermocoagulation

Thermocoagulation (endocoagulation) differs from electrosurgery in that the electrical current heats up the electrode itself, and this heat is then transmitted to the surrounding tissue by convection. No electricity comes in direct contact with the tissues. This method of hemostasis was initially suggested by Semm[6] in an attempt to circumvent the purported problem of electrical arcing with monopolar current that causes injury to adjacent organs. It was first designed as a method of sterilization, with the use of alligator forceps.

Three different instrument tips are now available for use with the thermocoagulation unit. Point coagulation can be achieved using the Endocoagulator® (Wisap Co., Saurlach, Germany), a rodlike instrument whose tip heats up to 100°–120°C. The point coagulator has a blunt tip of approximately 4 mm that heats slowly but works well if large areas need to be coagulated. It is principally used for myomectomies, treatment of diffuse endometriosis, or ablation of ovarian cyst walls. However, this point is much too large for microsurgical work (Fig. 5.10). An alligator forcep, designed for tubal ligation, has an overhanging hook on one paddle. While this may facilitate grasping of fallopian tubes, this paddle cannot be effectively used to grasp bleeding vessels and achieve hemostasis. The myoma paddle has a flat bladelike design that is useful when dissecting a myoma from its bed. Because it does not depend on transmission of electrical current, it works well in a wet field, and thermocoagulation is most often used for laparoscopic myomectomies.

References

1. Reich H, Vancaille TH, Soderstrom RM. Electrical techniques. In: Martin DC, Holtz GL, Levinson CL, Soderstrom RM, eds. *Manual of Endoscopy*. Santa Fe Springs: American Association of Gynecologic Laparoscopists; 1990:105–112.

2. Sebben JE. *Cutaneous Electrosurgery*. Chicago: Year Book Medical Publishers; 1989.

3. Boesch PF. Laparoscopie. *Schweiz Z Krankenh*. 1936;6:62–67.

4. Levy BS, Soderstrom RM, Dail DH. Bowel injuries during laparoscopy: gross anatomy and histology. *J Reprod Med*. 1985;309:168–170.

5. Soderstrom RN, Levy BS, Engel T. Reducing bipolar sterilization failures. *Obstet Gynecol*. 1989; 74:60–64.

6. Semm K. Endocoagulation: a new field of endoscopic surgery. *J Reprod Med*. 1976;31:7–9.

6

Principles of Endoscopic Laser Surgery

Richard P. Buyalos

Laser Physics

Electrons orbit in the atom at different distances from the nucleus. When an atom is "excited" by an external energy (in the form of a photon), electrons are shifted to an orbit further from the nucleus. The more energy absorbed by the atom, the higher the resulting orbit level of its electrons. This excited state lasts approximately a few millionths of a second until the electron drops down (decays) to its usual level to maintain thermodynamic equilibrium. During this decay the energy absorbed by the electron is emitted in the form of a photon, a process termed *spontaneous emission*. If an atom is in the excited state and is struck with another photon of the same energy as the one already absorbed, the decay process is accelerated. When this happens, two photons of identical energy, frequency, and direc-

tion are released, in a process termed *stimulated emission*. This principle is the basis for the production of LASER (Light Amplification Stimulated Emission of Radiation) light. The energy released by an atom during spontaneous or stimulated emission represents the difference between the initial and final energy of that atom, which in turn depends on the particular species of atom and its various electron orbits. Thus, different materials will produce lasers of different wavelenghts or energy (Fig. 6.1).

Laser energy follows principles of both light and electromagnetic radiation. Light consists of packets of energy (photons) that travel in a sinusoidal (wavelike) motion. Electromagnetic energy (E) (measured in joules) is calculated as $E = hf$, where f = frequency and h = Planck's constant or 6.63×10^{-34} joule $\cdot$ sec. Substituting c/λ for f gives $E = h \times c/\lambda$, where

FIGURE 6.1. The electromagnetic spectrum demonstrating various types of lasers and their associated wavelengths. (Reproduced with permission from Keye WR Jr. *Laser Surgery in Gynecology and Obstetrics.* Chicago: Year Book Medical Publishers; 1990.)

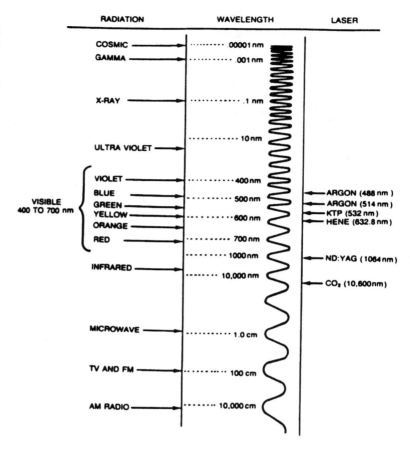

c = speed of light (186,000 miles/sec) and λ is the wavelength of the electromagnetic wave. The laser energy emitted is therefore inversely proportional to its wavelength and directly proportional to its frequency. Hence, the smaller the wavelength, the greater the energy.

Generation of Laser Light

Different atomic species in the forms of solids, liquids, and gases are used to create laser light (Fig. 6.1). To maintain the laser effect the majority of the atomic population of the laser medium must be in an excited (higher energy level) state. This is referred to as "population inversion." To maintain this state of excitability, external energy must be constantly infused into the atom population, for example, from continuous flashes from a xenon lamp. For the production of lasers the atom population (or active laser medium) is contained in an optical or resonant cavity. Atoms in the excited state spontaneously emit photons in all directions within the optical cavity. However, most travel along the longitudinal tube axis and are reflected by carefully aligned mirrors at both ends of the resonant cavity. These photons stimulate further emissions from already excited atoms (photon multiplier effect) and generate photon pairs of equal wavelength, frequency, and energy. These photon pairs are reflected within the optical cavity, are further amplified, and finally emerge through a partially transmitting mirror at the end of the tube as the laser beam. The properties of laser light are noted in Table 6.1.

TABLE 6.1.   Properties of laser light.

Coherent	Laser waves are always precisely in phase with one another, temporally and spatially
Collimated	All laser waves are parallel to each other. This facilitates transmission of the laser beam over relatively long distances with minimal scatter
Monochromatic	Laser consists of waves of essentially the same wavelength and energy level. This accounts for the reproducible effects on target tissue by a particular laser energy
Highest luminosity	It is the brightest existing light

Power Density and Exposure Time

Maximal power setting for most surgical laser units ranges from 20 to 100 W at the exit point of the optical cavity. Despite the relatively low power in watts, the magnitude of the beam energy is amplified immensely by adjusting the focus of the beam with special lenses or con-

trols. The area of the focused beam is referred to as the spot size. The magnitude of power concentration is usually referred to as the power density or power per unit area of beam. Power density is a property of both beam power (wattage) and spot size (determined by the focusing lens) such that:

$$\text{Power density} = \frac{\text{power at the focal spot}}{\text{area of the focal spot}}$$

Power density is therefore directly proportional to beam wattage and inversely proportional to spot size (Fig. 6.2). At a constant beam power, increasing the spot size decreases the beam concentration per surface area, achieving a lower power density. Conversely, a smaller spot size will achieve a significantly higher power density for a given beam power. If we assume an ideal beam with a perfect circular spot shape and uniform energy distribution in this circle, the surface area (A) is $A = \pi r^2$, where r is the beam radius. Because the radius is half the beam diameter ($r = D/2$) then

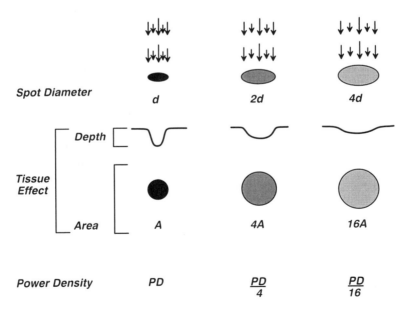

FIGURE 6.2.   Power density (*PD*) is proportional to beam wattage and inversely proportional to spot size (**d**). At a constant beam power, increasing the spot size decreases the beam concentration per surface area, achieving a lower power density. Doubling the beam diameter reduces the power density to one-fourth, while halving the spot diameter increases the power density by a factor of 4.

FIGURE 6.3. The cells absorbing the laser beam directly will be vaporized via intracellular boiling. Nonabsorbed photons will be reflected, scatter to surrounding tissues, or transmit through, resulting in either necrosis caused by cellular protein coagulation or reversible cellular damage. The extent of these tissue effects will vary according to the specific type of laser used, its power density and exposure time, and the characteristics of the tissue.

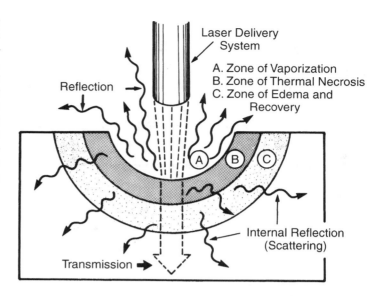

$A = \pi \ [D/2]^2$ or $A = \pi \ D^2/4$. Thus, doubling the beam diameter reduces the power density to one-fourth while halving the spot diameter increases the power density by a factor of 4. However, lasers do not have uniform power distribution throughout the beam spot area, and the actual calculation of power density varies depending on the shape of the power distribution of the beam. Nevertheless, the direct relationship of power density to power output and its inverse square relationship to spot size remains of paramount importance in laser use.

Although power density is the principal determinant of the effect of a laser beam on target tissue, exposure time is also an important determinant. Ideally, the largest volume of tissue should be exposed for the shortest period of time (i.e., using high power density), without compromising hemostasis. Shortened exposure time reduces thermal conduction, minimizing coagulation of surrounding tissue.

The Effects of Laser Light on Tissue

Living cells directly exposed to laser light of an appropriate wavelength are generally vaporized through the boiling of intracellular water.

As excess photons scatter into the adjacent tissues, some of the surrounding cells are destroyed or damaged by thermal coagulation of intracellular proteins. The zone of thermal or coagulation necrosis is constant at any given power density but varies with exposure time. The longer the beam is in contact with a particular area, the more heat will be conducted into the tissue adjacent to the vaporization site (Fig. 6.3), resulting in greater surrounding tissue damage and subsequent fibrosis.

Thermal effects on tissue are contingent on the intracellular temperature achieved (Fig. 6.4). Intracellular temperatures less than 45°C are reversible and do not permanently impair tissue function. Between 45° and 60°C, intracellular enzymes are damaged and tissue viability is impaired. When intracellular tissues reach temperatures between 60° and 65°C, extensive coagulation occurs and results in tissue blanching. Temperatures between 65° and 90°C completely denature cellular proteins. This gives the exposed tissue a grey-white color and indicates complete cellular death. When the intracellular temperature reaches 100°C, intracellular water boils and causes rapid transformation of liquid to vapor. The high vapor pressure causes explosive stretching of cell membranes, which eventually rupture and release the cellular particles as the laser plume, resulting in tissue ablation.

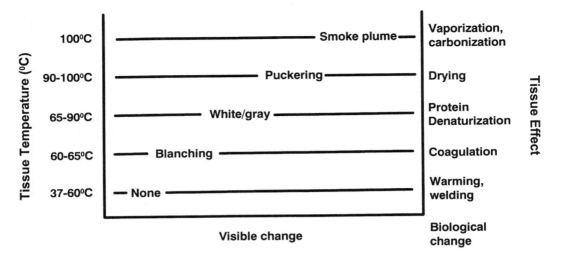

FIGURE 6.4.   The specific tissue effect of lasers, resulting in both visible and biological changes, depends on the tissue temperature generated.

Many laser-generating units today have the ability to produce beams in a continuous or pulsed fashion. Superpulse mode allows the beam to be delivered in a rapid series of pulses in a controlled repetitive fashion with short pauses between beam pulses. These micropauses reduce exposure time, allowing the tissue to cool between pulses, thus minimizing adjacent thermal damage. The efficacy of the superpulse mode declines when the pulse du-

ration is greater than 10% of the interval between beam micropulses.

Types of Lasers in Gynecology

Various media are used to produce laser light for use in gynecology today, including carbon dioxide-nitrogen-helium (CO_2) and argon gases, and neodymium:yttrium-aluminum-

TABLE 6.2.   Comparisons of the surgical lasers used in gynecologic endoscopy.

	CO_2	Nd:YAG	Argon	KTP
Active medium	CO_2, nitrogen, helium gases	Neodymium-yttrium-aluminum-garnet	Argon ion gas	Nd:YAG beam frequency doubled by a potassium-titanium-phosphate (KTP) crystal
Wavelength (nm)	10,600	1,064	418 and 514	532
Preferential absorbance (mm)	Water	Dark or black color	Hemoglobin	Hemoglobin, melanin
May pass through fluid	No	Yes	Yes	Yes
Hemostatic ability	Poor	Excellent	Excellent	Excellent
Depth of penetration (mm)	0.1–0.2	Contact: 0.3–2; Noncontact: 3–7	0.3–1[a]	0.3–1[a]

[a]Depth of penetration may be 4–5 mm in nonpigmented tissue.
Modified from Keye WR Jr. *Laser Surgery in Gynecology and Obstetrics.* Chicago: Year Book Publishers; 1990; and Houston: The Houston Laser Institute. *Laser Surgery Workshop Handbook,* 1989.

garnet (Nd:YAG) and potassium-titanyl-phosphate (KTP) crystals (Table 6.2).

Carbon Dioxide

Carbon dioxide and other laser energy in the infrared spectrum are preferentially absorbed by tissue that has a high water content (Table 6.2). Approximately 90% of the CO_2 laser energy is absorbed and transformed into heat within the initial 30 μm of exposed tissue. This induces instantaneous boiling of the intracellular water, resulting in cell disruption and vaporization. Therefore, the water content of impacted tissue determines its thermal response to the CO_2 laser. As epithelial cells possess a high water content (>90%), CO_2 laser energy can vaporize these superficial cells with minimal surrounding tissue damage. Alternatively, in cells with low intracellular water content the energy absorption is poor, resulting in more extensive coagulation. Precise cutting can be achieved with minimal peripheral cellular damage using the CO_2 laser.[1,2] However, it has limited hemostatic capacity in comparison to other commonly employed surgical lasers. If coagulation or superficial vaporization is desired, defocusing the beam (increasing the spot size) will decrease the power density while increasing the surface area treated.

Because the CO_2 beam wavelength is in the infrared spectrum (10,600 nm) and is invisible to the naked eye, a visible helium-neon (HeNe) laser (633 nm) is used as a parallel aiming beam. It is imperative that the two laser beams be well aligned. This alignment should be ascertained before each use (by firing the beam onto a moist tongue blade). The focusing mirrors and lenses of the CO_2 laser must be inspected regularly through scheduled maintenance to confirm precise alignment.

The CO_2 laser and HeNe aiming beam are delivered through an articulated arm that is attached to a coupling device containing mirrors and lenses to accurately focus and deliver the laser energy into the peritoneal cavity. The coupling device can be attached to the head of a laparoscopic operative channel, to a suprapubic channel, or to a suprapubic waveguide. The standard CO_2 laser laparoscopes use focusing lenses of 300 to 315 mm, with a focal point approximately 2 cm from the end of the delivery port and a focused spot diameter of 0.5 mm. CO_2 laser laparoscopes that have focusing lenses of both 250 mm and 300 mm have been introduced and provide greater system adaptability. The 250-mm lens, when used through the shorter probes employed through the suprapubic puncture, can generate smaller spot sizes and higher power densities. However, use of the 250-mm lens through the longer laparoscopic operating channel results in a defocused beam and reduced power densities. Efforts to design flexible fibers for delivery of the CO_2 laser beam have been unsuccessful thus far. Rigid hollow waveguides are currently available, many containing a focusing system at the distal end of the probe, allowing beam delivery via the operative channel of the laparoscope or a suprapubic second puncture.

Power densities of 2500 to 5000 W/cm² are usually employed in a continuous firing mode. Lesions close to vital structures such as the ureter, bladder, bowel, or large vessels may be effectively ablated using single-pulse or superpulse modes of 0.05 to 0.1 sec duration, which will provide tissue vaporization only 100 to 200 μm in depth. Additional protection of sensitive structures can be achieved by injecting saline underneath the peritoneum to elevate it off a ureter or large-caliber vessel. Because the CO_2 laser light is preferentially absorbed by water it cannot be transmitted through fluid medium. Therefore, the CO_2 laser cannot be used for operative hysteroscopy that uses liquid distension media.

Additional instruments are needed to evacuate the plume that forms from tissue vaporization, manipulate pelvic structures, and irrigate the operative field. Ancillary intraperitoneal instruments used during CO_2 laser surgery must be roughened to diffuse reflection. Instruments that are simply blackened are insufficient to dampen CO_2 laser energy, because black objects reflect infrared radiation and expose surrounding tissue to potential damage from a reflected beam. Backstops made of sandblasted or shotpeened titanium metal are preferred. These backstops can be flattened spatulas or rounded probes. When these instruments are moistened, they will enhance the safety margin as moisture trapped in the latticework of the instrument absorbs excessive CO_2 energy. Quartz rods should be avoided because they can conduct heat to adjacent tissue or absorb heat and potentially shatter in the pelvis. During surgery, additional protection can be obtained by frequent moistening and irrigation of pelvic surfaces.

Argon and KTP

The argon laser beam has combined wavelengths of 488 nm and 514.5 nm. The potassium-titanyl-phosphate (KTP) laser is produced by passing a Nd:YAG laser beam through a KTP crystal. This effectively doubles the frequency (or halves the wavelength) of the Nd:YAG laser (1064 nm) to produce the KTP laser beam (with a wavelength of 532 nm). The physical properties of the argon and KTP lasers are essentially identical.[3-5] Both can be delivered by flexible 0.3- to 0.6-mm fibers that remain cool during use and obviate the need for focusing devices or lens. Because the beam diverges as it exits the quartz fiber, maximum power density will be obtained within 2 mm of the fiber tip. The beams are easily visualized (green to blue-green), eliminating the need for a tracking beam. The KTP unit can be retrofitted to also produce Nd:YAG laser. Several companies market devices that can deliver both KTP and Nd:YAG laser from a single unit.

Red pigmented tissues rich in hemoglobin and hemosiderin preferentially absorb the argon and KTP lasers (Table 6.2), which accounts for their hemostatic properties. In addition to their ability to both coagulate and vaporize, these lasers have the additional advantage of being effective when fired within a clear fluid medium because the beam is not absorbed. The argon and KTP lasers are well adapted for use during laparoscopy; there is less plume production and minimal beam scatter compared to CO_2 laparoscopy. They have a depth of tissue penetration of 0.3 to 1 mm in pigmented tissues. In general, they provide a larger margin of safety because of their relatively shallow depth of penetration, short focal

lengths, and the selective absorption of these wavelengths by vascular tissue and endometrial implants. However, in less pigmented tissues the depth of tissue penetration can be as much as 4 mm.

The disadvantages of the argon and KTP lasers include the need for eye filters (because the beam wavelength is in the visible spectrum), possible breakage or damage of quartz fibers, and higher purchase costs. Although no flowing gases are needed for the production of these lasers, they require special electrical connections and running water, reducing their portability. Furthermore, these lasers have a limited capacity to incise tissue, but are quite useful for coagulation, particularly of heme-rich tissues.

To coagulate, the fiber is advanced within 1 to 4 mm of the target using a power setting of 2 to 5 W in a continuous mode. Vaporization is usually achieved by using a power setting of 5 to 10 W in continuous mode. Cutting can be achieved in a similar fashion, employing 10 to 15 W of power.

Nd:YAG

The wavelength of the neodymium:yttrium-aluminum-garnet laser (Nd:YAG) is 1064 nm, exactly twice that of the KTP laser. Its wavelength is in the infrared (invisible) spectrum, and a HeNe aiming beam is incorporated in these lasers for surgical use. As with the argon and KTP lasers, flexible fibers are used for delivery of the Nd:YAG laser, which are easily adaptable to laparoscopic and hysteroscopic use. Nd:YAG lasers are less readily absorbed by heme-rich tissue than are the argon or KTP lasers. In contrast to the argon or KTP units, Nd:YAG devices are available that are air cooled, do not require special plumbing, and can be easily moved between operating rooms. These units typically generate between 20 and 100 W.

The Nd:YAG laser has been used extensively in thoracic and urologic surgery. Because of its greater depth of penetration, the Nd:YAG laser was initially less popular for intraperitoneal use. Using "bare fiber" noncontact techniques, the depth of tissue penetration of the Nd:YAG laser is 3 to 4 mm (Table 6.2).[6] This depth of

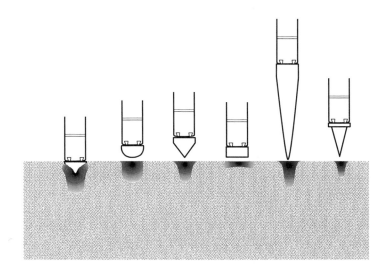

FIGURE 6.5. Sapphire tips for the Nd:YAG laser for laparoscopic surgery can be attached to quartz fibers and used endoscopically. The thermal effect on tissue is modified according to tip configuration by reducing beam scatter and modification of spot size.

penetration initially confined the gynecologic use of the Nd:YAG laser to hysteroscopic procedures, particularly endometrial ablation. However, many of these devices are air or gas cooled and carry the risk of air or gas embolization.[7] Furthermore, the rollerball and wire loop electrosurgical resectoscopes are probably superior for endometrial ablation (see Chapter 18).

The unfocused beam of a bare fiber can be modified to a variety of chisel and scalpel configurations with the use of attachable sapphire tips (Figure 6.5). The Nd:YAG beam heats the sapphire tip (photothermal effect) and allows more accurate control of both the depth of penetration and the configuration of the thermal effects on target tissue. This has greatly expanded the applicability of the Nd:YAG laser and increased its safety margin.[8] Additionally, the sapphire tips allow direct "contact" with the target tissue. This provides tactile feedback to the surgeon, unlike the noncontact techniques employed with the bare-fiber techniques of argon and KTP laser systems or in CO_2 laparoscopy, where the focal point of the laser energy is distal to the fiber or waveguide. Disadvantages of the sapphire-tipped probes include their relatively high costs, although with proper care sapphire tips can be used for multiple procedures. Also, care must be taken to avoid inadvertent contact with surrounding tissue because these probes remain hot for sev-

eral seconds after discontinuing activation of the laser.

Laser Safety

The safety of the patient and the operating team is of paramount importance. Trained, experienced assistants are invaluable during laser procedures. Many institutions have a technician familiar with laser equipment and safety who is available for all procedures utilizing surgical lasers. Operating theaters must be clearly labeled on the outside door indicating that a laser procedure is in progress; the type of laser must be specified on the "danger" sign. The window in the operating room must be covered. Some facilities have a warning light that is activated when the laser unit is operating.

The necessity for protective eyewear for all operating room personnel cannot be overemphasized. Permanent and serious ophthalmologic injuries from inadvertent ocular exposure to surgical lasers have occurred. The optical density for protective eyewear must be appropriate for the wavelength of laser employed. Ideally, protective eyewear appropriate for the given laser should be available outside the operating room. All operating personnel, including the anesthesiologist and assistants, must wear safety goggles or appropriate protective eyewear. Many surgical lasers have protective filters that fit over the eyepiece of the endoscope. The filter is activated and covers the lens when the laser is fired, and the laser cannot be engaged when the eye filter is dislodged or nonfunctional. Additional eye protection is also afforded by the use of video cameras that attach directly to the endoscopic eyepiece.

It is absolutely essential that flammable substances or explosive solutions be avoided in the operating room during laser usage. Special care must be taken when using paper drapes. When using CO_2 lasers the area surrounding the operative field should be draped with moist laps. The patient's eyes must also be appropriately protected with moist gauze or dressings.

Laser Plume

The production of smoke after tissue destruction with the lasers not only has led to respiratory complications but has been implicated as a possible source of mutagenicity. Approximately 75% of the solid particulate matter in a laser plume is less than 1 μm. When inhaled, this small particulate matter is capable of traveling directly to the distal tracheopulmonary tree and being deposited in individual alveoli. Using a dog tongue model it has been shown that 1 g of tissue generates 284 mg of particulate substance.

The rapid-flow (3–6 liters/min) CO_2 insufflating devices widely used for pelviscopic procedures are generally adequate for evacuating the laser plume. Although CO_2 laser laparoscopy is associated with more plume formation than the argon, Nd:YAG, or KTP lasers, adequate smoke evacuation systems are still mandatory when using the latter three wavelengths.

Efficacy

There are no prospective, blinded studies comparing laparoscopic use of lasers with conventional electrosurgery that have demonstrated an improvement in pregnancy rates or a reduction in adhesion formation.[9,10] Its use to date is based on the clinical impression or bias of the surgeon. Many surgeons advocate the use of lasers because of their controlled depth of penetration, the reduced thermal damage to adjacent tissue, and the reproducibility of tissue effects. These factors must be balanced against the increased equipment costs and operating room fees and the additional training required of the surgeon and supporting staff. Regardless of the availability of lasers, it is extremely important that the endoscopic surgeon master a wide variety of hemostatic and operative techniques.

References

1. Feste J. Laser laparoscopy: a new modality. *J Reprod Med*. 1985;30:413–417.
2. Martin DC. CO_2 laser laparoscopy for endometriosis associated with infertility. *J Reprod Med*. 1986;31:1089–1094.
3. Keye WR Jr, Dixon J. Photocoagulation of endometriosis by the argon laser through the laparoscope. *Obstet Gynecol*. 1983;62:383–386.
4. Keye WR Jr, Hansen LW, Astin M, et al. Argon laser therapy of endometriosis: a review of 92 consecutive patients. *Fertil Steril*. 1987; 47: 208–212.
5. Daniell JF, Meisels S, Miller W, et al. Laparoscopic use of the KTP/532 laser in nonendometriotic pelvic surgery. *Colposcopy Gynecol Laser Surg*. 1986;2:107–111.
6. Lomano JM. Photocoagulation of early pelvic endometriosis with the Nd:YAG laser through the laparoscope. *J Reprod Med*. 1985;30:77–81.
7. Perry PM, Baughman VL. A complication of hysteroscopy: air embolism. *Anesthesiology*. 1990; 63:546–547.
8. Corson SL, Unger M, Kwa D, et al. Laparoscopic laser treatment of endometriosis with the Nd:YAG sapphire probe. *Am J Obstet Gynecol*. 1989;160:718–723.
9. Sutton CJ, Ewen SP, Whitelaw N, Haines P. Prospective, randomized, double-blind, controlled trial of laser laparoscopy in the treatment of pelvic pain associated with minimal, mild, and moderate endometriosis. *Fertil Steril*. 1994;62: 696–700.
10. Tulandi T, Bugnah M. Operative laparoscopy: surgical modalities. *Fertil Steril*. 1995;63: 237–245.

7

Photo and Video Documentation in Endoscopic Surgery

Eric S. Knochenhauer and Ricardo Azziz

Instrumentation and Technique of Still Photography

The system required for endoscopic still photography includes the camera body, camera lens, flash generator, and photographic films.

Camera Body

For endoscopic still photography, almost any single-lens reflex (SLR) camera body with through-the-lens (TTL) viewing can be used. SLR refers to cameras that have one mirror showing the focused image to the viewer. Nevertheless, a camera with interchangeable focus-ing screens is preferred because the general-purpose ground glass focusing screen should be replaced with a circular clear glass screen specifically designed for endoscopic photography. The exception would be the need for a double-crossline focusing screen for use with lenses of longer focal length, requiring more careful focusing.

The camera body should be lightweight. Additional accessories such as remote shutter control, autowinder, and data recorder may be added, although the weight of the camera increases as well. The authors prefer an Olympus OM-1N or an SC-35 camera body with a type 1-9 focusing screen, databack recorder, and autowinder (Fig. 7.1).

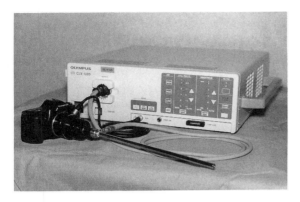

FIGURE 7.1. Endoscopic still photography system consisting of an SC-35 camera body and autowinder, an SM-EFR 3 combined dedicated lens/light sensor unit, and a variable video light source with a xenon vapor arc lamp (CLV-U20, Olympus Corp., Roswell, GA).

Camera Lens

In general, the longer the focal length of the camera lens the greater the amount of film filled by the image. Alternatively, the visual field seen is determined by the endoscopic optics and not by the camera. To completely fill a standard 35-mm film frame (36 × 24 mm), a lens with a focal length between 120 and 150 mm is required. Unfortunately, increasing the focal length of the lens also increases the demand for light and reduces picture brightness. It also decreases the depth of field, which requires more careful focusing, and may yield photos of varying sharpness, because pelvic organs are usually not in the same plane.

Fixed or telephoto lenses of 85 to 120 mm in focal length can be used, although telephoto lenses usually require more light. With these lenses an SLR camera will have a film image to actual size ratio of 1:3 to 1:5, depending on the endoscope. The f-stop is left wide open (3.5, 2.8, or the lowest possible number) because the size of the aperture is actually determined by the diameter of the endoscopy optic system, which is always smaller than that of the lens. The shutter speed varies with the intensity of the light source and ranges from ¼ to 1⁄15 sec.

Greater magnification, and thus a larger image on film, can be achieved using a "macro"-

type lens ("micro" if NIKON brand lenses are used), achieving a 1:1 or 1:2 ratio of film image to actual size. Greater degrees of magnification can also be obtained by using zoom lens of greater focal length or special teleconverter adapters. The Olympus Corp. produces two integrated lens and TTL light sensor systems, the SM-EFR 2 or 3 lens, which have no effective f-stop. The SM-EFR 2 is basically a 105-mm lens, producing an image of approximately 25 mm in diameter on standard 35-mm film. The focal depth is relatively narrow which may require a double-crosshair focusing screen to improve the sharpness of the image. The authors prefer the SM-EFR 3, which has a shorter focal length (82.8 mm) and provides an image that is 18 mm in diameter on film but is brighter and usually in focus throughout (Fig. 7.1).

Focusing During Endoscopic Still Photography

The longer the lens focal length, the narrower the focal plane (i.e., depth of field). Lens with shorter focal lengths (SM-EFR 3 or standard 85-mm lens) require minimum focusing and most of the image on film is seen clearly. Focusing can also be accomplished by setting the camera lens focusing ring on infinity and moving the laparoscope back and forth until the desired image is clearly seen. Unfortunately, this focusing technique changes the field's size and illumination. When viewing through an endoscope, the lens of the human eye (unlike the lens of a camera) automatically focuses images slightly closer or farther than this distance. Therefore, objects that would be slightly out of focus by photography are often not perceived as such by the viewer. Finally, the observer's eyesight should be corrected to as close to 20/20 as possible, otherwise he/she may be mislead while focusing.

Flash Generators

Flash generators can provide extremely potent extra illumination for still-photography. Early laparoscopic photography was obtained using a "distal flash." This system consisted of an in-

FIGURE 7.2. Distal incandescent lamp at the tip of a Decker culdoscope. Note size of replacement bulb.

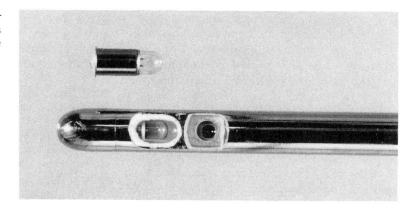

candescent light bulb placed at the distal end of the endoscope (Figure 7.2). Although this system provided extremely good pictures, it emitted a large amount of heat with the potential risk of organ burn or intraabdominal bulb breakage, and is not currently used. Currently there are two flash systems available for still photography:

1. *Intermediate or miniflash:* a small flash light source is attached to the light cable directly, and synchronized to the camera via a light meter (Fig. 7.3). It is fairly effective and economical, although somewhat cumbersome. It is available from Eder Co., or as Tiny-Flash® from Elmed or Reznick Instruments. (Skokie, IL).

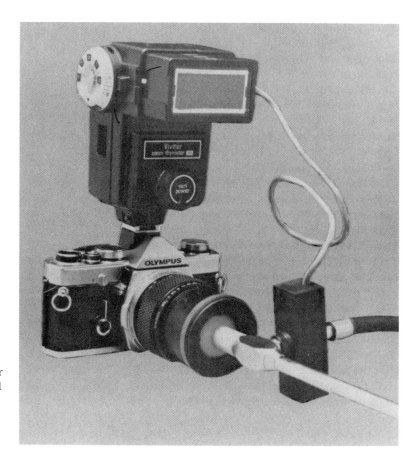

FIGURE 7.3. Intermediate or miniflash mounted on OM-1 camera body.

2. *Proximal flash generator:* this consists of an external light source that may form part of the same light source used for diagnostic purposes. This flash system is the one most widely used in the United States at this time. The light source is usually a 300-W mercury halide or xenon vapor arc lamp. Some of these flash generators can be synchronized to the camera-shutter. For example, as noted the Olympus Corp. currently has a dedicated TTL light sensor unit (SM-EFR 2 or 3) that automatically determines the shutter speed and duration of the flash from a dedicated (either the CLE-F10 or CLV-10) light source. In this system the flash can produce an image in $\frac{1}{100}$ to $\frac{1}{3000}$ sec with a recycling time of 2 to 3 sec (see Fig. 7.1). Some newer xenon light sources have a semiflash system that can increase the maximum illumination 1.5 fold the peak constant level (e.g., Olympus CLV-U20).

Photographic Film

Either Ektachrome® or Kodachrome® film can be used for slide photography. Kodachrome® lasts longer, although it has a reddish hue and is more difficult to develop because it must be processed directly by Kodak Co. Ektachrome film is easier to process and has a tendency to appear neutral or slightly blue. Both these films are available in "daylight" types, balanced for the blue spectrum (K° 5000–6000) light most frequently emitted by currently available flash systems. A film size of 35 mm is usually preferable. Occasionally 16-mm slide film is used as it requires less light for recording, although the image is relatively grainier.

The sensitivity of the film to light is designated by ASA (American Standards Association) or DIN (Deutsche Industrie Norm, primarily in Europe) scores. More recently the ISO (International Standards Organization) has provided a compilation of these two standards. For most endoscopic photography, film that is 160 to 400 ASA/ISO is preferred.

Slide film is easier to handle and process. However, if there was a possibility of requiring photographs for printing or publishing, it is preferable to use color or black and white print film initially; the quality of the picture is slightly better when slides are made from color print than visa versa.

Still Photography Technique in the Operating Room

The equipment for still photography must be present and ready in the operating room at all times because it is difficult to plan ahead and determine which operative cases may require photo documentation. When taking photographs it is important to maintain a record of the patient's name, date, number of exposures, and any other pertinent information. In addition, a data recording back, which imprints the film with the date or a code number, is extremely useful in later identifying the images. During processing slides are usually numbered in consecutive exposure order by the developing company. A photo of the patient's nameplate or pertinent information written out can be obtained before beginning endoscopy photography, although this may be difficult to perform well with some lens systems. To obtain quality slides or photographs, particularly for teaching or publication, a large number of pictures should be obtained.

The technique preferred by the authors for taking photographs in the operating room is to double glove, load the camera onto the endoscope, remove the left-hand double glove, and position the operative instruments with this hand while controlling the camera with the right. In this manner, contamination of the operative field is minimal and control over the photograph maximum.

For additional information on endoscopic still photography, see references 1–5.

Instrumentation and Techniques for Endoscopic Video Imaging, Recording, and Printing

The couplers, video camera, control unit, TV monitor, and video cassette recorder, along with the light source and endoscope, comprise the video imaging and recording system.

Light Source

As discussed previously, a high-intensity light source should be available. Although some systems provide continuous and nonvariable illumination, others can vary their intensity based on the amount of light reaching the camera head (e.g., Olympus Corp. CLV-10 light source). This tends to decrease glaring of the video image. Nonetheless, the resultant reduction in illumination may be annoying, particularly if the tissue of the interest is not the source of the glare.

Camera Couplers

Cameras can attach directly to the endoscope viewpiece through a straight coupler, which has the advantage of allowing all available light to be received by the camera chip. While this is preferred method for video imaging today, it has the disadvantage of obligating the surgeon to perform the entire operation from the monitor screen or to constantly remove the camera. For those surgeons who feel more comfortable directly viewing the operative field through the endoscope, an alternative is the use of a beam splitter. This device splits the light received from the endoscope 30%/70%, 20%/80%, or 10%/90%, the lesser portion being transmitted to the surgeon's eye and the remainder to the camera.

When using a beam splitter, it is more convenient if the camera head is able to rotate without unscrewing. This makes it possible to change the position of the beam splitter on the endoscopic head while keeping the video monitor image upright. Many beam splitters were originally designed for arthroscopy or gastroenterology. Compared to gynecology, these applications require a much narrower field of view and visualize a smaller, more light-reflective cavity. Thus, each make and type of beam splitter should be tested before being used in gynecology. Both beam splitters and direct couplers are usually furnished with a focusing ring. They may also provide a small degree of magnification. The diameter of the coupler will be the primary determinant of the size of the video image as projected into the video chip. Other coupling systems (mostly for arthroscopic/gastroenterologic applications) yield small round images on the video monitor. Nonetheless, most current systems do fill the entire screen with the image, using greater diameter couplers (e.g., 35 mm).

Video Camera

Early endoscopic cameras consisted of single or triple television tubes.[6] The single-tube (single-frequency, color-coded, and phase-integrated) cameras electronically split the image transmitted to the color monitor into component colors according to empirical values. Consequently, color resolution was often less than optimal. The triple-tube cameras split the image colors into the three primary colors via a prism that was then processed by three different television tubes. The color resolution of this type of camera was very good; however, the system was very bulky and usually required a counter-balance suspension system.

During the past decade, improvements to endoscopic video cameras have included the use of solid-state systems using a charge-coupled device (CCD) chip and a decrease in camera size and weight. With improved technology, these chip cameras, although smaller, have improved color fidelity, light sensitivity, resolution, and dynamic range compared to their earlier counterparts. Many common heads today provide remote control for video recording and photography (e.g., record/pause), which gives the surgeon direct control over the recording process. Preferably, the camera should be small and connecting cables should be fully sterilizable.

Currently, CCD chips (Fig. 7.4) are composed of approximately 380,000 to 410,000 light-sensitive elements or "pixels." Many of the video cameras contain a single CCD chip and can deliver between 300 and 450 horizontal lines of resolution. To further improve the quality of the video image, recent camera innovations have included three chip cameras, high-definition video, three-dimensional (3-D) imaging, digital signals, and distally placed video chips. Three chip cameras employ a prism to separate the three primary colors (red, green, blue), similar to the older three-

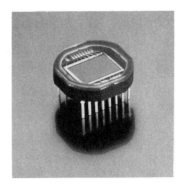

FIGURE 7.4. Close-up of charge-coupled device (CCD) chip. (Courtesy of Olympus Corp., Roswell, GA.)

tube cameras. The three primary colors are recorded individually, producing improved color and resolution. Some of these newer three-chip cameras can provide up to 750 lines of resolution (Endovision®, Storz; OTV-S4, Olympus; Microdigital®, Circon). The disadvantage of the three-chip compared to the one-chip camera is its increased cost, weight, and size. The use of high-definition video (video format for high-definition television or HDTV) effectively results in a fivefold increase in the number of pixels and an improvement in the image.[7] HDTV systems, although available, are not generally practical because they are not compatible with current television video standards (see resolution and standards sections, following). In addition to being much bulkier, HDTV systems are heavier and far more expensive than current CCD cameras. Three-dimensional imaging is currently in the experimental stage and if successful (and practical) may lead to improved hand-to-eye coordination. However, current efforts have been disappointing.

The first single-chip *digital* camera was introduced by Circon in 1992. Digital systems innately have the ability to improve and manipulate the image compared to analog systems. Image manipulation includes possible automatic white balance (to compensate for the blueing of the light source), black balance,

edge enhancement, and auto gain control. Finally, some newer systems place a CCD chip at the end of a flexible or rigid shaft, completely eliminating the need for the glass lens system (e.g., Hopkin Lens System®). Placement of the video "camera" into the abdominal cavity allows use of flexible endoscopes and results in lower light requirements.

Control Unit

The control unit is the power supply and signal processing center for the camera. In some control units the hue of the picture can be adjusted manually, adapting the image to the type of light and altering the light sensitivity. More current models are fully automatic, providing a uniform color setting based on a total white image received (i.e., "white balance"). They may also feature a "color bar" setting to fine-tune each primary color as it appears on the monitor. These camera/control units may also have an automatic shutter for minimization of possible glare. Different camera heads and control units are usually not interchangeable, with a specific model control unit for each camera. Digital control units are required for digital cameras and provide improved signal-to-noise ratio, improved resolution and color accuracy, contrast enhancement, detail enhancement, and edge correction.

Video input into the control unit is through the camera. Video output may and often does consist of multiple jacks of usually more than one of the following—composite, Y/C (separate channels for chromants and brightness), and RGB (separate channels for Red, Green, and Blue signals; see Resolution and Standards)—which allows the most flexibility while in use. A standard setup involves use of RGB outputs to the monitor(s) or video printer and Y/C output to the super VHS (S-VHS) video recorder. A monitor may receive its signal directly from the control unit or from another monitor's output. Each camera/control unit requires its own monitor for continuous viewing, unless a digital image processor is used to place both video images onto one screen (Twinvideo®, Storz).

Resolution and Standards

Before presenting the rest of the video system components, a discussion of resolution and standards is necessary. Horizontal resolution is the number of separate vertical lines available for the image. Accordingly, vertical resolution is the number of possible horizontal image lines. Thus, the greater the lines of resolution the sharper the image. The resolution of a complete system of video imaging (endoscope, camera, control unit, monitor) is set by its weakest link or the piece of equipment with the lowest resolution. Consequentially, if your camera produces 700 horizontal lines of resolution but the monitor can only handle 300 lines, the image will only have 300 lines of horizontal resolution. Resolution is also affected by the electronic noise of the system. Thus, the greater the signal strength to noise ratio, the better the image.

The most common video standard (used in the United States, Canada, Japan, most of Asia, and South America) is based on the television standard set by the National Television Systems Committee (NTSC). The image at each pixel is electronically converted to two signals combining both the chromants and luminance. Each signal (either for television or closed-circuit video) utilizes a composite signal of 4.3 MHz comprising both the luminance and the chromants information. Combining the two separate signal components into a single signal leads to some image (signal) degradation secondary to interference. With a limited bandwidth of 6 MHz, video systems based on NTSC have limited resolution. The NTSC standard is 525 lines/frame and 30 frames/sec, with only 485 lines used for the image and 40 for framing. Two other composite standards currently are available: the Phase Alternation Line (PAL), used in western Europe and South America, and the Se'quential Couleur a' Memoire (SECAM), used in France, eastern Europe, and the former Soviet Union. Both systems are based on 625 lines/frame and 25 frames/sec. All three systems are considered composite systems but are not compatible with each other.

Newer HDTV systems have a bandwidth of 30 MHz, compared to the 6 MHz of NTSC systems, which yields more than 1000 horizontal lines. While this may improve the image, replacement of existing equipment is expensive because NTSC, PAL, and SECAM monitors and cameras are not compatible.

Two other closed video systems have been utilized to improve image resolution. These systems require a compatible camera, control unit, and monitors to maximize the benefit. Briefly, NTSC utilizes a one-signal–one-channel approach while Y/C and RGB utilize a one-signal–multiple channels approach.

Y/C systems consist of two channels or separate signals, one for the luminants or brightness (Y) and the other for chromants or color (C). They also have an improved signal-to-noise ratio when compared to composite systems. Super-VHS utilizes a Y/C system and increases the video tape lines of resolution from 200 (NTSC) to 400. However, a S-VHS player must be used to gain this advantage in playback. The RGB system separates the signal into separate red (R), green (G), and blue (B) signals: brightness is a combination of these signals. The RGB system provides a sharp image and distinct color separation. This system is excellent for use with monitors, printers, and computers. No practical RGB-VHS is currently available. Subjectively, RGB is better than Y/C, which is superior to NTSC for image quality when compared on similar cameras of similar resolution.

Color Monitor

The color monitor rarely affects image quality. Most good home television screens today are only able to handle 350 horizontal lines of resolution, while video monitors can handle from 450 to 700 lines of resolution. The use of a larger screen size does not increase the brightness or resolution of the image, but the image may appear more blurred to those observing from a close distance. It is most important to completely fill the monitor screen with the projected image because this will increase the number of scanning lines used and improve the overall resolution. This can be achieved with use of different (20- to 35-mm) couplers as noted previously. However, the brightness of the image is reduced by the square of its size on the screen. Assuming the same illumination, a 40% larger image on the television screen will appear half as bright, despite improved resolution. Monitors usually accept input from at least two of the following formats: composite (i.e., NTSC), Y/C, and RGB signals. Images on monitors using RGB and Y/C usually yield a clearer image than monitors using only composite signals. Some newer monitors include features such as overscan enlargement, which can enlarge the received image by 117% (OEV201 monitor, Olympus Corp., Roswell, GA).

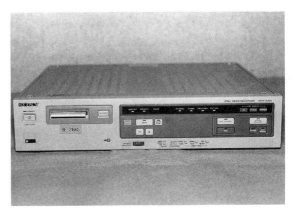

FIGURE 7.5. Digital 2-in. floppy storage system (MVR-5300, Sony Corp, Park Ridge, NJ).

Video Recorders

Video recorders are available in many formats. Remote controls and character generators are optional equipment. Three-quarter-inch tape is used preferentially for producing films for teaching, demonstrations, or television. This tape is more durable and less subject to distortion as it has a greater surface area-to-signal ratio than the standard half-inch format. Furthermore, most editing systems are geared to this format. Nevertheless, S-VHS (half-inch) videotape editing systems are becoming increasingly more sophisticated. S-VHS tape has approximately 60% the resolution of most three-CCD cameras and monitors (400 lines vs. 700 lines of resolution). This decreased resolution in tape storage results in decreased image quality when compared to live viewing. High-band 8-mm provides a similar increase in resolution when compared to regular 8-mm recorders (400 vs. 225 lines of resolution).

Video Printers

Video printers that convert video images to hard copy prints within seconds are available from various manufacturers and offer video photographic images with improved resolution (600-1500 horizontal line resolution). However, they still fall short of ocular resolution (approximately 1600 lines) and 35-mm still photography (to 2300 lines).[8] Several systems can store as many as 50 images digitally on a floppy disk (Figure 7.5) for later retrieval and processing. Although some printers require the video image to be frozen on the recorder, others do so automatically.

In the past, some systems used tiny jets to spray each primary color on paper. Today, most systems use a form of color thermal printing. Basically the image is composed of approximately 15 to 20 million dots of cyan, magenta, yellow, and black. Some systems produce black dots by superimposing the three primary colors. A heated printhead is used to melt dots of colored wax or plastic from long ribbons onto the paper. Dot density ranges from 5 to 9 dots/mm^2. Each color is laid down separately. The number of possible colors in each dot ranges from 2.1 million to 16.7 million in higher end models. One exception to color thermal printing is the Polaroid system (Cambridge, MA), which projects the video image onto a miniature internal color television screen. Using a color filter wheel, the image is then photographed three times and printed onto Polaroid paper. Higher end printers also have added features such as date, time, alphanumeric characters, strobe pictures of sequential events, picture in picture, multiple pictures (4–16/sheet), and reverse image for transparencies. Equipment is also available to produce 35-mm slides directly from the control unit. One such product (Surgislide®, Medgraphix International Imaging) has an RGB input connection and delivers 720 horizontal and 480 vertical lines of resolution.

Although video image print quality is still much poorer than that obtained from still photography, it is quite useful for clinical documentation and patient education.

References

1. Cohen MR. Photography. In: Phillips JM, ed. *Laparoscopy.* Baltimore: William & Wilkins; 1977: 300–305.
2. Marlow J. Endoscopic photography. *Clin Obstet Gynecol.* 1983;26:359–365.
3. Semm K. *Operative Manual for Operative Endoscopic Abdominal Surgery.* Chicago: Year Book Medical Publishers; 1987:46–53, 57–58, 242–248.
4. Hulka JF. *Textbook of Laparoscopy.* New York: Grune & Stratton, 1985:7–21.
5. Borten M. *Laparoscopic Complications: Prevention and Management.* Philadelphia: BC Decker; 1986: 430–441.
6. Circon. *Circon Micro Video Cameras Operating Manual.* Santa Barbara, CA: Circon Corp.; 3.1–3.2.
7. Circon. *The Circon Medical Video Revolution.* Santa Barbara, CA: Circon Corp.; 1–5.
8. Mathias H, Patterson R. *Electronic Cinematography.* Belmont, CA: Wadsworth; 1985.

Part II
Operative Laparoscopic Procedures

8

Technique and Instrumentation in Operative Laparoscopy

Sujatha Reddy, Arlene Morales, and Ana Alvarez Murphy

Introduction

The ability to perform complex operative procedures with the laparoscope is dependent on the skill of the surgeon and the availability of appropriate surgical instruments. In this chapter, we discuss the general instrumentation and technique needed to complete most laparoscopic procedures. Successful laparoscopy combines the skills of the surgeons, anesthesiologists, and operating room personnel with well-chosen and well-maintained endoscopic instruments and equipment. This team should bring an organized and thought-out approach to the operating room setup of equipment and instrumentation.

The Operating Room

Every operating room designed for operative laparoscopy should meet the criteria for a general operating room with full anesthesia, laboratory, blood bank support, and imaging. Major complications are unusual in operative laparoscopy, but vascular, urologic, intestinal, and other injuries may occur. Not only must one be skillful enough to recognize the injury, but the capabilities for immediate diagnosis and repair should be available. A sterile laparotomy pack should be available in the operating room before any endoscopic abdominal operation is started,[1] although it is not necessary to have it opened.

The laparoscopy cart provides drawers and space for the storage of laparoscopes and instruments as well as the automatic CO_2 insufflator, cylinders, electrosurgical unit, cold light source, and suction/irrigation unit. If it is large enough, the video camera and monitor can also be placed in the cart. Units from the same manufacturer can usually be stacked for more efficient use of space.

Patient Positioning

The operating table must be able to allow the various patient positions that are essential for gynecologic surgery from supine to lithotomy, including level, Trendelenburg, or reverse, and lateral tilts and varying heights. It must comfortably and securely support the patient in all these positions. Electrically powered tables meet these requirements best. To optimize the surgeon's mobility and facilitate the positioning of support equipment, the patient's arms are padded and placed on the table at her side, rather than extended on lateral arm supports (Fig. 8.1). Leg supports may vary. We prefer stirrups that allow the legs to be in the semiextended position and well supported, such as the Allen's Universal stirrups (Allen Medical Systems, Inc., Mayfield, OH) (Fig. 8.2). Additionally, the legs are maintained as flat as

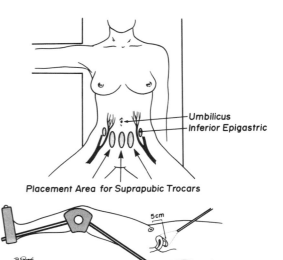

Placement Area for Suprapubic Trocars

FIGURE 8.1. Proper positioning of the patient for operative laparoscopy includes placing the legs in a frog leg position, with the thighs almost parallel to the longitudinal axis of the body. The left arm (if the operator is right handed) should be tucked alongside the patient's body because the surgeon usually operates from the patient's left shoulder area. The ancillary sites should be placed as high as possible above the pubis, but not less than 5 cm. Generally, these ports are placed medial to the inferior epigastric artery and vein, taking care to identify these vessels.

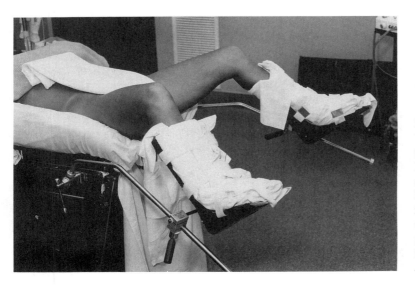

FIGURE 8.2. Using the Allen Universal Stirrup (Allen Medical Systems, Inc., Mayfield Heights, OH), the legs are well supported while keeping the knees out of the surgeon's field. (Reproduced with permission from Garzo VG, Murphy AA. Operative laparoscopy instrumentation. *Semin Reprod Endocrinol.* 1991;9:109–116.)

possible to maximize the operator's space and mobility of instruments (Fig. 8.1). Careful attention is given to adequate padding of the undersides of the legs, arms, and hands to minimize peripheral vascular or nerve injury.[2]

After proper positioning, prepping, and draping, instruments for uterine manipulation and chromotubation are placed. Uterine manipulators are essential to almost all laparoscopic procedures except those in which there is a suspicion of intrauterine pregnancy or when gamete intrafallopian transfer is planned.[3] Uterine manipulation facilitates the visualization of pelvic structures and is essential for operative exposure. The most common instruments available for manipulation and chromotubation include the Cohen olive-tipped cannula (Fig. 8.3), the Hasson balloon uterine elevator, the Harris uterine manipulator-injector (HUMI), and the Semm vacuum cannula (Fig. 8.4). Many others are available, including the Valtchev, which consists of a head with an intrauterine cannula and a body with a metal bar and tube that pivots on the head (see Fig. 21.1).[4] This feature allows changing the angle of the intrauterine portion

of the instruments in relation to the intravaginal portion and anteverts the uterus to a maximum of about 120°. The desired angle can be maintained with a screw. This uterine manipulator is particularly useful for laparoscopic-assisted vaginal hysterectomy, when maximum uterine displacement is required in all directions.

Placement of Ancillary Ports

The proper placement of the ancillary ports is of critical importance in reducing the incidence of vascular injuries, in addition to making laparoscopic surgery possible. Once the laparoscope has been inserted into the abdominal cavity, the operator must choose the site and number of ancillary ports. Rarely, if ever, should the surgeon attempt to perform a significant operative (even diagnostic) procedure using a single-puncture technique. Usually the first auxiliary site that is placed is a port in the midline suprapubic area. It is extremely important that the surgeon place this puncture as high as cosmetically possible, but

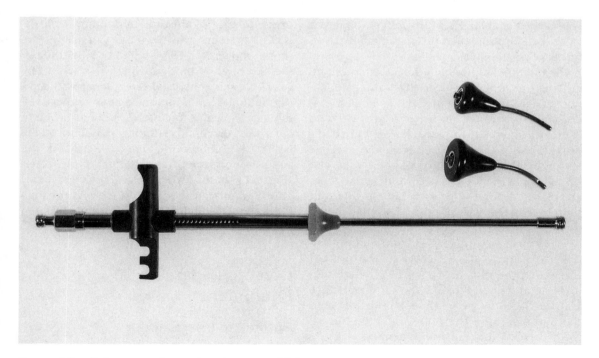

FIGURE 8.3. Cohen cannula: uterine elevator and injector.

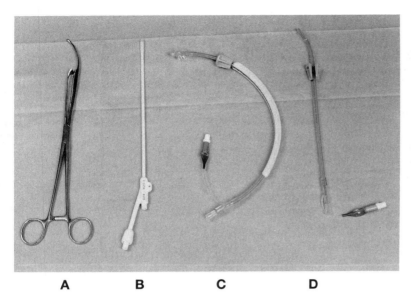

FIGURE 8.4.   Uterine elevators and injectors. *From left to right:* **A:** Hulka tenaculum (Allis Tip). **B:** Hasson balloon uterine elevator cannula. **C:** ZSI 4.5-mm uterine manipulator. **D:** ZSI 4.0-mm uterine injector. (**A** and **B** from Weck Eder Instrument Co., Chicago, IL; **C** and **D** from Zinnanti Surgical Instruments, Chatsworth, CA. Reproduced with permission as in Fig. 8.2.)

A   B   C   D

never less than 5 cm above the symphysis pubis (see Fig. 8.1). This will allow maximum access to the cul de sac and posterior uterus. During placement the bladder should be continuously drained. In the patient who has undergone prior surgery, an attempt should be made to identify the bladder edge laparoscopically, taking care to place the suprapubic puncture cephalad to it. This operator prefers to place a valveless 5-mm sheath at this site to facilitate removal of small biopsy specimens.

Once the pelvis has been fully examined, including the appendix, liver edge, and gallbladder, a decision must be made as to whether additional suprapubic punctures are needed. Generally, it is best to place the next auxiliary port opposite the area requiring the greatest amount of surgery. A third puncture site can be added as needed. These additional ports are placed along the suprapubic hairline, but there are a few exceptions. The small punctures required for the placement of the laser delivery fiber may be placed slightly more caudally to improve laser access to the ovarian fossa and posterior ovarian surface. When performing an appendectomy the third puncture may be placed in the midline, halfway between the umbilicus and the pubis, directed toward the cecal-ileal junction and appendix.

To gain the maximum degree of instrument maneuverability, it is important to place the ad-ditional suprapubic trocar as far lateral as safely possible without injuring the inferior epigastric or external iliac vessels (see Fig. 8.1). Translumination of the abdomen will occasionally reveal the inferior epigastric vessels, although most often the silhouette seen corresponds to more superficial vessels. To transluminate, the room must be darkened and the laparoscope pressed gently against the abdominal wall. Excessive pressure will decrease vascular perfusion and decrease vessel visibility. Nonetheless, the best method of identifying the inferior epigastric vessels consists of direct laparoscopic visualization. The abdominal course of these vessels usually begins just lateral to the insertion of the round ligament, running parallel and lateral to the umbilical ligaments. Generally, the auxiliary ports are placed lateral to these vessels (Fig. 8.1). Before trocar placement, the exact entry point can be established by pressing down on the abdominal wall with a finger, while viewing through the laparoscope.

General Laparoscopic Equipment

Automatic Insufflator

The development of the modern automatic pressure-limited insufflators and the use of

CO_2 rather than air or NO_2 has greatly aided our ability to establish endoscopic access to the peritoneal cavity. Because of its lipid solubility, CO_2 is more quickly absorbed from the peritoneal cavity than NO_2 and postoperative shoulder and chest discomfort from diaphragmatic irritation is minimized. The rapid absorption of CO_2 also allows for accurate interpretation of postoperative x-rays, as in the case of suspected bowel inuries. In these patients, a flat and upright x-ray of the abdomen can be useful even 1 day postoperatively with a minimum risk of false-positive findings of air under the diaphragm.

The key to insufflation safety is our ability to monitor intraabdominal pressure.[5] A useful feature for insufflators to have is separate gauges to distinguish true intraabdominal pressure from total insufflation pressure. Automatic sensors that shut gas off when the intraabdominal pressure reaches 15 to 20 mmHg can avoid overinflation and compromised venous return. In addition, a visual gauge of gas flow is essential at the time of initial insufflation. Most insufflators have a basal flow rate of 1 liter/min with maximum rates of 3 to 20 liters/min. An electronically controlled high-flow mode that maintains the pneumoperitoneum despite gas loss, which frequently occurs during fluid aspiration, instrument changes, and laser plume evacuation, will significantly decrease operating time. The insufflator response time to intraabdominal pressure changes should be rapid.

Pneumoperitoneum is established through insufflation using either a Veress or Touhy needle. The latter, used for epidural anesthesia, is rarely used today. The Veress needle has a blunt inner point that retracts as it penetrates the abdominal wall, springing out to avoid organ puncture when inside the abdominal cavity. Disposable Veress needles are also available. During insufflation the surgeon should percuss the right-upper quadrant over the liver edge. Loss of dullness to percussion, indicating free distension of the peritoneal cavity, generally occurs with less than 1 liter CO_2 insufflated. Obese individuals may need slightly more gas volume. However, if no loss to percussion occurs with 2 liters CO_2 then either the liver edge is severely adherent to the anterior abdominal wall (Fitz–Hugh–Curtis syndrome), or the insufflating needle is not placed properly (e.g., is insufflating preperitoneally).

Light Source

Fiberoptic technology has revolutionized endoscopy. Essentially, it brings light into the abdominal cavity without the heat generated by the light source. Light is captured from a chamber and carried to the pelvic cavity by a bundle of flexible fibers.[6] The amount of light delivered is therefore proportional to the number of intact fibers available for transmission of light. The ability of the surgeon to view the pelvic organs is a function of the intensity of the external light source, the quality of the light cord, and the quality of the optics system of the laparoscope. The amount of light required is also a function of the object being viewed. More light is necessary for panoramic views of dark objects, and much less is required for viewing close or light-reflective objects.

A 150-W halogen light source is sufficient for laparoscopy if video is not used. Light intensity is usually manually adjusted with a rheostat. Light sources for endoscopic photography or video systems utilize high intensity light, usually a 300-W xenon or halogen glass bulb, with automatic light intensity control. Additional desirable features in a light source include convenient access to the light bulb for ready replacement and a dual-bulb unit providing a backup in the event of primary bulb failure. Cables of different sizes and makes are accommodated by a turret of multiple female couplers. Inspection of fiberoptic light cables should be performed routinely because, with use, light-transmitting fibers are lost. The nonfunctioning fibers appear as dark spots when the cable is examined on end. Although more expensive, liquid light cables do not present this problem although they do demonstrate darkening over time as the inner gel carbonizes. See Chapter 4 for additional information on light cables and sources.

Video Imaging

Operative laparoscopy is a team effort. Proper assistance requires that others be able to see what the surgeon is seeing and thereby anticipate his/her needs. The camera used is composed of one or more small, lightweight, highresolution charge-coupled device (CCD) chips.[3] A high-resolution color monitor is necessary and permits the surgeon to operate from the screen, allowing the operator to stand upright and thus decreasing back strain and eye fatigue. A video cassette recorder, preferably with a color hard copy video printer, should be available to provide documentation of the surgical findings.

Most surgeons prefer to place the video monitor at the foot of the operating table, providing the surgeon and his/her assistant with an equal view. It also eliminates the hand-to-eye coordination problem that can arise from trying to maneuver in one direction while looking in another plane. General surgeons operating in the upper abdomen prefer the monitor at the head of the table for similar reasons. Alternatively, if two video monitors are available, they may be placed across the table from the surgeon and assistant such that each has a direct view of the pelvis. See Chapter 7 for additional discussion of video imaging systems.

Trocars and Sheaths

The umbilical trocar and sheath are inserted after appropriate insufflation has been achieved. Sheaths are available with either a trumpet (piston) or a flapper (trap) valve. Trumpet valves decrease the loss of gas with instrument changes but make movement of the instruments up and down the trocar more difficult and are primarily used for the umbilical (laparoscopic) sheath (10–12 mm in diameter). Smaller diameter (3–7 mm) trocars and sleeves are available for the ancillary puncture sites.

Trocars are available with either a pyramidal or conical tip, although most surgeons prefer the pyramidal tip because its three sharp edges require less force to perforate the anterior abdominal wall.[7,8] However, using the Z-puncture technique a conical trocar can be inserted through muscular tissues with minimum risk and effort.[9] The greater the force required for trocar insertion, the greater the risk of vascular or visceral injury. Thus, the trocar tip should be as sharp as possible. This is one of the ad-

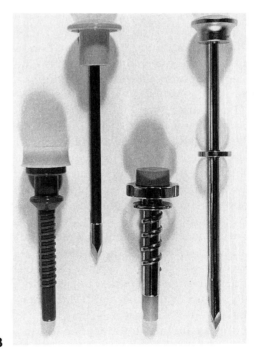

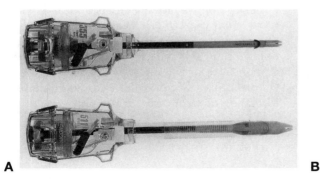

A   **B**

FIGURE 8.5.   Disposable trocars (Ethicon, Somerville, NJ).

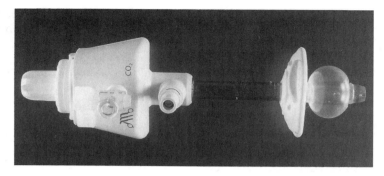

FIGURE 8.6. Trocar with inflatable balloon to anchor the trocar (Origin Medical Systems, Inc., Menlo Park, CA).

vantages of the disposable trocars (Fig. 8.5), which also have a protective sheath that springs out after trocar insertion to decrease the possibility of further intraabdominal injury. Nevertheless, these trocars are unlikely to prevent injury to organs (e.g., bowel) that are closely adherent to the area of insertion.

Sheaths are now available that have an inflatable balloon at the end to anchor the trocar in place (Fig. 8.6). An additional benefit of these trochars is that the balloon can be used to tamponade bleeding from a vessel injury at the trochar site. Other methods of anchoring the umbilical/ancillary port are available, the most common being the screw-type sheath (see Fig. 8.5B).

Laparoscopes

Diagnostic and operative laparoscopes are available in a variety of sizes and with different angles (see Chapter 4). Diagnostic or straight laparoscopes are widely used for operative laparoscopy as they provide the most light and field of view for any given size (see Fig. 4.4A). Additionally, many surgeons claim insertion of instruments through ancillary sites provides increased depth perception and a wider field of vision.[9]

Operating laparoscopes have a straight channel parallel to the optical axis for the introduction of operating instruments or the laser. The most commonly used operating laparoscope is the Jacob–Palmer model, which is offset with two right angles so that the eyepiece is parallel to the axis of the laparoscope (see Fig. 4.4C). The view is identical to that of a straight for-

ward laparoscope. The operating laparoscope can provide a unique view that at times cannot be achieved with an instrument placed through an ancillary site.[1]

Improved technology has allowed the miniaturization of the laparoscope. Flexible optical catheters (1.8 mm in diameter) are available that may be inserted through a Verres needle, midway between the umbilicus and the pubic symphysis. The optical quality of the view provided is surprisingly good. Instruments, 2 to 3 mm in diameter, including probes, graspers, and biopsy forceps, are also available (see Chapter 24). In most patients, diagnostic laparoscopy may be performed with local anesthesia and intravenous sedation if necessary. In selected patients this may be performed in an office setting.

Operative Laparoscopic Instrumentation

In choosing operative laparoscopic equipment, the surgeon usually must select from various vendors as no one company will provide all the instruments needed. Fortunately, despite the number of equipment vendors, the number of manufacturers is limited so that instruments are usually compatible. It is particularly important to remember that 10-mm or 5-mm-diameter sheaths will not easily accommodate 11- to 12-mm or 5.5-mm instruments, respectively. It is preferable to place a trocar that accommodates the largest diameter instruments used. Following are some of the principal categories of operative laparoscopic instruments.

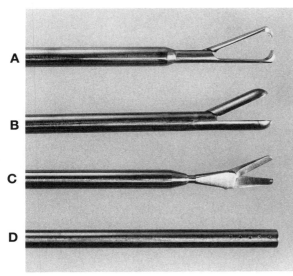

FIGURE 8.7   Ten-millimeter instruments. *From top to bottom:* **A:** Claw grasper. **B:** Spoon forceps. **C:** Straight scissors. **D:** Suction cannula. (All instruments by WISAP, Sauerlach, Germany, with the exception of suction cannula by Reznick Instrument, Inc., Skokie, IL.)

For Aspiration and/or Irrigation

Cannulas of different gauges are available for aspiration of cysts or injection of saline or di-lute vasopressin. Spinal needles introduced directly through the abdominal wall can serve the same purpose. Small-caliber (20- to 22-gauge) needles are preferred for injection of fluid into the pelvic sidewall or adnexa, as there is less leakage and risk of bleeding from the puncture site.

Large-bore cannulas are available for aspiration and irrigation of the pelvic cavity. Such devices are necessary, for example, to evacuate a hemoperitoneum quickly, remove contents of endometriotic cysts, or remove char during laser surgery. For example, a straight 10-mm tube connected to wall suction is extremely useful for the evacuation of a hemoperitoneum containing clots (Fig. 8.7D). The ability to evacuate a hemoperitoneum and identify the source of bleeding during surgery for ectopic pregnancy can make the difference between laparoscopic and laparotomy management of the pregnancy.

Suction/irrigation cannulas may simply be a valveless tube connected to a 60- or 100-cc syringe via an IV tubing connector. Irrigation can be achieved through a similar tube by hooking it up to a bag of intravenous fluid, placed inside a blood pressure cuff to increase flow. However, automatic units for irrigation and aspiration are commercially available and

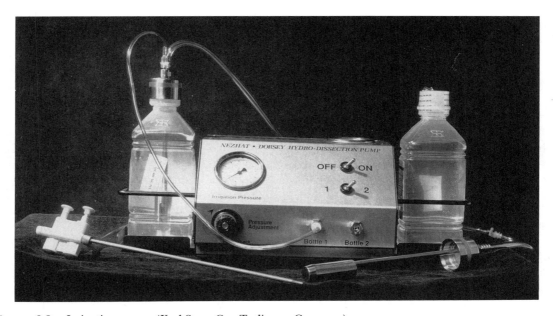

FIGURE 8.8.   Irrigation pump (Karl Storz Co., Tutlinger, Germany).

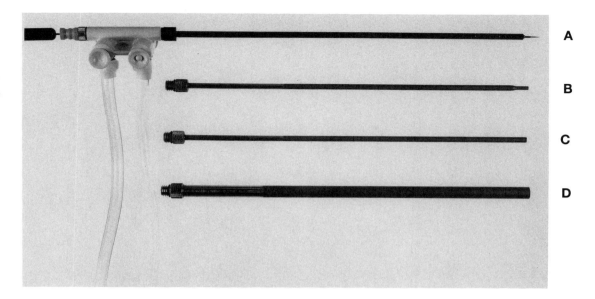

FIGURE 8.9. Different cannulas for aspiration/irrigation handle. *From top to bottom:* **A:** Sump tip with microtip unipolar cautery. **B:** Narrow single tip. **C:** Medium single tip. **D:** Large-bore single tip. (Karl Storz Co., Tutlingern, Germany.)

are an essential part of the operative laparoscopy set (Fig. 8.8). Standard operating room wall suction is preferable to the suction provided by combination suction/irrigation units. In addition, some of the irrigation/aspiration units have a pneumatic pump available that can create dissection planes by instilling fluid at high pressures (i.e., hydrodissection).

Various suction/irrigation cannulas are available for use with these automatic irrigators, some with interchangeable tips or for use with the unipolar needle or laser fiber (Fig. 8.9). Instruments that combine suction/irrigation with a port for a unipolar needle electrode are particularly helpful to pinpoint bleeding. A variation is the Nezhat suction/irrigation cannula, which has an adaptor for placement of a laser fiber (Fig. 8.10). Because of the 90° angle between the trumpet valve and the shaft of the cannula, blood clots and other debris may occlude this device. Cannulas with a single distal opening are more precise but easily obstructed by clots or tissue. Multiple holes at the suction tip make obstruction and loss of suction less likely.

Probes

Blunt probes are one of the most frequently used instruments (Fig. 8.11). They are very useful for manipulation of organs or adhesions in the pelvis, and are usually marked in centimeters. This is quite useful for marking sites of structures, as the laparoscope tends to magnify depending on the distance from the object viewed. Some probes are available with tapered ends, so as to examine fallopian tubes with stenotic ostia or agglutinated fimbria (Fig. 8.11). Many other instruments can be used as probes, including a closed grasping or biopsy forceps or an irrigation cannula. However, the blunt probe remains the least traumatic.

Forceps and Graspers

The ideal graspers hold tissue atraumatically, without significant damage. Unfortunately, such an ideal is rarely reached. Manipulation of tissue with metal instruments can be very traumatic. One should be careful not to crush tissue by applying excessive force in an attempt

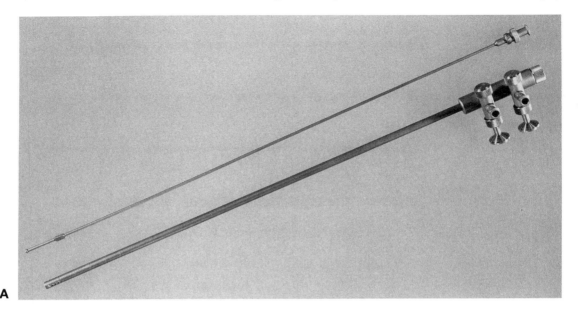

A

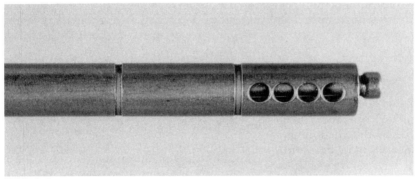

B

FIGURE 8.10. **A:** Nezhat 5-mm suction/irrigation cannula with trumpet valves *(bottom)* and guide for laser fiber placement *(top).* **B:** Tip of aspiration/ irrigation cannula with guide for laser fiber inserted and protruding slightly. (Cabot Medical Corp. Langhorne, PA.)

to maintain it in a fixed position. Several grasping forceps are available (Figs. 8.12, 8.13, and 8.14). The ampulla dilator or grasping tongs are most commonly used to dilate phimotic ampulla (Fig. 8.12). The instrument is placed inside the fallopian tube and withdrawn in the open position at various angles. In contrast, we believe that the traditional "atraumatic" grasping forceps is actually quite traumatic (Fig. 8.13) and should not be used, with the possible exception of placement on the utero-ovarian ligament to stabilize the ovary. Thin straight graspers with grooves and no spring are relatively atraumatic yet adequately hold tissue

(Fig. 8.12). Particularly useful are the tubal and adhesion graspers (Fig. 8.13). Hasson has designed a three- and four-pronged grasper with and without teeth (Fig. 8.14) useful for grasping the ovary.[10] The force applied by the prongs can be controlled and maintained by tightening a screw on the handle.

Large (10-mm or 11-mm-diameter) spoon forceps are commonly used to extract tissue from the pelvis (see Fig. 8.7B), particularly any trophoblast remaining in the cul de sac after surgery for an ectopic pregnancy. Large traumatic claw forceps are quite useful to grasp and stabilize tissue that is to be removed, such

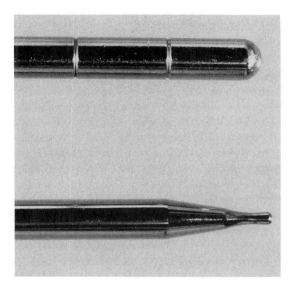

FIGURE 8.11. Blunt *(top)* and conical *(bottom)* probes.

as myomas or ovaries (see Fig. 8.7A). The hinged jaws allow large pieces to be grasped. A 5-mm version is available (Fig. 8.13). Biopsy forceps, with a single tooth on each jaw, can be used to remove small portions of tissue or to fix structures, such as the cyst wall of an endometrioma during enucleation (Fig. 8.13). The single tooth on each jaw prevents tissue from slipping. If the instrument is to be used to obtain a biopsy, the edges should be kept sharp so that tissue is cut and not avulsed. Hemostasis should be obtained *after* the specimen has been removed to avoid coagulation damage to the tissue being examined pathologically. However, biopsy forceps rarely provide a clean excision of tissue and it is often easier and more accurate to obtain a biopsy with a scissors or knife.

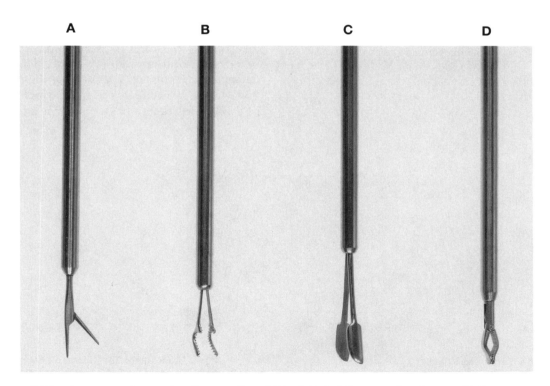

FIGURE 8.12. Laparoscopic grasping forceps. *From left to right:* **A:** Micrograsping forceps. **B:** Sponge or suturing graspers. **C:** Spatula forceps. **D:** Atruamatic grasper or ampulla dilator. (Karl Storz Co., Tutlingern, Germany.)

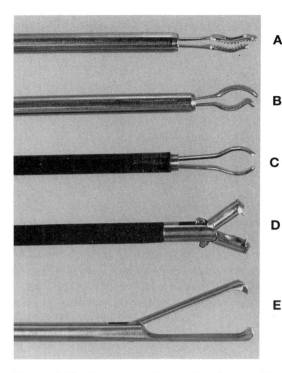

FIGURE 8.13.   Laparoscopic grasping forceps. *From top to bottom:* **A:** Adhesion graspers. **B:** Tube grasper. **C:** "Atraumatic" grasper. **D:** Biopsy forceps. **E:** Claw forceps. (Karl Storz Co., Tutlinger, Germany.)

Scissors and Scalpels

Scissors are available in many designs that include hook, micro, and serrated (Fig. 8.15). Scissors must be kept sharp or they will avulse rather than cut tissue. Microsurgical dissections may be performed using the microscissors, which are very versatile and quite useful when sharp. However, they tend to lose their cutting edge quickly. Hook scissors can be used for much the same purpose, as well as for cutting tissue and suture. The serrated scissors (either 5-mm or 10-mm-diameter) are not often used as they have little advantage over the afore-mentioned designs and tend to avulse tissue and dull quickly. Disposable scissors have the advantage of always being sharp and for this reason are increasingly popular. Scalpels are also available that can be used to make linear incisions, such as on ovaries and tubes.

Some scissors and scalpels are available with an insulated shaft and can be connected to unipolar current for electrocoagulation. The combination of electrocoagulation with cold cutting may be useful for adhesiolysis of vascularized adhesions. Nonetheless, it should be remembered that the indiscriminant use of unipolar current can result in significant tissue damage and distortion and a loss of the dissection planes. A recent advent is the tripolar forceps. This instrument has a bipolar head so tis-

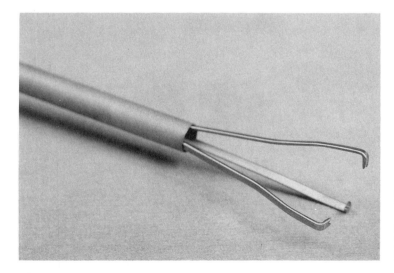

FIGURE 8.14.   Hasson three-prong (Bulldog) forceps (Weck-Eder Instrument Co., Chicago, IL). (Reproduced with permission as in Fig. 8.2.)

FIGURE 8.15. Laparoscopic scissors. *From top to bottom:* **A:** Hook, insulated for unipolar cautery. **B:** Straight serrated. **C:** Micro (*top,* by Richard Wolf Medical Instruments Corp., Rosemont, IL; *bottom two,* by WISAP, Sauelach, Germany). **D:** Bipolar shears with rotating tip (Ethicon, Somerville, NJ).

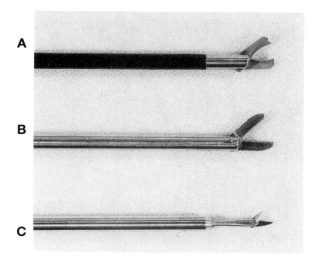

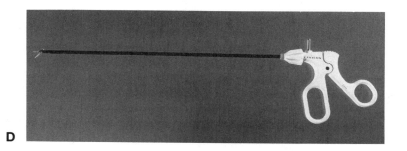

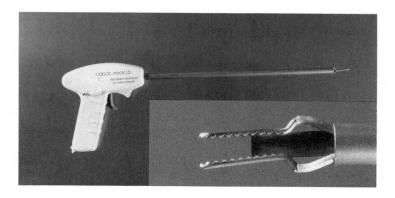

FIGURE 8.16. Tripolar cutting forceps. The *inset* shows bipolar grasping tips with a releasable cutting blade. Tissue can be coagulated and bisected with the same instrument (Cabot Medical Corp., Langhorne, PA).

sue can be coagulated between its paddles and then cut with the blade that jets out between the jaws of the forceps when the trigger is pulled (Fig. 8.16). Also available is a scalpel that uses ultrasonic waves for tissue coagulation and cutting (Fig. 8.17).

Instruments for Tissue Removal

Removal of large pieces of tissue from the abdomen at laparoscopy can be cumbersome and time consuming. Tissue may be cut into pieces no larger than the diameter of the puncture

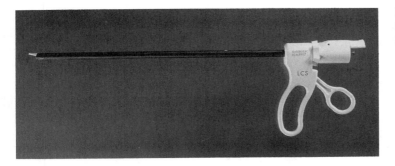

FIGURE 8.17. Endoscopic Harmonic scalpel (Ultracision, Inc., Smithfield, RI).

site and removed through 5-mm or 10-mm sleeves with grasping forceps. Alternatively, a suprapubic ancillary puncture site may be enlarged for removal of tissue. If the tissue is difficult to cut or if it should be removed intact, such as an ovary with a possible cancer, a posterior colpotomy incision can be made. This incision may be performed laparoscopically or transvaginally (see Chapter 16).

A 10- or 11-mm punch biopsy instrument with a storage sheath, the morcellator, may also be useful (Fig. 8.18). This instrument is particularly effective for the removal of ovaries or fibroids, although it is much less useful for very fibrotic or calcified fibroids or for very soft tissues, such as the tube. Unfortunately, the man-

ual morcellator is tiring and time consuming. An automated morcellator is now available. To remove the uterus, as in a supracervical laparoscopic hysterectomy, or large fibroids, morcellating trocars are available. These trocars have serrated edges and a double-tube mechanism that cores out strips of tissue, which are then removed through the center of the trocar.

When tissue is to be evacuated without spillage, tissue removal may be accomplished with the Endocatch (Fig. 8.19) (Ethicon, Somerville, NJ) or Endopouch (Autosuture Co., Norwalk, CT), two different types of tissue removal bags. Each bag is attached to a metal ring that is flattened to allow passage through a 10-mm port. Once in the abdomen, the ring

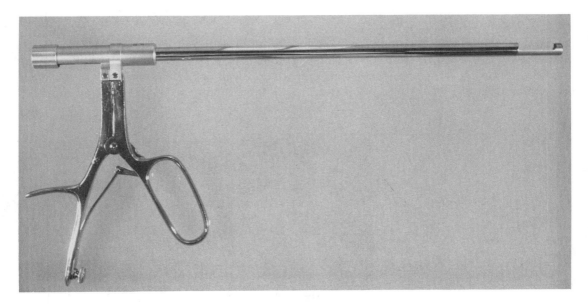

FIGURE 8.18.   Morcellator, 10 mm in diameter (WISAP, Sauerlach, Germany).

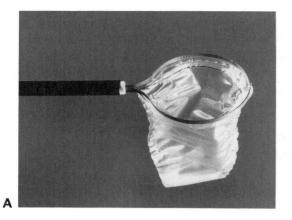

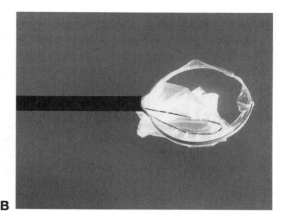

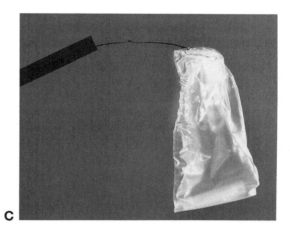

FIGURE 8.19. Endocatch is a tissue-extracting device. As the handle is pushed in, the plastic bag is released **(A)**. Once tissue is placed in the bag, the purse string is pulled and the bag is closed **(B)**. The metal ring can be pulled back by pulling on the handle until only the speciman and bag remain **(C)**. The bag can then be brought up through the sheath or through the incision (Autosuture Co., Norwalk, CT).

and attached bag are allowed to open and the tissue to be removed is placed into the bag. A pursestring suture around the bag is closed to prevent spillage and the ring is recompressed and pulled up through the port with the bag attached. Occasionally the port itself may need to be removed along with the bag. If the tissue is too large to pass through the incision, it may be necessary to extend the incision. If this is done the surgeon must take great care to close the fascia of the incision because the patient will be more suceptible to trocar hernias.

Enlargement of the ancillary puncture site can be achieved by two methods. The smaller trocar can be withdrawn and a larger one inserted through the previous site, after enlarging the skin incision. An attempt is made to introduce the trocar through the previous tract into the peritoneum. Semm has described an alternate method using a dilatation set. A dilator rod is first inserted into the smaller sleeve, which is then withdrawn and replaced with a larger cone-shaped sleeve, which has a screw tip.

Summary

Although a vast array of equipment is available for gynecologic operative laparoscopy, more innovative instruments need to be designed that will allow us to achieve our surgical goals more effectively and efficiently. With proper instrumentation, operative laparoscopy will become less surgical "gymnastics." The recent explosion of operative laparoscopy for the general surgeon has generated more interest in instrument development.

References

1. Murphy AA. Operative laparoscopy. *Fertil Steril.* 1987;47:1–18.
2. Garzo VG, Murphy AA. Operative laparoscopy instrumentation. *Semin Reprod Endocrinol.* 1991; 9:109–116.
3. Boyers SP. Operating room setup and instrumentation. In: Diamond MP, ed. *Clinical Obstetrics and Gynecology—Pelviscopy.* Philadelphia: Lippincott; 1991:373–386.
4. Valtchev KL, Papsin FR. A new uterine manipulator. *Am J Obstet Gynecol.* 1977;127:738–740.
5. Murphy AA. Diagnostic and operative laparoscopy. In: Thompson JD, Rock JA, eds. *TeLinde's Operative Gynecology.* Baltimore: Lippincott; 1991:361–384.
6. Quint RH. Physics of light and image transmission. In: Phillips JM, ed. *Laparoscopy.* Baltimore: Williams & Wilkins; 1977:18–25.
7. Gomel V, Taylor PJ, Yuzpe AA, Rioux JE. *Laparoscopy and Hysteroscopy in Gynecologic Practice.* Chicago: Year Book Medical Publishers, 1986: 1–21.
8. Borten M. *Laparoscopic Complications: Prevention and Management.* Toronto: Decker; 1986:1–414.
9. Semm R. *Operative Manual for Endoscopic Abdominal Surgery.* Chicago: Year Book Medical Publishers; 1984:1–484.
10. Hasson HM. Ovarian surgery. In: Sanfilippo JS, Levine RL, eds. *Operative Gynecologic Endoscopy.* New York: Springer-Verlag; 1989:19–37.

Additional Reading

1. Hulka J, Reich H. Facilities and equipment. In: *Textbook of Laparoscopy.* Philidelphia: Saunders; 1994:51–63.
2. Nezhat CR, Nezhat FR, Luciano AA, Siegler AM, Metzger DA, Nezhat CH. *Equipment in Operative Gynecologic Laparoscopy: Principles and Techniques.* New York: McGraw-Hill;1995: 15–45.

9

Sutures, Clips, and Staples

Ana Alvarez Murphy and Sujatha Reddy

Introduction

The ability to achieve hemostasis is integral to any laparoscopic procedure. This is probably the single most important factor that delayed the evolution of diagnostic and, certainly, of operative laparoscopy. Many laparoscopic operations require the surgeon to be skilled in laparoscopic suturing techniques if surgery is to be successful. The modalities to achieve hemostasis essentially mirror those of laparotomy surgery.

Basic suturing skills are essential at laparotomy. It is therefore logical that suturing be modified to allow it to be used at laparoscopy. These modifications must account for the altered access to the operative field. Unfortunately, the flexibility with which suturing is carried out at laparotomy is partially lost at laparoscopy. Endoscopic suturing was first demonstrated by Semm who adapted the Roeder loop, previously used for tonsillectomy, for endoscopic use. Laparoscopic sutures may be used to obtain hemostasis or approximate tissue. They may be placed such that the knot is tied (or pretied) extracorporeally or tied intraabdominally. Applicators for laparoscopic clips, both absorbable and nonabsorbable (titanium), are available and have added a new dimension to laparoscopic hemostasis. This chapter discusses suturing, clips, and staples. Lasers are discussed in Chapter 6 and electrosurgery and thermocoagulation are discussed in Chapter 5.

Suturing

Extracorporeal Loops and Knot Tying

The Roeder loop was the first reliable method of laparoscopic suturing consisting of a suture loop with a pretied slip knot. A commercially preformed loop, the Endoloop, is available as O-chromic, O-plain catgut, O-Vicryl, and O-PDS from Ethicon (Somerville, NJ), or as O-plain Endoschlinge (Fig. 9.1) from WISAP (Sauerlach, Germany). The ligature is formed into a loop using a fisherman's knot and the

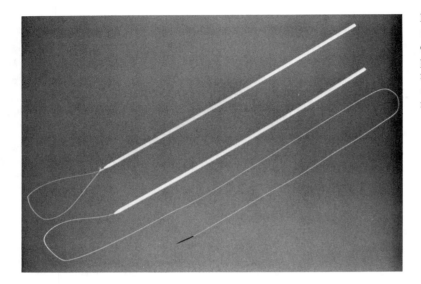

FIGURE 9.1. *Top:* Endoloop (aka Endoschlinge) 0-plain catgut loop ligature. *Bottom:* 2-plain Endosuture (aka Endonaht) on a 3-cm Keith needle (WISAP Co., Sauerlach, Germany).

free end passes up the hollow core of a plastic push guide to be embedded at its distal tip. Once the loop is placed around the tissue of interest, the plastic guide rod is snapped off from the embedded tip and used to push the slip knot closed.

The loop is most easily placed into the abdomen by loading into an Endoloop applicator (Fig. 9.2), which is then placed through a suprapubic port. A forceps is usually necessary to help place the loop correctly around the tissue to be ligated. The knot is tightened by pushing down on the plastic guide as the suture is pulled up. Tensile strength studies have shown the importance of one or at most two pushes of the plastic guide[1]; more than two pushes significantly decreases knot strength. Depending on the size of bleeding points, only one loop may be necessary. Alternatively, it has been recommended that three ligatures be used when performing an oophorectomy, salpingectomy, or adnexectomy.[2,3] As an alterna-

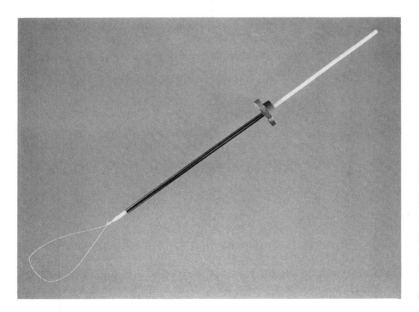

FIGURE 9.2. Endoloop is loaded into the applicator by pushing the plastic push rod up through the distal tip of the applicator and pulling the suture loop up into the shaft of the applicator. The loaded applicator is then placed through a 5-mm suprapubic sleeve.

FIGURE 9.3. Diagram of extracorporeal knot tying using the Roeder loop technique.

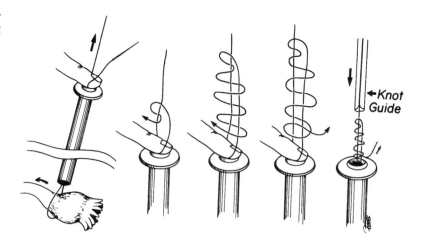

tive to commercially manufactured loops, sutures of different materials and sizes can be used to make a loop ligature. Either a Roeder knot (Fig. 9.3) or a Duncan loop (Fig. 9.4) can be made and slipped down the ancillary port using a metal knot guide[4] (Fig. 9.5). This metal knot guide is available commercially or can be made by making a large notch into the end of a laparoscopic probe.[5] If braided suture is used, a Duncan knot is generally easier to use than a Roeder knot. Marrero and Corfman[4] noted that the slipping strength of both loops may be increased if a half hitch is added to the knot (Fig. 9.6).

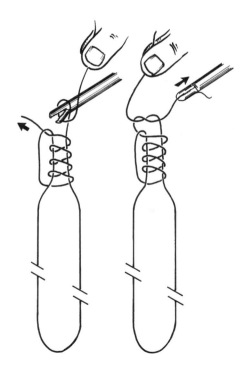

FIGURE 9.4. Diagram of Duncan slip knot. (Adapted from reference 4.)

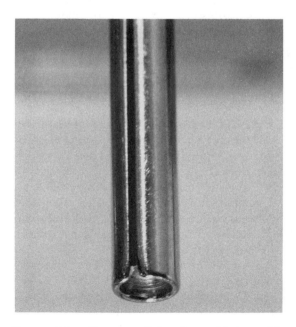

FIGURE 9.5. Close-up of tip of metal knot guide (WISAP Co., Sauerlach, Germany).

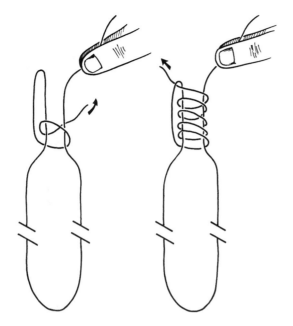

FIGURE 9.6. Diagram of a Duncan loop plus a half hitch. (Adapted from reference 4.)

Extracorporeal Suturing

The preformed loop ligature is used mainly to secure pedicles and to obtain hemostasis. However, if tissues need to be approximated, a suture on a needle may be used and the knot tied extracorporeally (see Fig. 9.3). The knot is then pushed into the abdomen with a metal or plastic knot guide. The Endopath (WISAP Co., Sauerlach, Germany) consists of a 3-cm needle on an 80-cm 2-plain suture with a plastic snap-off push rod (see Fig. 9.1). Also available are O-chromic and O-Vicryl Endosutures from Ethicon (Sommerville, NJ). As an alternative to commercially manufactured sutures, one can use a variety of sutures and needles using the metal knot guide to advance the knot. Some curved needles can be bent slightly to allow introduction into the abdomen through a 3- or 5-mm port.

To suture intraabdominally using an extracorporeal knot, a 3- or 5-mm needle holder (Fig. 9.3) is placed through an Endoloop applicator. The suture is grasped near the hilt of the needle and drawn up into the shaft of the applicator. The loaded applicator is then intro-

duced into the abdomen through a 5-mm ancillary port. The needle is pushed into the abdomen, regrasped using the needle holder, and the tissue sutured. After the needle is passed through the tissues to be approximated, the suture is grasped near the needle and brought out of the abdomen through the applicator. A knot, either Roeder or Duncan is tied extracorporeally, and either the plastic push rod (with the Endosuture) or the metal knot guide is used to tighten the knot in the abdomen.

Intraabdominal Knot Tying

Intraabdominal knot tying is usually reserved for 3-0 or finer gauge suture. This is most com-

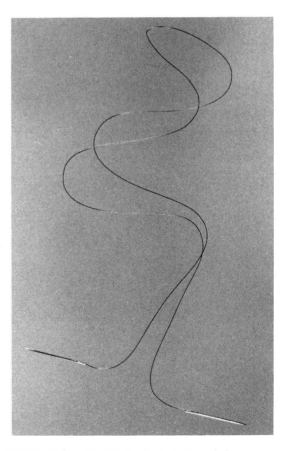

FIGURE 9.7. Double-barbed 4-0 polydioxanone (PDS) suture (Ethicon, Somerville, NJ) for intraabdominal laparoscopic knot tying.

FIGURE 9.8. Close-up of jaws of a needle holder. Note deep transverse grooves designed to accommodate the straight needle of the Endosuture.

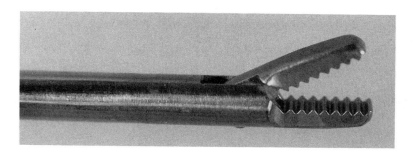

monly used to secure a neosalpingostomy or other microsurgical work. Suture of this caliber is too fragile to withstand reintroduction into the cavity with a knot guide. Thus, two techniques of intraabdominal knot tying have been described for use with these sutures. Although a variety of sutures can be used, a 35-cm 4-0 PDS suture (Z-420, Ethicon, Somerville, NJ) with an ST-4 tapered needle at each end is available and is quite useful (Fig. 9.7). This suture was initially designed for tendon repair but can be used at laparoscopy after the suture is cut in half. Each needle is straight, making it easier to push through tissues. Appropriate microsurgical technique should be used at all times (see Chapter 1) and the tissues treated as atraumatically as possible.

The first technique for intraabdominal knot tying is essentially the same as for a standard microsurgical knot. The suture is grasped near the hilt of the needle with a needle holder and introduced into the abdominal cavity by drawing it up into a suture applicator, which is then placed through a 5-mm suprapubic sleeve. Alternatively, the suture can be pushed directly into the abdomen through a 5-mm suprapubic valveless port using a micrograsper that allows the needle to slide down alongside its jaws. After being pushed into the abdomen, the needle is regrasped, making sure that it lies in one of the transverse grooves lining the needle-holder jaws (Fig. 9.8), and is driven through the tissue. A second needle holder or other grasper is used to immobilize the tissue through which the needle is driven. The needle is grasped at right angles to the suture and a surgeon's knot made (Fig. 9.9). The right angle keeps the suture from slipping off easily.

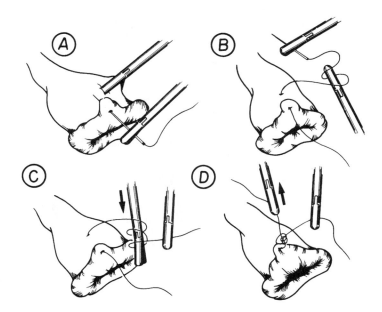

FIGURE 9.9. Microsurgical intraabdominal knot-tying technique.

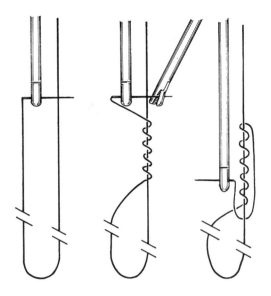

FIGURE 9.10. Alternative technique for intraabdominal knot tying using a modification of an intracorporeal fisherman's knot, as described by Thompson and Reich.[6]

Two other knots are placed using standard microsurgical technique. The needle is cut off and withdrawn from the abdomen by grasping the suture and pulling it out through the applicator. This type of suturing requires a great

deal of training as it can be technically demanding and generally frustrating. A pelvic trainer, obtained commercially or manufactured in house (see Fig. 3.2), is helpful for developing these skills.

An alternative method of knot tying has been described[6] that is essentially an intracorporeal technique using a fisherman's knot (Fig. 9.10). A long swagged-on needle is introduced into the abdomen in the same manner as previously and the other end of the suture is held outside the abdomen. The needle is grasped at right angles and rotated around the long end being held. Another needle holder is used to grasp the needle, which is then passed through the loop closest to the tissue. By retracting the long end, which is being held, the knot is formed and tightened. This technique is somewhat easier to perform than the previously described microsurgical knot technique.

The Endostitch (Ethicon, Inc.) is a suturing device that has a special needle which is passed from one paddle to the other (Fig. 9.11, also see Fig. 17.3B). As the paddles of the instrument are closed, the needle and attached suture are passed from one paddle, through the tissue between the paddles, to the opposite side. This method of passing the double-sided needle from side to side also simplifies intraab-

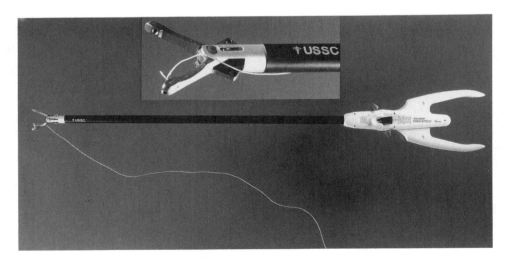

FIGURE 9.11. Endostitch device with needle and suture. *Inset:* close-up of one arm of the Endostitch with the needle and attached suture in one receptacle. The opposite receptacle is also visible. (Autosuture Co., Norwalk, CT.)

dominal knot tying. To tie a knot with this device, a loop is made in the abdomen and one side is held between the jaws of the stitch. Next the needle is passed from one paddle to the other and thus a single hitch is thrown. If this is repeated, a surgeon's knot can be tied. Once proficiency with the Endostitch is achieved, one suture and attached needle can be used for several ties.

Knot Strength

With the development of modern laparoscopic instrumentation, it is possible for the skilled surgeon to use most of the suture materials available for open abdominal surgery in operative laparoscopic procedures. Dorsey et al.[7] recently compared the knot strength of standard laparoscopic knots with standard knots used at laparotomy using a variety of suture technique. The variability in knot strengths can be explained partly by knot geometry and partly through the interaction of the knot and material. The laparoscopic Roeder knot was significantly weaker than all other knots tested. The extracorporeal sliding square knot was only significantly weaker than the conventional surgeon's flat square knot and the laparoscopic intracorporeal two-turn flat square knot. The conventional sliding square knot was significantly weaker than the conventional flat square knot and the conventional surgeon's square knot.

It is important to understand that there are significant differences between laparoscopic and traditional knots that may affect the suc-

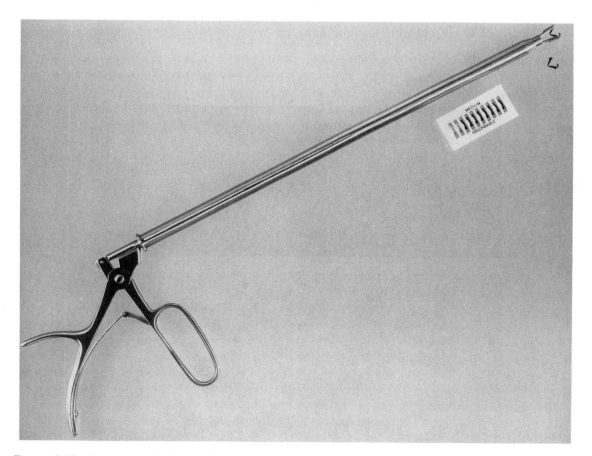

FIGURE 9.12. Laparoscopic clip applicator (Karl Storz, Culver City, CA; 11 mm in diameter) and medium PDS ligating clips (AP-200, Ethicon, Somerville, NJ).

cess or failure of a surgical procedure. Knot strength is of obvious importance in colposuspensions, retropubic urethropexy, repair of bowel or bladder injuries, and others. While the well-known Roeder loop has the obvious advantage of ease, it lacks the knot strength that may be required in some situations. On the other hand, the extracorporeal square knot that is "sliding" is significantly stronger than the Roeder loop. The extracorporeal sliding square knot is tightened with several throws using a knot pusher as opposed to only a single throw used in the Roeder knot. The intracorporeal two-turn flat square knot is the strongest laparoscopic knot. This knot is made by making two loops around an instrument, repeated three times. The surgeon's knot has two turns in the first throw, followed by a single turn in the second throw. Obviously, the knot chosen will depend on the intended use and the ultimate function of the suture as some knots will be subjected to greater tension than others.

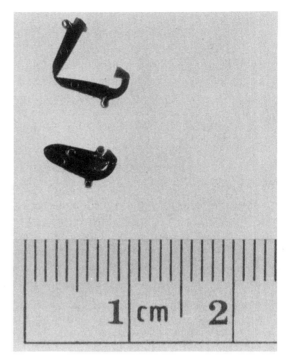

FIGURE 9.13. Close-up of open and closed medium AP-200 ligating clip (Ethicon, Somerville, NJ).

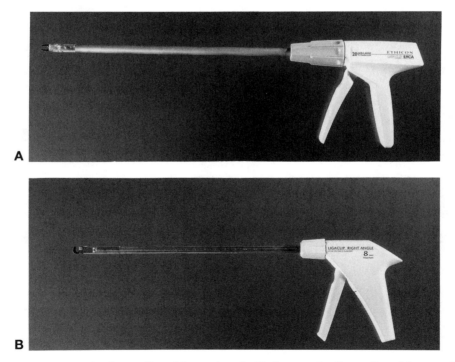

FIGURE 9.14. **A:** Automatic clip applier with rotating tip. **B:** Automatic clip applier with a rotating right-angle tip. (Both from Ethicon, Somerville, NJ.)

FIGURE 9.15. Stapler with replaceable cartridge. *Inset:* close-up with multiple rows of staples visible. (Ethicon, Somerville, NJ.)

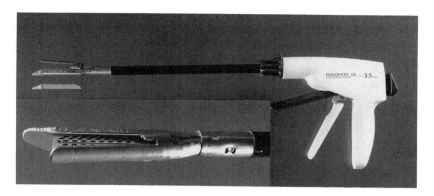

Clips and Staples

Clips have long been used in general surgery and less frequently in gynecology to obtain hemostasis. Clips for endoscopic use are available. An endoscopic clip applicator (Fig. 9.12) is available from Karl Storz (Culver City, CA). The PDS ligating clips are available from Ethicon (Somerville, NJ) and are broken down approximately 7 weeks after placement (Fig. 9.13). The clips come in different sizes which can be placed through a 5-mm or a 10-mm port and are loaded singly. Unfortunately, because these clips close based on a latch mechanism (Fig. 9.13), they can only be used on small isolated vessels or pedicles. Furthermore, they tend to fall off the applicator when holding the instrument straight down.

Titanium clips are most useful for obtaining hemostasis of moderate-size pedicles or vessels. These clips have no latch and are therefore more versatile. A reusable single-clip applier is available from Ethicon (Somerville, NJ). The AE-214 uses medium-size clips (TI200), which are 5.2 mm long when closed, and the AE-314 uses medium-long clips (TI314, 8.8 mm in length). A newer disposable multiple-clip applicator (EM-320, Ethicon, Somerville, NJ) comes preloaded with 20 medium-long titanium clips. Similar devices are available from Auto Suture Co. (Norwalk, CT). These are disposable and are available in straight and right-angle applicators (Fig. 9.14). These automatic clip appliers are loaded with 20 medium or medium-large titanium clips and are available in either a standard pistol-handle or a bicycle-handle grip. Both the multiple- and single-clip applicators fit through a 10-mm trocar. In general, clips have limited usefulness in laparoscopy because the relative lack of maneuverability may make it difficult to obtain the correct placement angle.

Automatic stapling devices, similar to those used in general surgery for bowel resections, are available from Ethicon (Endo-Cutter) (Fig. 9.15) and Auto Suture Co. (Endo-GIA). These place two or three rows of titanium clips on either side of the area to be incised (Fig. 9.16). When fired, the instrument automatically staples and then incises. Endo-Cutter has staple lines available in 30-, 60-, and 90-mm

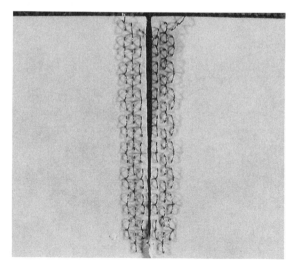

FIGURE 9.16.   Close-up shows three rows of staples on either side of incision.

lengths. A knob on the device controls tissue compression and can be adjusted for varying tissue thickness. The Endo-GIA is available in two sizes to accommodate tissue thickness. The tissue thickness may be measured using a device provided by the manufacturer that indicates which size instrument to use. These devices may be useful for laparoscopic hysterectomy or adnexectomy. Hernia staplers have heads that rotate 360° to facilitate staple placement.

Summary

The ability to achieve hemostasis is the key to any endoscopic procedure. The wide variety of methods available for hemostasis makes it imperative that we be aware of these and their limitations. No method is perfect, and surgeons should strive to master a combination of different techniques to achieve the versatility necessary to meet their surgical aims. The development of new instruments and techniques for achieving hemostasis will greatly advance endoscopic surgery.

References

1. Hay DL, Levine RL, von Fraunhofer JA, Masterson BJ. The effect of the number of pulls on the tensile strength of the chromic gut pelviscopic loop ligature. *J Reprod Med.* 1990;35:260–262.
2. Semm K. New methods of pelviscopy (gynecologic laparoscopy) for myomectomy, ovariectomy, tubectomy, and adnexectomy. *Endoscopy.* 1979;2:85–87.
3. Semm K. Tissue puncher and loop ligation: new aids for surgical-therapeutic pelviscopy (laparoscopy)-endoscopic intra-abdominal surgery. *Endoscopy.* 1978;10:110–114.
4. Marrero MA, Corfman RS. Laparoscopic use of sutures. In: Diamond MP, ed. *Clinical Obstetrics and Gynecology-Pelviscopy.* Philadelphia: Lippincott; 1991;34:387–394.
5. Levine RL. Instrumentation. In: Sanfillipo JS, Levine RL, eds. *Operative Gynecologic Endoscopy.* New York: Springer-Verlag; 1989:19.
6. Thompson RG, Reich H. Intra-abdominal laparoscopic suturing: a new technique. 46th Annual Meeting of the American Fertility Society, Washington, DC, 1990. Abstract # FP-09.
7. Dorsey JH, Sharp HT, Chovan JD, Holtz PM. Laparoscopic knot strength: a comparison with conventional knots. *Obstet Gynecol.* 1995;86:536–540.

10

Laparoscopic Anatomy

William W. Hurd and Jean A. Hurteau

Introduction

A good working knowledge of abdominal and pelvic anatomy is probably the most important single element necessary to minimize laparoscopic complications and to effectively handle complications when they arise. Although several of the important anatomic features are readily visible, many important structures cannot be seen directly but must nevertheless be avoided.

In general, anatomic considerations are especially important for two aspects of laparoscopic surgery. The first is the placement of trocars through the anterior abdominal wall. Understanding the anterior abdominal wall anatomy and the relative location of retroperitoneal vessels is extremely important for blind placement of the primary umbilical trocar. Knowledge of the abdominal wall vasculature is equally important for placement of secondary trocars both in the midline (commonly used for all diagnostic laparoscopy) and lateral to the midline (often necessary for operative endoscopy).

The second instance in which anatomy becomes important is when the laparoscopic surgery involves manipulation of the peritoneal surfaces or the retroperitoneal area. The importance of anatomic knowledge for advanced operative laparoscopy is obvious. However, because of decreased tactile feedback and depth perception associated with laparoscopic surgery, even the simplest cases of endometriosis and lysis of adhesions require a thorough understanding of those structures that may lie hidden just beneath the peritoneum.

With these general areas in mind, this chapter considers specifically (a) the anatomy of the anterior abdominal wall, especially as it changes with body weight, (b) the vessels of the anterior abdominal wall, and (c) the location of the retroperitoneal structures.

Anterior Abdominal Wall Thickness

Common to all laparoscopic procedures is the placement of a 10-mm port through the abdominal wall in or immediately below the umbilicus. Knowledge of the various tissue layers at this level is important not only for closed laparoscopy but also for open laparoscopic techniques to ensure successful and easy trocar placement. Immediately below the umbilicus, the subdermal layers include, in descending order, the subcutaneous tissue, the anterior rectus sheath, the rectus abdominis muscles, the posterior rectus sheath, and the peritoneum of the abdominal cavity. At the base of the umbilicus these layers coalesce so that the skin is often attached to the anterior rectus sheath, which is in turn attached to the posterior rectus sheath and peritoneum. At this level, there is no subcutaneous tissue or rectus abdominis muscle. In obese patients, however, some adipose tissue may be found between the parietal peritoneum and the rectus fascia.

In patients of all weights, the base of the umbilicus represents the thinnest part of the anterior abdominal wall (Fig. 10.1).[1] This observation is especially important in the obese patients in whom the abdominal wall under the umbilicus may be several centimeters less in thickness than the rest of the abdominal

wall. This relationship of increasing abdominal thickness with increasing weight has implications for both the open and closed laparoscopic technique. Probably the most important variable of the laparoscopic technique is the angle of placement of the Veress needle and primary trocar. Traditionally, both these instruments are placed through the anterior abdominal wall at the lower margin of the umbilicus at approximately 45° from vertical. This approach is believed to minimize injury to major retroperitoneal vessels and to lessen the chance of placing the needle and trocar in the preperitoneal space. More recently, a vertical intraumbilical incision has been utilized to improve the cosmetic result and take advantage of the thinnest part of the anterior abdominal wall.

In thin patients, placement of the instruments through the base of the umbilicus at a 45° angle appears to be ideal because the abdominal wall is relatively thin and the retroperitoneal vessels are relatively close to the anterior abdominal wall (Fig. 10.1A). In overweight patients, because the anterior abdominal wall is thicker, the angle of insertion should be increased to 60° to decrease the chance of preperitoneal placement while not significantly increasing the chance of retroperitoneal vessel injury (Fig. 10.1B). Finally, in patients who are obese, placing the

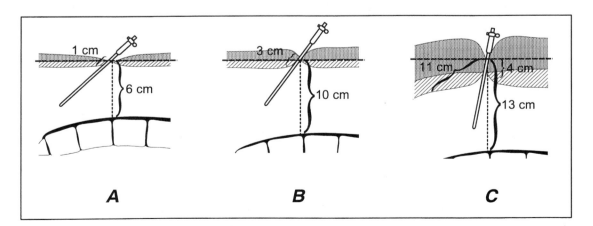

FIGURE 10.1. Diagram of representative sagittal views of patients from three groups. **A:** Thin, body mass index (BMI) <25 kg/m². **B:** Normal weight, BMI 25–30 kg/m². **C:** Obese, BMI >30 kg/m². An 11.5-cm Veress needle is superimposed on each view for comparison. (Adapted from Hurd et al.[1])

Veress cannula and primary trocar through the base of the umbilicus at 75°–80° from the horizontal appears to be the most appropriate way to minimize the chance of preperitoneal placement (Fig. 10.1C). Because there is a significantly greater distance between the umbilicus and the vessels, the chance of injuring these vessels appears to be decreased. However, because vessel injury is one of the most serious complications of trocar placement, it is recommended that great care be taken with its placement. Use of a disposable trocar with a safety shield may increase the margin of safety, although this is yet to be proven in clinical trials.

Abdominal wall anatomy also has important implications for open laparoscopy. When open laparoscopy is performed, especially in obese patients, the distance from the skin to the fascia is often significant. It is apparent from our data that the closer to the base of the umbilicus that the open laparoscopy is performed, the shorter this distance will be. Likewise, if the skin incision is made in the lower half of the umbilicus and the fascia is grasped beneath the umbilicus (i.e., at an angle toward the head of the patient), the distance from skin to fascia will be minimized.[2]

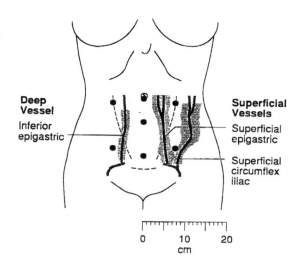

FIGURE 10.2. Location of the deep and superficial vessels of the anterior abdominal wall, frontal view. *Gray shadows following blood vessels (in black)* represent mean ± SD for data from abdominal computer tomograms. The *dashed lines* indicate the relative location of the rectus abdominis muscle lateral margin and the symphysis pubis. The *solid circles* indicate standard sites for midline laparoscopic trocar placement and for lateral trocar placement 8 cm from midline at levels 8 cm above symphysis and at the level of the umbilicus. (Adapted from Hurd et al.[4])

Anterior Abdominal Wall Vessels

Injuring unseen abdominal wall blood vessels has always been a risk associated with the placement of additional trocars required for operative laparoscopy. In the past, vessel injury was minimized by placing these trocars primarily in the midline. However, with the advent of advanced operative techniques that required placement of multiple ports of increasing size lateral to the midline, abdominal wall vessel injury has become an increasing problem.[3] For this reason, knowledge of anterior abdominal wall vasculature and techniques for avoiding injury to these vessels is essential.

The major vessels in the anterior abdominal wall can be divided into deep and the superficial.[4] The deep vessels consist of the inferior epigastric artery and vein (Fig. 10.2).[4] This artery originates from the external iliac artery and courses along the peritoneum until it dives deeply into the rectus muscle, midway between the symphysis and the umbilicus. The superficial vessels include the superficial epigastric artery and the superficial circumferential iliac artery, which are both branches of the inguinal artery, and their corresponding veins. These arteries course bilaterally through the subcutaneous tissue of the abdominal wall, branching as they proceed toward the head of the patient.

Several techniques exist for identifying the location of these vessels. One of the oldest techniques is transillumination. While this technique is excellent for visualizing the superficial vessels in thin patients, it appears to be of little help for identifying the inferior epigastric artery in any patient as this vessel runs beneath or within the rectus abdominis muscle.[5] Laparoscopic visualization, when possible, is the most appropriate technique for identifying the inferior epigastric vessels. In many patients, these vessels can be seen adjacent to the peritoneum as they lie near the inguinal canal (Fig.

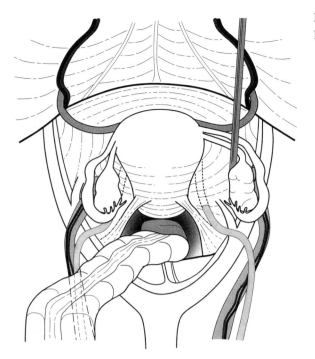

FIGURE 10.3. Laparoscopic view of the female pelvis.

10.3). From this point, the vessels run cephalad and medial. In patients in whom these vessels cannot be seen, their approximate origin can be assumed to be where the round ligament enters the inguinal canal just above the external iliac vessels. Another useful landmark is the medial umbilical fold (also known as the obliterated umbilical artery), because the inferior epigastric vessels uniformly lie lateral to these folds.

A final technique for avoiding the inferior epigastric vessels, especially in patients in whom they are not visible, is to know the average location of the vessels and to avoid this location.[4] At a level approximately 3 cm above the symphysis, the inferior epigastric vessels are located approximately 5.5 cm from the midline (see Fig. 10.2). From this point, they course cephalad and somewhat more medially.

Unfortunately, the location of both the inferior and superficial epigastric vessels varies widely. Immediately above the symphysis, they may be found as far as 8 cm from the midline. For this reason, we recommend that when lateral trocars are required they be placed at a location more cephalad and more lateral. Our preferred location is approximately 8 cm above

the symphysis and 8 cm from the midline (Fig. 10.2). This relatively lateral location will give a reasonable margin of safety in most patients. An extremely important point to remember when using this location is that the external iliac vessels often lie directly beneath, and thus trocars must be placed at 45° toward the midline under direct visualization.

Because of the wide anatomic variation of both the major vessels and their branches, other methods should be considered for minimizing the risk of injury to abdominal wall vessels. Probably the most important consideration is to use the smallest diameter trocar possible when lateral placement is required. A 10-mm trocar is approximately eight times more likely to injure a vessel than a 5-mm trocar placed in the same position.[6] A 12-mm trocar would be even more likely to injure a vessel in the same relative area. We routinely limit the placement of trocars larger than 5 mm to the relatively avascular midline position whenever possible. When larger ports are required laterally, dilatation of a 5-mm incision to a 10- or 12-mm incision using a commercially available system or a blunt trocar may minimize the risk of vessel injury.

Another helpful technique is the use of conical rather than pyramidal trocars for lateral port placement as these smooth trocars appear to be less likely to lacerate vessels.[6] Unfortunately, conical trocars take somewhat more pressure to place and thus are only useful when 5-mm ports are being placed.

Retroperitoneal Structures

Several retroperitoneal structures are at risk for injury during both trocar placement and during pelvic surgery. For extensive laparoscopic procedures, a thorough knowledge of the pelvic anatomy, and of the relationship of major organs to the laparoscopically visible landmarks, is imperative.

Bladder

The dome of the bladder usually lies several centimeters below the symphysis and, when empty, should be relatively difficult to injure during trocar insertion. To minimize the risk of bladder injury, routine catheterization is recommended before trocar placement.

In patients who have had previous laparotomy, the dome of the bladder may extend more cephalad secondary to postoperative scarring, even when the bladder is empty. Unfortunately, the empty bladder is usually not easily visualized laparoscopically. For this reason, we recommend routinely placing midline trocars at a level at or above the site of any previous low transverse skin incisions to minimize the risk of bladder injury. In patients with no previous surgery, or those who have had previous midline incisions, the trocar should be placed slightly off the midline and at least 3 to 4 cm above the symphysis.

Ureter

The ureters are in danger of being injured, not principally during trocar placement, but rather during those intraabdominal procedures requiring ablation, lysis of adhesions at the pelvic side wall, or extensive retroperitoneal dissections or division of the infundibulopelvic liga-

ment. To reduce the risk of ureteral injury, the surgeon should be aware of its general location within the retroperitoneal space and its relationship to other major landmarks.

The ureter is approximately 30 cm long and is divided into abdominal and pelvic segments. The abdominal segment extends from the renal pelvis to the pelvic brim. This ureteral segment courses along the anterior and medial aspect of the psoas muscle until it crosses over the common iliac vessels, approximately 1.5 cm above the bifurcation of the internal and external iliac vessels. Because of the consistency of this relationship, this serves as an excellent method for locating the mid-ureter.

The second segment, the pelvic ureter, starts at the pelvic brim and terminates in the bladder. The pelvic ureter courses anterior to the hypogastric vessels, crossing the obturator muscle and turning medial at the level of the ischial spines. It then passes lateral and superior to the uterosacral ligaments and courses below the uterine vessels. After running obliquely through the cardinal ligament, ventral to the anterior vaginal fornix, the ureter angles upwards (forming a "J") and inserts into the bladder trigone.

During laparoscopy, the ureter can often be identified through the semitransparent peritoneum in thin patients.[7] When possible, it is best to identify the ureter at the bifurcation of the common iliac vessels and trace it into the pelvis by observing its peristaltic activity. If surgical dissection is necessary in this area and the ureter is not visible, intravenous injection of indigo carmine or methylene blue can be used to color the urine blue and thus allow identification of the ureter through the peritoneum. Unfortunately, in the presence of adhesions between the ovaries and the lateral pelvic side walls, or with a high sigmoid colon obscuring the common iliac vessels, transperitoneal identification of the ureters may not be possible. In these cases, the best way to avoid injury to the ureter may be to open the retroperitoneal space.

The retroperitoneal space can best be entered using the same techniques used during laparotomy. The initial incision is made either by dividing the round ligament or by incising the peritoneum above the psoas muscle. The pararectal and paravesical spaces are then carefully developed and the ureter identified coursing along the medial leaf of the broad ligament peritoneum at the level of the bifurcation of the iliac vessels.

A common type of laparoscopic case in which the ureter can be injured is the treatment of endometriosis.[8] Endometriosis commonly involves the uterosacral ligament and the peritoneum between the uterosacral and the broad ligaments. Because the ureter is in intimate contact with the peritoneum in this area (see Fig. 10.3), it is at risk for injury during either laser ablation or electrocautery.

Another common procedure that may result in ureteral injury is the laparoscopically assisted vaginal hysterectomy (LAVH).[9] The most likely site of ureteral injury during these procedures may be near the cardinal ligament at the time of uterine vessel transection.[10] If the uterine vessels are to be approached laparoscopically, retroperitoneal dissection to identify the ureter is required to reduce the risk of injury. The second most common site of ureteral injury during LAVH may be near the infundibulopelvic ligament, during ligation of the ovarian vessels. If adequate distance cannot be achieved between the pelvic side wall and the site of ligature, ureteral visualization by retroperitoneal dissection should be performed in this area as well.

When extensive ureteral adhesions have been lysed, a potential injury can be ascertained by observing for leakage after intravenous injection of indigo carmine. In questionable cases, an intraoperative retrograde pyelogram will demonstrate even the smallest injuries.

Iliac Vessels

The major vessels in the pelvis include the external iliac and the hypogastric, or internal iliac, vessels that arise as bifurcations from the common iliac vessels at the pelvic brim. The external iliac vessels, with the artery running lateral to the vein, course along the pelvic side wall and exit the pelvis below the inguinal ligament. The round ligament disappears into the peritoneum as it enters the inguinal canal immediately above the external iliac vessels (see Fig. 10.2). This consistent relationship is a useful anatomic landmark for locating these vessels.

The hypogastric vessels course downward into the pelvis along with the ureter. Both the hypogastric and the external iliac vessels can sometimes be identified through the semitransparent peritoneum. However, in the presence of peritoneal adhesions or scarring, especially in the presence of endometriosis, the vessels may not be readily visible. If extensive dissection is required in this area, the retroperitoneal space should be opened as just described to avoid injury to both the major vessels and the ureter. In difficult cases, identification of major retroperitoneum structures before the resection and removal of surgical specimens may reduce morbidity. If this is not possible laparoscopically, conversion to laparotomy is indicated.

Obturator Nerve

Although not commonly encountered in most gynecologic cases, the obturator nerve must be considered when performing pelvic lymphadenectomy. Injury to this nerve will cause both motor impairment to the adductor muscles and sensory deficiency to the medial thigh. The obturator nerve originates from the anterior division of the second, third, and fourth lumbar nerve and emerges into the pelvis through the psoas muscle. It courses along the obturator fossa, within the obturator lymphatic fat pad, to exit through the obturator foramen. During laparoscopic dissection beneath the hypogastric vein, the obturator nerve should be identified as a white band within the yellow obturator lymphatic fat pad.

Rectosigmoid

A final structure at risk for injury during laparoscopic surgery is the rectosigmoid. This structure can imperceptibly blend into the peritoneum along the posterior vagina. In cases of severe endometriosis, dissection into the rectovaginal space is sometimes required.

This potential space, which is usually easy to enter with blunt dissection, can be obliterated along with the cul de sac by dense fibrotic adhesions between the rectosigmoid, the vagina, the cervix, and the lower uterine segment.

The pararectal space is another area where dissection is sometimes required. This triangular space is delineated anteriorly by the cardial ligament, laterally by the iliac artery, and medially by the ureter. The uterosacral ligament also transverses this space laterally. If extensive dissection is required in either of these areas, extreme care is needed to avoid injury to the bowel, ureters, or major blood vessels. In cases where dense bowel adhesions have been lysed, insufflation of the rectosigmoid colon with either a bulb syringe or a proctoscope can be helpful in identifying this structure. If the area of dissection is immersed in irrigation fluid at the conclusion of the case, even minute breaches in the bowel mucosa can be identified by the presence of escaping air.

Summary

The role of laparoscopic surgery in gynecology continues to expand. Although this approach may be associated with decreased incisional pain and risk of incision-related complications, significant surgical risks remain. Safe trocar placement is dependent on a thorough understanding of anterior abdominal wall and pelvic anatomy, because several vital structures remain unseen during placement. During pelvic procedures performed laparoscopically, a comprehensive knowledge of anatomy is necessary because of the decreased tactile feedback and depth perception associated with this technique. As laparoscopic experience increases, it has become apparent that a different appreciation of the location of vital structures is required to minimize the risk of surgical complications.

References

1. Hurd WW, Bude, RO, DeLancey JOL, Gauvin JM, Aisen AM. Abdominal wall characterization by magnetic resonance imaging and computed tomography: the effect of obesity on laparoscopic approach. *J Reprod Med.* 1991;36(7):473–476.
2. Hurd WW, Ohl DA. Blunt trocar laparoscopy. *Fertil Steril.* 1994;61:1177–1180.
3. Hurd WW, Pearl ML, DeLancey JOL, Quint EH, Garnett B. Laparoscopic injury of abdominal wall blood vessels: a report of three cases. *Obstet Gynecol.* 1993;82:673–676.
4. Hurd WW, Bude RO, DeLancey JOL, Newman JS. The location of abdominal wall blood vessels in relationship to abdominal landmarks apparent at laparoscopy. *Am J Obstet Gynecol.* 1994;171:642–646.
5. Quint EH, Wang FL, Hurd WW. Laparoscopic transillumination for the location of anterior abdominal wall blood vessels. *J Laparoendosc Surg.* 1996;6:167–169.
6. Hurd WW, Wang FL, Schemmel MT. Comparison of the relative risk of vessel injury using conical versus pyramidal laparoscopic trocars in a rabbit model. *Am J Obstet Gynecol.* 1995;172:1731–1733.
7. Grainger DA, Soderstrom RM, Schiff SF, Glickman M, DeCherney AH, Diamond MP. Ureteral injuries at laparoscopy: insights into diagnosis, management and prevention. *Obstet Gynecol.* 1990:75:839–843.
8. Cheng YS. Ureteral injury resulting from laparoscopic fulgarization of endometriotic implant. *Am J Obstet Gynecol.* 1976;8:1045–1046.
9. Davis GD, Wolgamott G, Moon J. Laparoscopically assisted vaginal hysterectomy as definitive therapy for stage III and IV endometriosis. *J Reprod Med.* 1993;38:577–581.
10. Hunter RW, McCartney AJ. Ureteric injuries at laparoscopic hysterectomy [letter]. *Am J Obstet Gynecol.* 1993;169:752.

11

Principles of Laparoscopic Microsurgery and Adhesion Prevention

Jacqueline N. Gutmann and Michael P. Diamond

Introduction

Pelvic adhesions are known to play a role in female infertility; additionally, adhesions may lead to complications including bowel obstruction and pelvic pain. Because postoperative pelvic adhesions following laparotomy have been reported to occur in 55% to 95% of cases,[1] the development of strategies to reduce adhesion formation and reformation is of paramount importance to the pelvic surgeon. In this regard, several advances have been made in reproductive surgery over the last quarter of a century, including the use of microsurgical technique, adhesion reduction adjuvants, and endoscopic surgery. This chapter presents our understanding of the pathogenesis of postoperative adhesion development and the surgical techniques and adjuvants currently used in attempts to minimize their formation.

Pathophysiology of Adhesion Formation

Normal Peritoneal Healing

Adhesion formation represents an aberrancy of normal peritoneal healing. Thus, to understand and subsequently prevent the formation of adhesions it is important to review the physiology of normal healing (Fig. 11.1). In response to peritoneal injury, there occurs a release of histamine and vasoactive kinins, leading to an increase in capillary permeability with the subsequent outpouring of serosanguinous fluid. Within 3 hr, and frequently within 15 to 30 min, this proteinaceous fluid coagulates, producing fibrinous bands between abutting surfaces.[2] These fibrinous strands (i.e., fibrin matrix) become infiltrated by monocytes, plasma cells, polymorphonuclear cells, and histiocytes. The bulk of fibrin accumulation is transient, and these strands are rapidly lysed as a result of endogenous fibrinolytic activity, usually within 72 hr of the insult (Fig. 11.2). The denuded area of peritoneum is then reepithelialized, with healing becoming complete within 3 to 4 weeks (Fig. 11.3).

Reepithelization of the peritoneal injury begins with mesothelial migration into the peri-

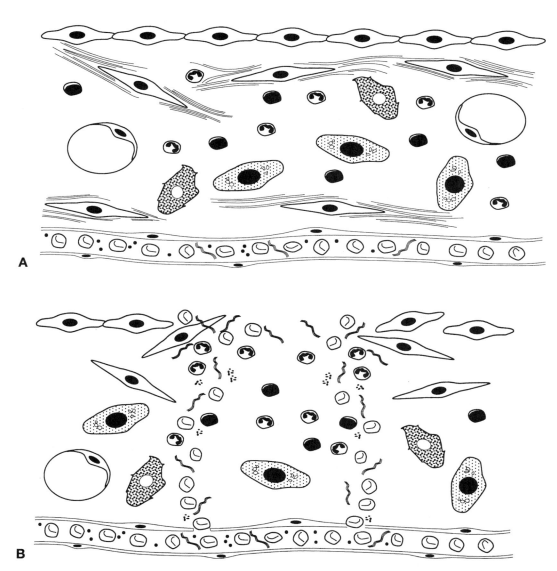

FIGURE 11.1. **A:** Normal peritoneum: mesothelial cells overlying loose connective tissue containing lymphocytes, macrophages, adiopocytes, fibroblasts, plasma cells, mast cells, and blood vessels. **B:** Serosal injury: connective tissue vasculature transports various cell types, including polymorphonuclear cells, platelets and fibrin, to the injured area. A sticky, fibrinous exudate forms that causes adherence of adjacent structures. (Modified with permission from Drollette CM, Badawy SZA. Pathophysiology of pelvic adhesions. *J Reprod Med.* 1992;37:107–121.)

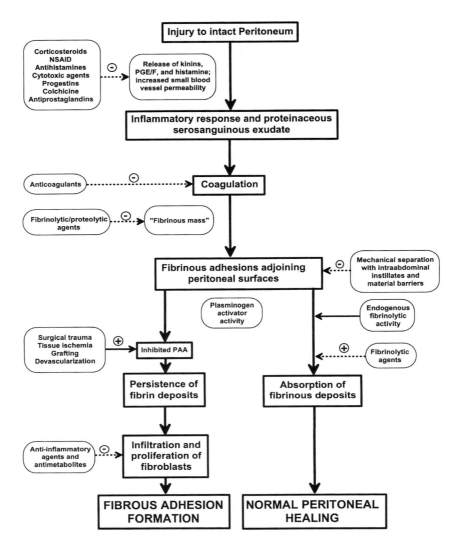

FIGURE 11.2. Mechanism of peritoneal healing and adhesion formation and sequential stages at which adjuvants exert their promotional (+) or inhibitory (−) effect. *NSAID,* Nonsteroidal antiinflammatory drug; *PGE/F,* prostaglandin E,F; *PAA,* plasminogen activator activity. (Modified from Schwartz L, Diamond M. Formation, reduction and treatment of adhesive disease. *J Reprod Med.* 1991;9:89–99.)

toneal supportive matrix. Possible sites of the new mesothelium include (1) primitive mesenchymal cells present at the periphery of the defect; (2) from primitive mesenchymal cells indirectly via differentiation into fibroblasts; and (3) subperitoneal fibroblasts, which in turn arise from differentiated, but resting, fibroblasts in the perivascular connective tissue.

As multiple sites of repair are initiated simultaneously, large peritoneal defects reepithelialize as quickly as do smaller lesions.[2]

Adhesion Formation

Disruption of the existing equilibrium between fibrin deposition and fibrinolysis leads to per-

FIGURE 11.3. Change in the relative number of cellular elements and fibrinolysis (fibrin) at the site of peritoneal injury in mature rats during the course of reepithelialization. (Reproduced with permission from diZerega GS. The peritoneum and its response to surgical injury. In: diZerega GS, Malinak LR, Diamond MP, Linsky CB, eds. *Treatment of Post Surgical Adhesions.* New York: Wiley-Liss; 1990:1–11.)

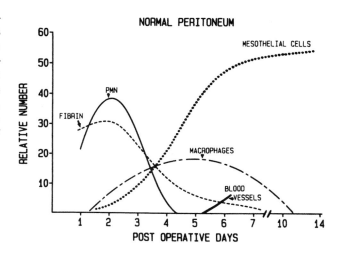

sistence of the fibrinous strands, which then become infiltrated by proliferating fibroblasts (see Figs. 11.1, 11.2). Subsequently, vascularization and cellular ingrowth occur and an adhesion is created.[2] Factors that disrupt this equilibrium are those which suppress fibrinolytic activity or those that lead to excessive fibrin deposition.

Inhibition of fibrinolysis often results from tissue ischemia.[3] Ischemia may also induce adhesion formation by stimulating the growth of blood vessels from a nonischemic to an ischemic site. Ischemia may result from excessive handling, crushing, ligating, suturing, cauterizing, or stripping the peritoneum. In addition, desiccation of the peritoneal tissue during prolonged procedures results in mesothelial cell desquamation with a resultant raw basement membrane and fibrin deposition,[3] which also predisposes to adhesion development.

Excessive formation of the fibrin coagulum, which is most commonly the result of foreign-body reaction, also stimulates the development of adhesions. Common foreign bodies include sutures as well as cornstarch powder and lint from drapes, caps, gowns, masks, and laparotomy pads. However, under today's surgical conditions, foreign bodies in the absence of peritoneal injury are an infrequent cause of adhesion formation[3] and thus inhibition of fibrinolysis appears to be the primary mediator of adhesion formation.

The presence of intraperitoneal blood has also been proposed to play a role in adhesion formation, although its actual contribution is unclear. The volume of blood, type of blood product used, and the presence or absence of peritoneal injury have all been demonstrated to influence adhesion formation.[3] Free blood in the peritoneal cavity generally does not lead to adhesions, except in the presence of tissue ischemia.[4]

It is generally believed that the mechanism responsible for adhesion reformation after surgical adhesiolysis is the same as that responsible for the de novo formation of adhesions after peritoneal insult, although there are no experimental data to support this theory. Nevertheless, investigators have demonstrated a greater propensity for adhesion reformation than for de novo formation in both animal models and clinical trials. This may result from either a greater extent of tissue damage and hence reduced fibrinolytic activity or from differences in the pathogenesis of healing and adhesion formation between previously damaged and never damaged peritoneum.[1] Potentially, these differences reflect varying degrees of tissue ischemia, with previously damaged tissue less able to perfuse and fibrinolyse the newly traumatized area.

Principles of Microsurgery at Laparoscopy

Microsurgical technique was initially applied to the performance of reproductive pelvic surgery by Swolin in 1967.[1] The tenets of operative laparoscopy are similar to those of gynecological microsurgery, and have the objective of preventing or reducing the formation of pelvic adhesions that could compromise the results of the procedure.

As with pelvic surgery performed at laparotomy, adequate visualization and access to the area of interest is of paramount importance. When the surgical procedure is performed laparoscopically, the Trendelenburg position and an adequate pneumoperitoneum displace the bowel from the operating field and aid in proper visualization. A multiple-puncture technique is encouraged to properly manipulate pelvic structures and maximize the operator's access to the pathology being treated. Appropriate instruments should be available and adequate surgical assistance, aided by a video monitor, is necessary. The surgical technique should be as atraumatic as possible. Hemostasis is also imperative, and is aided by adequate assistance, visualization, and appropriate instrumentation. Irrigation should be performed continuously, and also at the completion of the procedure to remove clots and debris and to detect any persistent bleeding. The use of adhesion reduction adjuvants is also possible. Additionally, the experience of the surgeon is likely to play a role in the successful outcome of operative laparoscopy. This has been demonstrated to be the case at laparotomy, in both an animal model and clinical experience.[1]

A wide variety of procedures performed by the reproductive surgeon at laparotomy can also be performed at laparoscopy. Operative laparoscopy has several undisputed advantages over laparotomy. Procedures performed at laparoscopy appear to be associated with decreased patient morbidity. Furthermore, patients are often discharged on the day of surgery and return to normal activities within 3 to 5 days, as compared with 3- to 5-day hospital stay and a 4- to 6-week convalescence period after laparotomy.

The issue that remains less clear is the efficacy of procedures performed by operative laparoscopy versus laparotomy. Intuitively, one would expect that endoscopic surgery is less precise than a formal microsurgical laparotomy; that is, there is a greater chance of injury to adjoining structures and that hemostasis is more difficult to achieve from a distance. On the other hand, during laparoscopic surgery, there is less tissue handling and fewer opportunities for foreign-body contamination, such as lint and suture. In addition, desiccation of tissue is far less likely to occur.

Animal studies have been performed to assess postoperative adhesion formation subsequent to both laparoscopy and laparotomy. In the rat, comparison of postoperative adhesion formation subsequent to standard uterine trauma using sharp scissors inflicted at laparoscopy or laparotomy revealed no significant difference in postoperative adhesion formation. Similar results were obtained using a CO_2 laser to inflict the uterine horn injury. Finally, in a rabbit model, postoperative adhesion formation was assessed after conservative ovarian surgery, in which an incision was made on the antimesenteric surface of the ovary using a microelectrode. Adhesion formation was not affected by the surgical approach.[5]

Clinical studies comparing laparoscopy and laparotomy in minimizing postoperative adhesion formation and reformation are scarce. In a rabbit model, Maier demonstrated that laparotomy, but not laparoscopy, was associated with the formation of de novo adhesions.[5] Diamond and colleagues noted adhesions in more than 50% of women undergoing a microsurgical laparotomy.[1] In contrast, in a separate study Diamond reported that the adhesion formation rate was only 12% following operative laparoscopy.[1] However, the adhesion reformation rate, which occurred to some degree in more than 90% of patients, did not differ significantly between patients undergoing laparotomy or operative laparoscopy.[1] In a randomized clinical trial, in the treatment of ectopic pregnancy adhesion formation after laparotomy was increased when compared to laparoscopy, as assessed by second-look laparoscopy.[6] Other studies that have evaluated adhesion formation and reformation after laparoscopic surgery have failed to include a laparotomy control, although it appears that fertility outcome after operative laparoscopy for lysis of adhesions is not different than after laparotomy[7] (Table 11.1).

One of the tenets of microsurgical techniques is "precise reapproximation of tissue planes".[1] This principle has recently been called into question. Studies in the rat have demonstrated that closure of a laparotomy incision without peritoneal suturing results in fewer adhesions. A large clinical trial has demonstrated no difference in postoperative complications, wound healing and adhesions to the laparotomy incision, regardless of whether or not the peritoneum was closed.[1] Reduction of adhesions when tissue is not reapproximated may relate to decreased tissue anoxia. Operative laparoscopy is associated with a reduced need and ability to reapproximate the peritoneal edges, which may play a factor in reducing postsurgical pelvic adhesions.

Avoidance of tissue reapproximation by suture has also been applied to pelvic viscera. It has been has recommended that the tubal incision after linear salpingostomy for ectopic pregnancy be allowed to close by secondary intention. Meyer and colleagues examined adhesion formation after ovarian wedge resection with and without reconstruction of the ovary using a polygalactin suture in a rabbit model.[8] Their data support the hypothesis that the incidence and severity of adhesion formation is increased after suture reapproximation of the ovarian cortex. Given the increased use of endoscopic treatment of ovarian and other adnexal pathology and the inherent difficulty in laparoscopic suture placement, this finding, if confirmed in clinical trials, will have important implications. Nonetheless, this is an area that requires much future assessment before definite conclusions regarding the value of tissue closure can be determined.

The use of the laser has become increasingly popular in reproductive surgery. It has been suggested that the CO_2 laser may result in de-

TABLE 11.1. Results of infertility surgery: laparotomy versus laparoscopy.

Author	Number of patients	Intrauterine pregnancy (%)
Laparotomy[a]		
Diamond (1979)[b]	140	57.1
Hulka (1982)[c]	47	25.5
Frantzen (1982)[d]	49	38.8
Kelly (1982)[e]	21	19.0
Lubor (1986)[f]	13	54.0
Total:	270	45.2
Laparoscopy		
Madelenat (1979)[g]	144	23.6
Mintz (1979)[h]	65	36.9
Bruhat (1983)[i]	93	51.6
Gomel (1983)[j]	92	58.7
Donnez (1987)[k]	54	57.0
Serour (1989)[l]	30	12.0
Total:	478	40.6

[a]All reports followed the tenets of microsurgery when performing infertility surgery via laparotomy.
Modified with permission from Hershlag A, Diamond MP, DeCherney AH. Adhesiolysis. *Clin Obstet Gynecol.* 1991; 34(2):395–402.
[b]Diamond E. Lysis of postoperative pelvic adhesions in infertility. *Fertil Steril.* 1979;31:287–295.
[c]Hulka JF. Adnexal adhesions: a prognostic staging and classification system based on a five-year survey of fertility surgery results at Chapel Hill, North Carolina. *Am J Obstet Gynecol.* 1982;144:1412.
[d]Frantzen C, Schlösser HW. Microsurgery and postinfectious tubal infertility. *Fertil Steril.* 1982;38:397–420.
[e]Kelly RW, Roberts DF. Experience with the carbon dioxide laser in gynecologic microsurgery. *Am J Obstet Gynecol.* 1982;146:585–588.
[f]Lubor K, Beeson CC, Kennedy JF, Villaneuva B, Young PE. Results of microsurgical treatment of tubal infertility and early second-look laparoscopy in the post-pelvic inflammatory disease patient: implications for in vitro fertilization. *Am J Obstet Gynecol.* 1986;154:1264–1270.
[g]Madelenat P, Palmer R. Etude critique des liberations per-coelioscopiques des adherences peri-annexielles. *J Fr Gynecol Obst Reprod.* 1979;8:347–352.
[h]Mintz M, Madelenat P, Palmer R. Aspect therapeutique de la coelioscopie dans les sterilities tubo peritoneales. In: Brosens I, Cognet M, Constantin A, Thibier M, eds. *Oviduse et fertilite.* Paris: Masson: 1979:279.
[i]Bruhat MA, Mage G, Manhes H, Soualhat C, Ropert JP, Pouly JL. Laparoscopy procedures to promote fertility: ovariolysis and adhesiolysis: results of 93 selected cases. *Acta Eur Fertil.* 1983;14:113–115.
[j]Gomel V. Salpingo-ovariolysis by laparoscopy in infertility. *Fertil Steril.* 1983;40:607–611.
[k]Donnez J. CO_2 laser laparoscopy in infertile women with endometriosis and women with adnexal adhesions. *Fertil Steril.* 1987;48:390–394.
[l]Serour GI, Badrouni MD, El Agizi HM, Hamed AF, Abdel-Aziz F. Laparoscopic adhesiolysis for infertile patients with pelvic adhesive disease. *Int J Gynecol Obstet.* 1989;30:249.

creased adhesion formation secondary to its ability to make precise incisions, maintain meticulous hemostasis, and reduce tissue handling.[1] Most of the studies using animal models report that postoperative adhesions are formed to the same degree with either CO_2 laser or electrocautery used at laparotomy. A difference in postoperative adhesions when laparoscopic lysis of adhesions was performed using laser (CO_2 or Nd:YAG), electrocautery, or a cavitron ultrasonic surgical aspirator was also not demonstrated.[9,10]

Clinical trials performed to date also fail to demonstrate a difference in adhesion formation and reformation at laparotomy using the CO_2 laser or electrocautery as assessed by second-look surgery or pregnancy outcome.[1] A small series evaluating laparoscopic tubal anastomosis found a tubal patency rate of 50% (four of eight tubes) and a crude pregnancy rate of 50%.[11] Although this does not compare favorably to tubal anastomosis at laparotomy, the results of this small study were encouraging (see Chapter 14). It has been suggested that adhesion formation following laparoscopic myomectomy appears to be less than that following abdominal myomectomy.[12] In that report, laparoscopic myomectomy was associated with adhesion formation in 66% of patients assessed by second-look laparoscopy; compared to other studies in which postoperative adhesions occurred in 82% to 100% of patients following abdominal myomectomy.

Adjuvants for Adhesion Reduction

Despite strict adherence to microsurgical principles, either at laparotomy or laparoscopy, adhesion reformation and de novo adhesion formation commonly occur. This observation, and the need to prevent this occurrence, have led to the development of adjuvants to decrease adhesion formation (Table 11.2). These adjuvants can act at one or more of the stages of adhesion formation: reduction of the initial inflammatory response and the subsequent outpouring of sanguinous material, inhibition of the formation of a coagulum from this exu-

TABLE 11.2. Classes of adhesion-reduction adjuvants.

Fibrinolytic agents
Fibrinolysin
Papain
Streptokinase
Urokinase
Hyaluronidase
Chymotrypsin
Trypsin
Pepsin
Plasminogen activators
Anticoagulants
Heparin
Citrates
Oxalates
Antiinflammatory agents
Corticosteroids
Nonsteroidal antiinflammatory agents
Antihistamines
Progesterone
Calcium channel blockers
Antibiotics
Tetracyclines
Cephalosporins
Mechanical separation
Intraabdominal
Dextran
Crystalloid solutions
Carboxymethyl cellulose
Barriers
Endogenous tissue
Omental grafts
Peritoneal grafts
Bladder strips
Fetal membranes
Exogenous material
Oxidized cellulose
Oxidized regenerated cellulose
Polytetrafluoroethylene (PTFE)
Fibrin sealant
Poloxamer 407

date, stimulation of fibrinolytic activity, mechanical separation of abutting surfaces, and inhibition of fibroblast proliferation.[2]

Antiinflammatory Agents

Corticosteroids have been used in an attempt to reduce the inflammatory response to peritoneal injury. These agents are theorized to reduce the inflammatory response by decreasing vascular permeability, stabilizing lysosomes, and inhibiting the synthesis and release of histamines. Additionally, they have been reported to inhibit the proliferation of fibroblasts, although more recent evidence does not support this finding.[2] Small animal studies have demonstrated the efficacy of intravenous corticosteroids in adhesion prevention, although only when large doses were administered either before or shortly after the peritoneal injury. Use of steroids in these studies was associated with increased morbidity, including infection and wound disruption. Primate studies failed to confirm the efficacy of corticosteroids in adhesion reduction. Promethazine, an antihistamine, has been reported to inhibit histamine-induced vascular permeability and stabilize lysosomal membranes.[3] Replogle in 1966 described the use of glucocorticoids in conjunction with promethazine as a means to reduce adhesion formation.[13] Nonetheless, other studies have failed to demonstrate a direct benefit of the use of this combination therapy in the prevention of adhesions.[3]

Prostaglandins are known to play a role in adhesion formation. Indeed, the instillation of the prostaglandins $F_{2\alpha}$ and E_2 in the peritoneal cavity enhanced adhesion formation in animals.[2] Nonsteroidal antiinflammatory drugs (NSAIDs) have been shown to inhibit prostaglandin biosynthesis, platelet aggregation, secretory activity, leukocyte migration, and phagocytosis, and also to suppress lysosome release.[3] Iloprost (Berlex Laboratories, Cedar Knolls, NJ), a prostacyclin analog, has demonstrated vasodilatory, antiinflammatory, fibrinolytic, and antithrombotic properties. Perioperative iloprost therapy given subcutaneously has been shown to reduce adhesions in a rodent model.[14] Many animal studies have shown a reduction in the formation of peritoneal adhesions with the use of NSAIDs, including oxyphenbutazone, ibuprofen, and meclofenamate.[2,3] A reduction in postoperative adhesions was seen with both systemic and intraperitoneal administration. Theoretically, however, the devascularized sites at which adhesions are most likely to occur are less available to systemically administered medications. Therapy with pharmacologic adjuvants such as NSAIDs thus may require the use of a local drug delivery system.[2]

Progesterone has been demonstrated to have antiinflammatory and immunosuppressive activity. It has been reported that adhesion formation is decreased after ovarian wedge resection if the ovary operated upon contains a progesterone-secreting corpus luteum. Subsequently, it has been shown that intraperitoneal instillation of aqueous progesterone decreased adhesion formation in the guinea pig, although other studies have failed to confirm this finding.[3]

Calcium channel blocking agents have been demonstrated to modulate sequential aspects of the peritoneal repair process, such as decreasing cellular injury, inhibiting the release of vasoactive substances such as histamine and prostaglandins E and F, decreasing exudation of fibrin-rich plasma as substrate for clot formation, reducing phagocyte activation, and inhibiting fibroblast penetration into fibrin matrices. In animal studies, Steinleitner and colleagues have demonstrated a reduction in pelvic adhesions after postoperative intraabdominal instillation of diltiazem, nifedipine, and verapamil.[3] Intramuscular administration, however, was not associated with reduction in adhesions. In these studies, administration of these calcium channel antagonists was not associated with any increased morbidity.

Hyaluronic acid is a glucosaminoglycan that plays a role in maintenance of the structural integrity of tissues, fluid regulation, and cell protection. In a randomized, blinded rat cecal model, adhesions were significantly reduced by precoating the tissue before injury with a hyaluronic acid solution.[15] Clinical trials using hyaluronic acid solutions are currently under way.

Anticoagulants

The use of anticoagulants, specifically high-dose heparin given intraperitoneally and systematically, has been associated with a decrease in adhesion formation. However, wound disruption and hemorrhage have precluded its use in this manner. In contrast, peritoneal irrigation with a dilute heparin solution, while not associated with these side effects, has not been demonstrated to be effective in adhesion prevention.[3]

Fibrinolytic Agents

Plasminogen activator (PA), a serine protease, converts plasminogen to plasmin, which causes fibrin degradation. It was postulated that replacement of the deficient PA activity associated with adhesion formation would result in a decrease in adhesions. In fact, in animal models, application of recombinant tissue plasminogen activator (TPA) has been shown to reduce adhesion formation and reformation. No wound healing or bleeding complications were noted.[16] Interestingly, intraperitoneal verapamil and recombinant TPA acted synergistically to reduce adhesion formation in a rabbit model.[17] At present there are no data available regarding administration of recombinant TPA to humans.

Pentoxyfylline, a methylxanthine analog, has been shown to decrease granulocyte-mediated tissue damage, improve perfusion of damaged structures, and augment PA activator production, thereby enhancing fibrinolysis. Adhesion reformation after subcutaneous injection of pentoxyfylline was shown to be reduced in rabbits.[3]

Antibiotic Therapy

Systemic antibiotics, either broad-spectrum cephalosporins or tetracyclines, are often given as prophylaxis against postoperative infection and subsequent adhesion formation. There are few data to support this practice, which may, in part, result from the low incidence of postoperative infection during procedures. In contrast, peritoneal irrigation with antibiotic-containing solutions (cefazolin and tetracycline) has been shown to increase peritoneal adhesion formation in the rat model. Thus, their intraabdominal use is not suggested.

Mechanical Separation

Mechanical separation of pelvic structures is another mechanism by which adhesion formation

can be reduced. This class of adjuvants includes abdominal instillates and material barriers.

The adjuvant most commonly used to reduce adhesion formation is crystalloid solution, administered as an instillate at the end of the surgical procedure. Crystalloid instillation is hypothesized to decrease adhesion formation through the separation of raw peritoneal surfaces and by dilution of fibrin and fibrinous exudate released from the injured surfaces. Nonetheless, it has been shown that crystalloids are absorbed from the peritoneal cavity at a rate of approximately 35 ml/hr. Thus, a 200-ml solution would be absorbed in 6 hr and a 5000-ml solution in 6 days. The process of peritoneal repair, fibrin deposition, and adhesion formation extends well beyond the time during which a reasonable volume of crystalloid persists. Theoretical consideration of peritoneal fluid dynamics thus suggests that crystalloids would not prevent adhesion formation, a suggestion that has been confirmed by clinical trials.[2] In addition, leaving a large volume of fluid in the peritoneal cavity may reduce the ability of the host to eliminate infection.[2]

A 32% solution of dextran-70 (Hyskon®, Pharmacia Corp., molecular weight 70,000) in saline is a commonly used adhesion-reducing instillate. It has been suggested that Hyskon® acts as a siliconizing agent, coating raw surfaces, and as an osmotic agent, resulting in hydroflotation of pelvic viscera. In addition, there are data suggesting that this solution has immunosuppressive effects in vitro. Much of the literature evaluating the efficacy of 32% dextran-70 in animals demonstrates that its use is associated with a significant decrease in adhesion formation,[2] although it is more efficacious in preventing adhesion formation than reformation. However, the results of large-scale clinical trials evaluating the efficacy of 32% dextran are conflicting.[2] Complications from its use in humans have been reported, including anaphylaxis, pleural effusion, vulvar extravasation, and transient liver function abnormalities.[2] Hyskon® can be used laparoscopically, and 200 ml of Hyskon® should be instilled through an irrigation cannula into the posterior cul-de-sac. It is generally well tolerated, although patients should be forewarned of abdominal bloating.

Expanded polytetrafluoroethylene (PTFE, Gore-Tex®), a mechanical barrier, has been used for several years in vascular and cardiovascular surgery. It has been found to be nonreactive, nontoxic, and antithrombogenic.[2] When formulated as a surgical membrane (0.1 mm thick and pores less than 1 μm in diameter, thinner and less porous than the material used for grafts, etc.), it retards penetration by the inflammatory cells and fibroblasts, thereby minimizing adhesion formation. Animal studies evaluating the use of Gore-Tex® surgical membrane are conflicting, although recent studies appear to support its use in reducing adhesion formation.[2,3,16]

In a clinical trial, the use of Gore-Tex® surgical membrane was effective in reducing adhesion formation after myomectomy[18] and in lysis of adhesions performed at laparotomy as assessed by second-look laparoscopy.[19] Gore-Tex® surgical membrane is not without its shortcomings, however; it must be secured in place and, because it is not water soluble, it does not easily conform or adhere to irregular peritoneal surfaces. Finally, because it is nonabsorbable, the membrane likely requires removal at a second surgical procedure unless it is going to be left in place. The long-term implications of leaving Gore-Tex® surgical membranes in the peritoneal cavity are unknown.[17] The membrane is generally easy to remove if this is done 2 to 6 weeks after the initial procedure. It is removed laparoscopically by cutting the sutures holding it in place and then gently pulling on the membrane until it is free. At a limited number of third-look procedures, adhesions were not found at the site where the membrane was removed.[18]

Oxidized regenerated cellulose, Interceed® (TC7), which exhibits bacteriostatic properties, also acts as a mechanical barrier. It forms a gelatinous mass within hours of placement; it is metabolized into glucose, glucuronic acid, and other oligosaccharides within a short time period (usually 4 days) and has been shown to be nonreactive. The data regarding the use of Interceed® in preventing adhesion formation

and reformation in several animal models are conflicting.[2,3,16] In addition, a complicated randomized trial with multiple variables using monkeys demonstrated that Gore-Tex® surgical membrane, when applied at laparotomy, prevented adhesion formation and reformation to a greater degree than did Interceed®.[20] To improve the ability of Interceed® to prevent adhesion formation, at least in animal models, a heparin solution was added to the fabric. A significant reduction in adhesion formation and reformation was noted in this rabbit uterine horn model. Neither alterations in clotting parameters nor hemorrhagic complications were found.[16]

It was postulated that Interceed® acted as a carrier delivering heparin directly to the affected peritoneal surfaces.[16] It is known that the presence of blood diminishes the effectiveness of oxidized regenerated cellulose in adhesion prevention. Hence, meticulous hemostasis is required to maximize its efficacy. In fact, using a rabbit uterine model, achieving hemostasis with thrombin before the application of Interceed® barrier appears to be more effective than placing Interceed® alone on bleeding or oozing surfaces.[2] The efficacy of Interceed® applied after achieving hemostasis with thrombin was further improved by moistening it with heparin.[2]

Despite the conflicting results obtained in animal models, several randomized clinical trials have shown that Interceed® is efficacious at preventing adhesion formation and reformation when placed at laparotomy. The TC-7 Adhesion Barrier Study Group II evaluated 134 patients at 13 centers and found that the placement of the barrier reduced the incidence, extent, and severity of postoperative adhesions when assessed at second-look laparoscopy (Table 11.3). Overall, 90% of patients at risk for adhesions benefited from the use of the Interceed® barrier.[21] In a similar study, Sekiba and colleagues confirmed these findings (Table 11.3). In addition, they demonstrated that Interceed® was highly effective in preventing adhesion formation after removal of severe endometriosis (28 patients).[22] Interceed® has also been found to decrease the incidence of

TABLE 11.3.   Side-wall adhesions at the time of second-look laparoscopy.

					Matched pair comparison of treatment effect: side walls with no adhesions		
Interceed side wall[a]	+	−	+	−	Interceed (n)	Control (n)	Interceed benefit
Control side wall	+	−	−	+			
Azziz et al.[20] (n = 134)	42%	16%	8%	34%	46 (82%)	10 (18%)	×4.6
Sekiba et al.[21] (n = 63)	36%	19%	5%	40%	25 (89%)	3 (11%)	×8.3
Total (n = 197):	40%	17%	7%	36%	71 (85%)	13 (15%)	×5.5

[a]+, Adhesions present; −, adhesions absent.
Modified with permission from diZerega G. Contemporary adhesion prevention. *Fertil Steril.* 1994;61(2):219–235.

ovarian adhesions after lysis of ovarian adhesions, ovarian cystectomy, removal of endometrioma, and oophoroplasty.[2] In addition, Interceed® has been shown to reduce the incidence and severity of adhesion reformation to the ovary, fallopian tube, and fimbria after infertility surgery.[23]

Interceed® can also be easily placed at the time of laparoscopy. Unfortunately, few data are available on the efficacy of laparoscopic placement of Interceed® in reducing adhesion formation and reformation. A reduction in ovarian adhesions after laparoscopic ovarian drilling was found by wrapping the ovaries with Interceed®.[2] Nonetheless, further data on the value of Interceed® placement at laparoscopy are required.

Poloxamer 407 has been shown to reduce adhesion formation and reformation in animal models.[16] In one rat uterine horn model, poloxamer 407 compared favorably to Interceed® in reducing adhesions.[24] Poloxamer 407 is a liquid at room temperature but changes to a solid gel at body temperature. This property, which is known as "reverse thermal gelation," makes it an ideal material for use at the time of operative laparoscopy.

Fibrin sealant is a solution containing fibrinogen, aprotinin, thrombin, and calcium chloride. This solution has been shown to enhance the normal healing process by increasing the influx of macrophages that produce factors causing angiogenesis, fibroblast proliferation, and collagen production. It has also been demonstrated to reduce the formation of postsurgical adhesions when used during laparoscopic surgery in a rabbit uterine horn model.[25]

Second-Look Laparoscopy

Swolin introduced second-look laparoscopy (SLL) to assess the result of certain surgical procedures.[1] As postoperative adhesions are commonly encountered at the time of SLL, the procedure also provides an opportunity to perform adhesiolysis. It is believed that because pelvic adhesive disease plays a role in infertility, lysis of these adhesions may also improve pregnancy rates. Trimbos-Kemper and colleagues performed a "third-look laparoscopy" in patients who had undergone an early second-look procedure with lysis of adhesions at that time. They reported that more than half of the adhesions that were separated at the first laparoscopic procedure did not recur.[26] Similarly, Jansen reported that second-look laparoscopy was associated with a significant reduction in adhesions at the time of "a third-look" procedure.[27] Trimbos-Kemper reported a reduction in the incidence of ectopic pregnancies in women who had undergone second-look laparoscopy, although the intrauterine pregnancy rate was unchanged.[26] Surrey et al. reported a 52% intrauterine pregnancy rate in 31 patients who had undergone early SLL after reconstructive pelvic surgery.[28] They had no control group, but noted that this pregnancy rate was greater than that reported in the literature for comparable procedures.

Swolin recommended that SLL be performed 6 weeks after the initial surgery to allow treatment of the forming adhesions[29] (Table 11.4). Adhesions found at laparoscopy 1 to 16 weeks after surgery were primarily filmy and avascular when compared to those encountered at laparoscopy 18 months or more

TABLE 11.4. Pelvic adhesions noted at second-look laparoscopy.

Source	Time from initial procedure	Total number of patients	Number with adhesions (%)	Predominant type of adhesion
Diamond et al. (1984)[29]	1–12 weeks	106	91 (86)	Filmy
DeCherney and Mezer (1984)[30]	4–16 weeks	20	15 (75)	Filmy
	1–3 years	41	31 (76)	Dense
Surrey and Friedman (1982)[27]	6–8 weeks	31	22 (71)	Filmy
	6 months	6	5 (83)	Dense
Pittaway et al. (1986)[31]	4–6 weeks	23	23 (100)	Thick
Trimbos-Kemper et al. (1985)[25]	8 days	188	104 (55)	Filmy
Daniell and Pittaway (1983)[32]	4–6 weeks	25	24 (96)	Filmy
McLaughlin (1984)[33]	6–12 weeks	25	14 (58)	Filmy
Jansen (1988)[26]	1–3 weeks	73[a]	42 (58)	Filmy
		183[b]	168 (92)	Filmy
Tulandi et al. (1989)[34]	1 year	36	21 (58)	N/A[c]

[a]No preoperative adhesions
[b]Preoperative adhesions present
[c]N/A, not available.
Modified with permission from Diamond MP. Surgical aspects of infertility. In: Sciarra JJ, ed. *Gynecology and Obstetrics*. Philadelphia: Harper & Row; 1995:1–26.

after the primary procedure. It has similarly been noted that bleeding is more commonly encountered if the second-look procedure is performed more than 12 weeks after the initial procedure.[27] Alternatively, it has been suggested that early SLL, i.e., that performed less than 2 weeks after the initial surgery, results in increased bleeding from granulation tissue encountered during adhesiolysis.[1] Other investigators, in large series, have not described this problem.[26] Finally, Diamond et al. have demonstrated that there appears to be no difference in the type of adhesions observed at SLL when laparoscopy is performed within 1 to 12 weeks after the initial procedure.[1] Overall, while it is probable that early SLL reduces postoperative pelvic adhesions, to date no appropriately designed studies have demonstrated a benefit on subsequent pregnancy rates in women undergoing infertility surgery.

Summary

There appears to be a wide array of adhesion-reducing adjuvants available to the reproductive surgeon. However, the results in the literature on the efficacy of these substances are often conflicting, with a limited amount of human data available for most adjuvants. Currently, there is evidence to support the use of Interceed® and Gore-Tex® surgical membrane to reduce adhesion formation during gynecologic surgery by laparotomy. The data regarding their efficacy during laparoscopic surgery are limited. Other adjuvants, such as plasminogen activator instillation, appear promising but await further evaluation and clinical trials. Nevertheless, the use of adjuvants must not be considered a replacement for meticulous surgical technique, which remains the most significant deterrent to adhesion formation.

References

1. Diamond MP. Surgical aspects of infertility. In: Sciarra JJ, ed. *Gynecology and Obstetrics*. Philadelphia: Harper & Row; 1995:1–26.
2. diZerega GS. Contemporary adhesion prevention. *Fertil Steril*. 1994;61:219–235.
3. Drollette CM, Badaway SZA. Pathophysiology of pelvic adhesions. *J Reprod Med*. 1992;37:107–121.
4. diZerega GS. The peritoneum and its response to surgical injury. In: diZerega GS, Malinak LR, Diamond MP, Linsky CB, eds. *Treatment of Post Surgical Adhesions. Progress In Clinical and Biological Research*. Vol. 358. New York: Wiley-Liss; 1989:1–11

5. Marana R, Luciano AA, Muzii L, Marendino VE, Mancuso S. Laparoscopy versus laparotomy for ovarian conservative surgery: a randomized trial in the rabbit model. *Am J Obstet Gynecol.* 1994;171:681–864.

6. Lundorff P, Hahlin M, Källfelt B, Thorburn J, Lindblom B. Adhesion formation after laparoscopic surgery in tubal pregnancy: a randomized trial versus laparotomy. *Fertil Steril.* 1991;55:911–915.

7. Hershlag A, Diamond MP, DeCherney AH. Adhesiolysis. *Clin Obstet Gynecol.* 1991;34:395–402.

8. Meyer WJ, Grainger DA, DeCherney AH, et al. Ovarian surgery in the rabbit: Effect of Cortex closure on adhesion formation and ovarian function. *J Reprod Med.* 1991;36:639–643.

9. Luciano AA, Frishman GN, Maier DB. A comparative analysis of adhesion reduction, tissue effects, and incising characteristics of electrosurgery, CO_2 laser, and Nd:YAG laser at operative laparoscopy: An animal study. *J Laparoendosc Surg.* 1992;2:287–292.

10. Hurst BS, Awoniyi CA, Stephens JK, Thompson KL, Riehl RM, Schlaff WD. Application of the cavitron ultrasonic surgical aspirator (CUSA) for gynecological laparoscopic surgery using the rabbit as an animal model. *Fertil Steril.* 1992;58:444–448.

11. Katz E, Donesky BW. Laparoscopic tubal anastomosis. A pilot study. *J Reprod Med.* 1994;39:497–498.

12. Hasson HM, Rotman C, Rana N, Sistos F, Dmowski WP. Laparoscopic myomectomy. *Obstet Gynecol.* 1992;80:884–888.

13. Replogle RL, Johnson R, Gross RE. Prevention of postoperative intestinal adhesions with combined promethazine and dexamethasone therapy: Experimental and clinical studies. *Ann Surg.* 1966;163:580–588.

14. Steinleitner A, Lambert H, Suarez M, Serpa N, Robin B. Reduction of primary posttraumatic adhesion formation with the prostacyclin analog iloprost in a rodent model. *Am J Obstet Gynecol.* 1991;165:1817–1820.

15. Goldberg EP, Burns JW, Yaacobi Y. Prevention of postoperative adhesions by precoating tissue with dilute sodium hyaluronate solutions. *Prog Clin Biol Res.* 1993;381:191–204.

16. Pados GA, Devroey P. Adhesions. *Curr Opin Obstet Gynecol.* 1992;4:412–418.

17. Dunn RC, Steinleitner AJ, Lambert H. Synergistic effect of intraperitoneally administered calcium channel blockade and recombinant tissue plasminogen activator to prevent adhesion formation in an animal model. *Am J Obstet Gynecol.* 1991;164:1327–1330.

18. The Surgical Membrane Study Group. Prophylaxis of pelvic sidewall adhesions with Gore-Tex surgical membrane: a multicenter clinical investigation. *Fertil Steril.* 1992;57:921–923.

19. The Myomectomy Adhesion Multicenter Study Group. An expanded polytetrafluoroethylene barrier (Gore-Tex surgical membrane) reduced post-myomectomy adhesion formation. *Fertil Steril.* 1995;63:491–493.

20. Grow DR, Seltman HJ, Coddington CC, Hodgen GD. The reduction of postoperative adhesions by two different barrier methods versus control in cynomolgus monkeys: a prospective, randomized, crossover study. *Fertil Steril.* 1994;61:1141–1146.

21. Azziz R, INTERCEED (TC7) Adhesion Barrier Study Group II. Microsurgery alone or with Interceed absorbable adhesion barrier for pelvic sidewall adhesion reformation. *Surg Gynecol Obstet.* 1993;177:135–139.

22. Sekiba K, Obstetrics and Gynecology Adhesion Prevention Committee. Use of Interceed (TC7) absorbable adhesion barrier to reduce postoperative adhesion reformation in infertility and endometriosis surgery. *Obstet Gynecol.* 1992;79:518–522.

23. Nordic Adhesion Prevention Study Group. The efficacy of Interceed (TC7) for prevention of reformation of postoperative adhesions on ovaries, fallopian tubes, and fimbriae in microsurgical operations for fertility: a multicenter study. *Fertil Steril.* 1995;63:709–714.

24. Rice VM, Shanti A, Moghissi KS, Leach RE. A comparative evaluation of poloxamer 407 and oxidized regenerated cellulose (Interceed [TC7]) to reduce postoperative adhesion formation in the rat uterine horn model. *Fertil Steril.* 1993;59:901–906.

25. De Iaco PA, Costa A, Mazzoleni G, Pasquinelli G, Bassein L, Marabini A. Fibrin sealant in laparoscopic adhesion prevention in the rabbit uterine horn model. *Fertil Steril.* 1994;62:400–404.

26. Trimbos-Kemper TCM, Trimbos JB, van Hall EV. Adhesion formation after tubal surgery: results of the eighth-day laparoscopy in 188 patients. *Fertil Steril.* 1985;43:395–400.

27. Jansen RPS. Early laparoscopy after pelvic operations to prevent adhesions: safety and efficacy. *Fertil Steril.* 1988;49:26–31.

28. Surrey MW, Friedman S. Second-look laparoscopy after reconstructive pelvic surgery for endometriosis. *J Reprod Med.* 1982;27:658–660.

29. Swolin K. Electromicrosurgery and salpingostomy long term results. *Am J Obstet Gynecol.* 1975;121:418.

30. Diamond MP, Daniell JF, Feste J, et al. Pelvic adhesions at early second-look laparoscopy following carbon dioxide laser surgical procedures. *Infertility.*1984;7:39–44.

31. DeCherney AH, Mezer HC. The nature of posttuboplasty pelvic adhesions as determined by early and late laparoscopy. *Fertil Steril.* 1984;41:643–646.

32. Pittaway DE, Daniell JR, Maxson WS. Ovarian surgery in an infertility patient as an indication for short interval second look laparoscopy: A preliminary study. *Fertil Steril.* 1986;4:611–614.

33. Daniell JF, Pittaway DE. Short interval second-look laparoscopy after infertility surgery. *J Reprod Med.* 1983;28:281–283.

34. McLaughlin DS. Evaluation of adhesion reformation by early second-look laparoscopy following microlaser ovarian wedge resection. *Fertil Steril.* 1984;42:531–537.

35. Tulandi T, Falcone T, Kafka I. Second-look operative laparoscopy 1 year following reproductive surgery. *Fertil Steril.* 1989;52:421–424.

12

Contemporary Management of Ectopic Pregnancies

Ana Alvarez Murphy and Sujatha Reddy

Introduction

The incidence of ectopic pregnancies has increased fourfold since 1970.[1] Ectopic pregnancy now accounts for roughly 1.2% to 1.4% of reported pregnancies.[2] This may be the consequence of our ability to treat pelvic inflammatory disease (PID) effectively before permanent tubal obstruction occurs or it may be a reflection of the general trend toward delayed childbearing. Early diagnosis and treatment have reduced mortality and morbidity, as well as probably improving subsequent fertility. Advances in ultrasound, particularly transvaginal imaging, and human chorionic gonadotropin (β-hCG) detection have considerably improved our diagnostic capability. Laparoscopy is an integral part of the diagnostic scheme and recently has become the preferred therapeutic method when surgery is required. Depending on the patient's desire for future fertility and the extent of her disease, conservative as well as radical surgery may be performed laparoscopically.

Diagnosis of Ectopic Pregnancies

If an ectopic pregnancy is diagnosed early, it can usually be treated before significant tubal destruction and hemorrhage occur. Those patients with significant risk factors, including previous pelvic inflammatory disease, tubal surgery, or history of ectopic pregnancy, should be screened early in the course of pregnancy with serial serum β-hCG measurements and transvaginal ultrasound to confirm the intrauterine location of the gestation. Patients of childbearing age who present with pelvic pain or abnormal vaginal bleeding should be screened with a rapid and sensitive monoclonal antibody urine β-hCG test. With test sensitivity currently averaging 20 mIU/ml, the false-negative rate is about 1%.[3,4] In a hemodynamically unstable and symptomatic patient with a positive urine pregnancy test and a positive culdocentesis for free-flowing nonclotting blood, one should proceed directly to laparoscopy or laparotomy, depending on the skill and experience of the surgeon.

In the hemodynamically stable patient with a positive β-hCG and pelvic pain, a transvaginal sonogram should be performed to evaluate the uterine and adnexal structures initially. If an intrauterine sac is not seen and a complex adnexal mass is noted on sonography, the patient is taken to laparoscopy, because this clinical picture is highly predictive of an ectopic pregnancy. Alternatively, patients suspected of having an ectopic pregnancy but who are pain free and do not demonstrate a gestational sac or complex adnexal structure by sonogram may be followed carefully with serial quantitated serum β-hCG measurements. Laparoscopy is usually indicated if the initial β-hCG is greater than 2000 mIU/ml and no intrauterine sac is seen on the transvaginal sonogram.[5-7] Transvaginal sonography can image a 3-mm intrauterine gestational sac, generally correlated to serum β-hCG levels as low as 1000 to 2000 mIU/ml (by the International Reference Preparation [IRP] standard). If the initial β-hCG is less than 2000 mIU/ml, the differential diagnosis includes an early intrauterine or ectopic pregnancy, and the β-hCG level is repeated in 48 hours.

Normally, at least a 66% rise in β-hCG level is observed if a normal intrauterine pregnancy is present. An abnormal increase, plateau, or decrease in the quantitated pregnancy test denotes an abnormal gestation—either a spontaneous or threatened abortion or an ectopic pregnancy. A dilatation and curettage (D&C) may be performed to detect the presence of intrauterine chorionic villi, either grossly (e.g., by flotation of the specimen in sterile water) or on frozen/permanent section. If no villi are found at D&C, laparoscopy is recommended unless the clinical setting is highly suggestive of a complete spontaneous abortion or the β-hCG levels continue to fall toward negative. With this algorithm most ectopic pregnancies can be diagnosed early, minimizing tubal damage and patient morbidity. The most common differential diagnosis for an ectopic pregnancy is a threatened abortion. The most common differential diagnosis when the ultrasound shows an adnexal mass is an intrauterine pregnancy with a bleeding corpus luteum cyst(s).

Patient Selection and Prerequisites for Laparoscopic Surgery

To perform laparoscopic surgery safely for ectopic pregnancy, one must have a skilled surgeon, an appropriately selected patient, and the appropriate instrumentation. The most important requirement for the laparoscopic treatment of ectopics is surgical experience. Because laparoscopic surgery involving small ectopic pregnancies is relatively easy to perform, many surgeons begin their training treating these pregnancies, which is quite appropriate in the stable patient so long as an experienced surgeon is on hand to supervise. However, it is inappropriate for a novice to operate on a hemodynamically unstable patient.

Contraindications to laparoscopic treatment, particularly in regard to size and location of the ectopic, are relative depending on the experience and skill of the surgeon. Nevertheless, an intramural ectopic may be more difficult to manage than an isthmic or ampullary tubal pregnancy. Although excessive size of the pregnancy has been mentioned as a relative contraindication, this depends more on the surgeon's ability to identify the pelvic anatomy clearly. Reich and colleagues reported on the laparoscopic treatment of 109 ectopic pregnancies[8]; 16 ectopic pregnancies were ruptured, 3 had unstable vital signs, and 3 were interstitial. There were no intraoperative complications, and no laparotomies were performed.

Techniques and Instrumentation

Instrumentation

Many operative laparoscopic instruments are available for the treatment of ectopic pregnancies.[9] However, a few specific instruments are key. An aspirator/irrigator is helpful in evacuating a hemoperitoneum quickly and effectively. The aspirator may be attached directly to wall suction. It must also be able to irrigate large volumes of fluid rapidly to ensure good visualization and to remove any remaining trophoblast from the pelvis. In addition, a 10-mm suction cannula connected to wall suction may be helpful in evacuating clotted blood.

Hemostasis of the operative site may be achieved using various modalities including ligature, electrocautery, thermocoagulation, or laser energy.[10] However, it is a good precaution always to have a bipolar coagulator available, as this instrument can achieve hemostasis quickly, safely, and effectively. In general, lasers, particularly CO_2, provide precise cutting but poor coagulation. Both traumatic and atraumatic forceps should be available. Additionally, methods of removing the resected tissue should be considered (see following).

Procedure Specifics

The patient should have general anesthesia with good muscle relaxation and be placed in the dorsal lithotomy position with the buttocks protruding from the table. As outlined in the *Diagnosis* section, a D&C may be performed first and the tissue examined grossly or sent for frozen section. Otherwise the uterus should not be instrumented if there is the possibility of a viable intrauterine gestation and the patient desires preservation of the pregnancy.

Once the diagnosis of an ectopic pregnancy is made at laparoscopy, a rigid metal or plastic cannula may be placed in the cervical os for manipulation. Video monitoring of the procedure is helpful for teaching purposes and to maximize assistant involvement. A straight 10- or 11-mm laparoscope is preferred, although an operating (offset) laparoscope can be used. Ancillary puncture sites are placed cephalad to the uterus, and generally in the midline and lateral on the side of the ectopic pregnancy. Most often only two ancillary sites are needed, although occasionally a third puncture site may be required.[10]

Total Salpingectomy

The treatment of choice for an ectopic pregnancy, when preservation of fertility is not an issue, is a total salpingectomy. Additionally, if the tube has been markedly destroyed by the ectopic or prior tubal disease, a conservative procedure may not be possible or advisable.[10]

A salpingectomy may be performed by successive coagulation and cutting of the mesosalpinx. Hemostasis can be achieved with unipolar and bipolar electrocoagulation or thermocoagulation. Cutting is usually performed using hook scissors (Fig. 12.1). The tubal isthmus proximal to the ectopic is coagulated before transection. Serial cautery of the mesosalpinx can begin either at the fimbriated end of the tube or proximal to the ectopic pregnancy. Surgical ease determines in which direction dissection proceeds; right-handed surgeons usually find it easier to operate from right to left. Care must be taken to coagulate and cut the mesosalpinx as close to the fallopian tube as possible to avoid excessive damage to the ovary and its blood supply. A tripolar device (see Fig. 8.15) has been created that has grasping jaws that are attached to bipolar current. It also has a blade that will transect the coagulated intervening tissue. This device eliminates the need to change instruments from the bipolar forceps to the scissors and consequently decreases operating room time.

The excised portion of the tube can then be removed through an enlarged ancillary puncture site using a 10-mm claw forceps or through the channel of an operating laparoscope with a 5-mm grasping forceps. As in all laparoscopic procedures for ectopics, care must be taken to not leave trophoblastic tissue behind, because peritoneal implantation and persistent β-hCG activity may be observed. Extensive irrigation and aspiration are useful in removing any remaining gestational tissue.

Salpingectomy may also be performed using loop ligatures (Endoloop, Ethicon Co., Somerville, NJ). Three loops are placed proximal to the ectopic pregnancy and the tube transected. However, the distal mesosalpinx may need to be partially coagulated and cut to minimize the amount of tube left behind.

FIGURE 12.1. Salpingectomy can be performed by successive coagulation (with either electrocautery or thermocoagulation) and cutting of the mesosalpinx. The proximal tube is coagulated and transected.

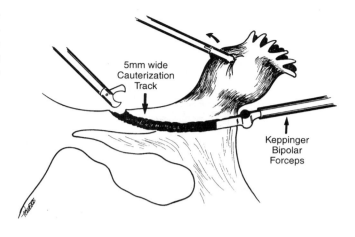

5mm wide
Cauterization
Track

Keppinger
Bipolar
Forceps

Conservative Procedures

It is appropriate to offer a conservative procedure to those patients desirous of further childbearing. Sherman et al. suggested that conservation of a tube with an ectopic pregnancy, when coexistent sterility factors are present, is associated with an increased subsequent pregnancy rate (76% vs. 44%).[11] The risk of recurrent ectopic pregnancy appears to be minimally increased in patients undergoing conservative procedure. Tulandi and Guralnick have noted that the repeat ectopic pregnancy rate approximately doubles in patients after conservative surgery for an ectopic pregnancy, and the patient must be carefully counseled in this regard.[12] Furthermore, before surgery patients must be advised regarding the possibility of persistent trophoblast that may require additional surgical or medical therapy. All patients undergoing a conservative surgical procedure must have a quantitated β-hCG level checked postoperatively on a weekly basis until negative. Patients undergoing conservative tubal surgery for an ectopic pregnancy must be reliable and able to return for their serial β-hCG measurements. Depending on the location of the ectopic and the surgeon's skill, both linear salpingostomy/salpingotomy and segmental resection are conservative surgical options for the treatment of ectopic pregnancies, as follows.

Linear Salpingostomy/Salpingotomy

Unruptured and selected ruptured isthmic and ampullary ectopic pregnancies may be treated with linear salpingostomy or salpingotomy. In the study by Pauerstein and colleagues,[13] 67% of ectopics were located within the tubal lumen while the remaining were extraluminal or mixed (Fig. 12.2) Thus, in approximately one-third of cases the tubal lumen may be intact at the time of salpingostomy/salpingotomy.

It should be noted that salpingostomy refers to the incision of the tubal ostia for removal of distal ectopics (Fig. 12.3A), while salpingotomy refers to the incision and opening of the tube away from its ostia (Figure 12.3B). It is usually preferable to perform a salpingotomy, preserving the integrity of the tubal ostia, than a salpingostomy for all except the most distal of ectopics. In the following, we refer to all these procedures as salpingotomy, unless specified.

In the past, all isthmic ectopic pregnancies were treated by segmental resection rather than linear salpingotomy. However, we believe that in those patients with an unruptured isthmic ectopic pregnancy desiring conservative surgery, a linear salpingotomy should be attempted first. Persistent β-hCG may then be treated medically or surgically. If bleeding is significant, a segmental resection (see following) is then performed. It is quite possible that

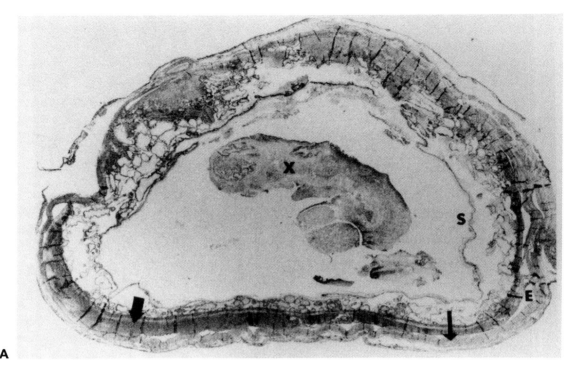

A

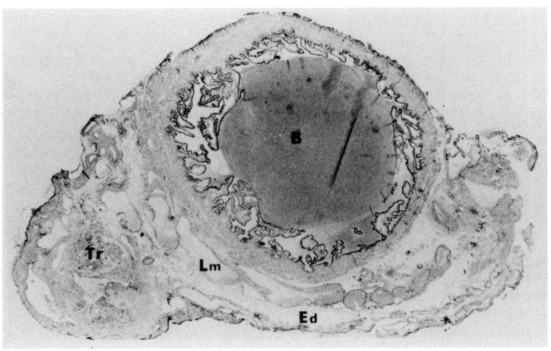

B

FIGURE 12.2. *Top:* Intraluminal ectopic pregnancy (*X,* embryo; *S,* gestational sac; *E,* endosalpinx; *thick arrow,* maternal blood within lumen interspersed with chorionic villi; *thin arrow,* myosalpinx). *Bottom:* Extraluminal ectopic pregnancy (B, maternal blood in lumen; *Lm,* lymphatic dilation; *Ed,* stromal edema; *Tr,* trophoblastic tissue). (Reprinted with permission from Pauerstein CJ. Anatomy and pathology of tubal pregnancy. *Obstet Gynecol.* 1986;67:301–308.)

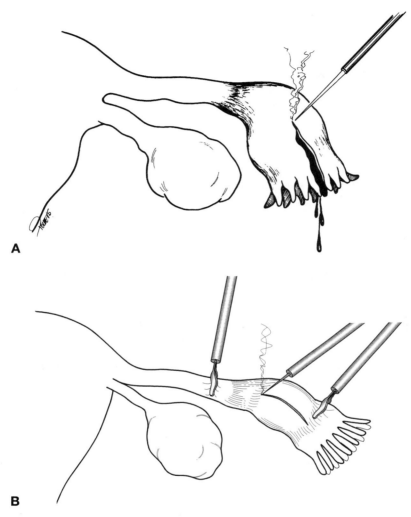

FIGURE 12.3. Laparoscopic linear salpingostomy/ salpingotomy. A linear incision is made along the antimesenteric border of the tube over the ectopic pregnancy, using a potassium-titanyl-phosphate (KTP), argon, or CO_2 laser, or unipolar needle cautery. The ectopic usually extrudes from the tube and is gently removed with adhesion of biopsy forceps. **A:** Salpingostomy refers to a tubal incision that includes the tubal ostial (ostomy). **B:** Salpingotomy refers to all incisions of the fallopian tubes, including those away from the ostia.

the treatment of isthmic ectopics with methotrexate therapy may eventually prove to result in the least morbidity and the highest tubal conservation and patency rates.

A linear incision is made with either a unipolar needle or a laser along the antimesenteric side of the tube dilated by the ectopic. Alterna-

tively, the tube can be opened using a knife or scissors. The site can be coagulated with electrocautery or thermocoagulation before incision if desired. In addition, the mesosalpingeal vessels beneath the site of the ectopic can be gently coagulated before performing the linear salpingotomy. Some surgeons use dilute vasopressin solution to minimize bleeding from the operative site. Concentrations of vasopressin (Pitressin) ranging from 0.05[14] to 2.0[15] units/ml can be injected into the mesosalpinx just below the ectopic, using a 20- or 22-gauge spinal needle placed through the abdominal wall. This may decrease bleeding not only from the incision but from the bed of the ectopic as well. Alternatively, the vasopressin solution may be injected directly over the area to be incised (Fig. 12.4).

On incision, the ectopic usually extrudes and can be gently removed with forceps or aspiration. Care must be taken not to damage normal tubal mucosa unnecessarily in an overzealous attempt to remove any remaining trophoblast. With the availability of methotrexate for the treatment of persistent ectopics (see following), the need for excoriation of the tubal lumen is even less. Occasionally it is helpful to irrigate the lumen forcefully through the antimesenteric incision, as this may dissect the ectopic gestation from the tubal wall and facili-

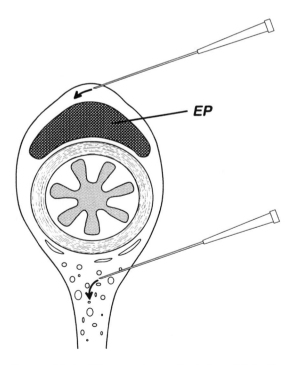

FIGURE 12.4. Vasopressin can be injected into the mesosalpinx just below the ectopic (*EP*) or injected directly over the area to be incised.

tate removal. The implantation site is observed closely for bleeding and any remaining trophoblastic tissue. With small early ectopic pregnancies one may encounter deep infiltration of trophoblast into the tubal wall resulting in persistent bleeding. Irrigation and coagulation with needle-point cautery or bipolar may be necessary. Coagulation of mesosalpingeal vessels supplying that portion of the fallopian tube may also be necessary. More simply, pressure on the surgical site can be applied using a grasper. If the blood loss cannot be stopped with these maneuvers, a segmental resection or partial salpingectomy may need to be performed.

The tubal incision is usually not closed. Fistula formation at the incision site is a possible complication, but does not appear to be common. If the defect appears to be very large or marked eversion of the mucosa is seen, an interrupted suture of 4-0 polydioxanone (PDS) may be placed using the techniques previously described (see Chapter 9). After conservative surgery by laparotomy, Tulandi and Guralnick[12] observed that pregnancies occur sooner after salpingostomy without tubal suturing than after those in which tubal suturing is performed.

Segmental Resection

In the patient with a ruptured isthmic or ampullary ectopic pregnancy who desires conservative surgery, segmental resection with subsequent reanastomosis may be the only choice. Segmental resection is reserved for ruptured ectopic pregnancies depending on the extent of tubal damage and, rarely, a failed isthmic or ampullary salpingostomy.

Segmental resection may be accomplished with electrocautery, thermocoagulation, laser, or loop ligature. Coagulation of the tube both proximal and distal to the ectopic is accomplished and the tube is then transected. The mesosalpinx just below the ectopic is successively coagulated and cut (Fig. 12.5). The tripolar described previously can be utilized for segmental resection (see Fig. 8.15). The procedure is facilitated by applying gentle traction to the segment of ectopic-containing tube to be removed. After complete transection, the

FIGURE 12.5. Laparoscopic segmental re-section. The normal fallopian tube on either side of the ectopic pregnancy is coagulated and transected. The mesosalpinx below the ectopic is coagulated and cut.

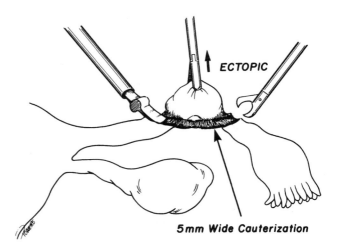

ECTOPIC

5mm Wide Cauterization

mesosalpinx is inspected carefully and all bleeding points coagulated.

A variation of the Pomeroy technique for tubal sterilization may also be used. The site of the ectopic pregnancy is placed under traction and an Endoloop is placed around its base. The ligated tubal segment containing the ectopic pregnancy is then transected and removed. This technique unfortunately results in a large amount of tubal destruction. Nevertheless, it is quick and easy to perform, particularly when tubal bleeding is brisk.

A variation of the cautery method of sterilization has also been used. The segment of tube containing the ectopic pregnancy is thoroughly coagulated with electrocautery or thermocoagulation. Obviously, the segment of tube is destroyed and no specimen can be sent to pathology. Furthermore, a significant portion of tube may be damaged.

With these conservative procedures, the potential for fertility remains after anastomosis. Nevertheless, segmental resection is infrequently used today because methotrexate or salpingotomy may be less damaging for the treatment of midtubal ectopics.

Ovarian Ectopic Pregnancy

Although ovarian pregnancies are rare, most can be treated through the laparoscope. An attempt should be made to excise the ectopic with either lasers or unipolar needle cautery if

a normal ovary can be discerned. After dissection, the ovary is carefully inspected to ensure good hemostasis and complete removal of trophoblastic tissue. The ovarian defect is not closed. If the ectopic gestation encompasses the entire ovary and normal ovary cannot be discerned, an oophorectomy is performed (see Chapter 16). Because ovarian vascularity is increased, this type of laparoscopic surgery should be performed only by an experienced surgeon.

Interstitial Ectopic Pregnancy

Removal of interstitial or cornual ectopic pregnancies may be attempted through the laparoscope, depending on ectopic size and the experience of the surgeon. The fallopian tube is transected distal to the ectopic pregnancy, and dissection of the mesosalpinx is extended toward the uterus. Dissection into the myometrium is performed with cautery or fiber laser. The myometrium may be infiltrated with Pitressin before dissection.

Removal of Resected Tissue

Removal of the products of conception or resected fallopian tube can, on occasion, be extremely tedious. Small pieces of tissue can be removed through the ancillary 5-mm puncture sites. Larger pieces of tissue may be removed through an ancillary 10-mm site. Alternatively, forceps may be introduced through the instrument channel of an operating laparoscope, and the tissue grasped and brought out through the sleeve. Holding the trumpet valve open, the laparoscope and grasped tissue are removed together. If the fallopian tube or gestational products are larger than 10 mm in diameter, relaxing incisions may be made into the specimen with scissors to decrease its size and allow removal through the 10- to 12-mm trocar in one piece. Alternatively, the tissue may be cut into pieces no larger than 10 mm in diameter. Removal may also be achieved by mincing the tissue using a 10-mm morcellator or by extracting intact tissue using a uterine polyp forceps introduced directly through the suprapubic site. Rarely is it necessary to perform a posterior colpotomy to remove a fallopian tube.

When large pieces of tissue need to be evacuated without spillage, the use of tissue removal bags, e.g., the Endocatch (see Fig. 8.18) or Endo pouch (Autosuture Co., Norwalk, CT), may be useful. Each bag is attached to a metal ring that is flattened to allow passage through a 10-mm port. Once in the abdomen, the ring and attached bag are allowed to open. The tissues to be removed are placed into the bag, a pursestring suture around the bag is closed to prevent spillage, and the ring is recompressed and pulled up through the port with the bag attached. Occasionally the port itself may need to be removed if the tissue is too large to be brought up through the lumen of the port. Furthermore, the skin incision may need to be extended. If the skin incision is enlarged, the surgeon must take great care to close the fascia, as the patient will be more susceptible to trocar hernias. After removal, thorough aspiration and irrigation or forceps may be used to remove any remaining tissue.

Alternative Techniques

With the increasing frequency of ectopic pregnancy, practitioners and patients strive to achieve cure through the least invasive measures. Laparoscopy has virtually replaced laparotomy in the treatment of ectopic pregnancy. Currently the use of methotrexate (MTX)

therapy for ectopic pregnancy is gaining widespread acceptance and soon will be the standard of care for selected patients.[16–19] Methotrexate is a folic acid antagonist that inhibits de novo synthesis of purines and pyridines and consequently inhibits trophoblast DNA synthesis, cell replication, and cell growth. MTX has been administered intramuscularly, intravenously, orally, and by local injection. Local injection of the ectopic with MTX has been reported laparoscopically, hysteroscopically, and by transvaginal ultrasound-guided injection.[20,21] The success rates of local injection have been similar to those reported with systemic therapy.[20,21] Local delivery of MTX unfortunately requires specialized training and equipment.

The most widely used method is the single- or multidose intramuscular (IM) regimen. The IM protocols are recommended because they require no special equipment and can be given on an outpatient basis. The single-dose schedule appears to be as effective as the multidose regimen.[17] The single-dose protocol begins with MTX 50 mg/m^2 IM on day 1. The β-hCG levels are checked on days 1, 4, and 7. If by day 7 the β-hCG has not dropped by at least 15%, a second dose of MTX is given. Serum β-hCG, complete blood count (CBC) with platelets, and liver enzymes are checked weekly. One algorithm for the medical or nonsurgical management of ectopic pregnancy is presented in Fig 12.6.

Side effects of MTX include impairment of liver function, stomatitis, gastritis, enteritis, and bone marrow suppression. These side effects are very infrequent with the single-dose regimen, but patients must be aware of these potential complications.[22] These effects are believed to be dose related and lessened by the administration of leucovorin. Contraindications to MTX include abnormal liver function, blood dyscrasias, pulmonary disease, patients who are not reliable and may not return for follow-up, an adnexal mass greater than 3.5 cm on ultrasound, patients who are hemodynamically unstable, and patients with fluid in the cul-de-sac and pain. Relative contraindications to MTX therapy include extrauterine cardiac activity and β-hCG greater than 10,000 mIU/

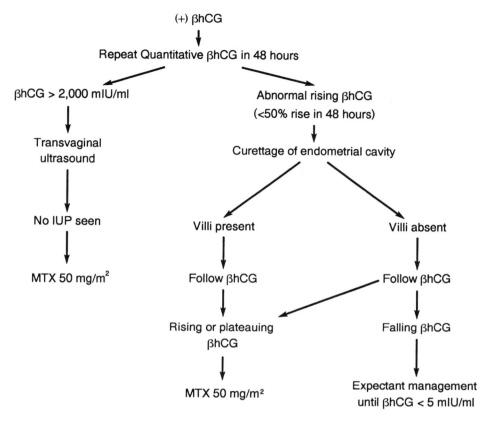

FIGURE 12.6. Algorithm for the medical management of ectopic pregnancies. β-*hCG*, Human chorionic gonadotropin; *MTX*, methotrexate; *IUP*, intrauterine pregnancy.

ml. Although patients with these relative contraindications have been successfully treated, failures occur more often in this group of patients.[17]

Success rates for single-dose regimens have been reported to be 85.7%, with a time to resolution of the ectopic (as manifested by nonpregnant β-hCG) of 23.1 days.[23] Stovall and Ling[24] reported a success rate of 94.2% using the single-dose schedule with a time to resolution of 35.5 days. A second dose was required in 5.7% of the patients treated by Glock et al.[23] and in 3.3% of the patients treated by Stovall and Ling.[24]

Subsequent pregnancy rates differ in the two studies, but this is probably the result of the differences in the populations studied. Glock et al. studied a predominately infertile population and reported a post-MTX pregnancy rate of 20%. Stovall and Ling studied all patients who presented to the emergency room and to outpatient clinics and noted a posttreatment conception rate of 79.6%, with an intrauterine pregnancy (IUP) rate of 69.4%. If MTX is used in only 30% of ectopic pregnancies and a success rate of 90% is assumed, a savings of $265 million is projected.[25]

Risks and Complications

The most common complication specific to the laparoscopic treatment of ectopic pregnancy is hemorrhage. Pregnancy increases the vascularity of these tissues, and blood loss may be significant. If excessive intraoperative bleeding is encountered, coagulation can be performed with electrocautery, laser, thermocoagulation, vasopressin injection, or application of direct pressure. If the hemorrhage becomes uncontrollable by laparoscopic methods, a laparotomy should be performed. Other complications include damage to adjacent structures, particularly when there are dense adhesions present.

As previously discussed, trophoblastic tissue may persist as the result of any conservative procedure for ectopic pregnancy. All patients undergoing a conservative procedure should be followed with β-hCG levels until the titer is negative. Patients with persistent ectopics tend to have an initial decline in β-hCG and progesterone levels 3 to 6 days after surgery, with a subsequent rise or plateau in these levels.[18] Persistent trophoblastic tissue may be treated surgically with either a repeat laparoscopy or a laparotomy. Nevertheless, persistent β-hCG levels do not mandate a total salpingectomy, and a segmental resection or repeat salpingostomy usually suffices.

The treatment of choice today for patients with persistent ectopic pregnancy however is methotrexate therapy. Rarely do these patients require more than one course of therapy. Seifer et al.[26] recently published their experience with reproductive outcome following surgical and medical treatment of persistent ectopic pregnancy. The cumulative clinical pregnancy rate following treatment was 59% at 36 months, which is similar to that of patients with primary surgical treatment of ectopic pregnancy.

Results

Shapiro and Adler performed the first surgery for ectopic pregnancy through the laparoscope in 1973.[27] Since then multiple studies have attested to the feasibility and safety of laparoscopic surgery for ectopic pregnancy. In the 1980s, in their large series Pouly and colleagues,[28] Mecke and colleagues,[14] and Reich and colleagues[8] found that subsequent pregnancy rates were historically comparable to those achieved via laparotomy. Pouly and colleagues,[28] in a series of 321 patients treated laparoscopically, reported a 57% intrauterine

pregnancy rate, a 22% recurrent ectopic pregnancy rate, and a 4.8% persistence rate. Di-Marchi and colleagues[29] also reported a persistent ectopic pregnancy rate of 4.8%; however, a 20% persistence rate has been reported in a small series.[14] Most studies note postoperative intrauterine pregnancy rates between 45% and 65%.[5] Overall, repeat ectopic rates range from 5% to 30%, with an average of approximately 15%.

Conclusions

The benefits of laparoscopy versus laparotomy are evident. Case control studies by Brumsted et al.[30] and randomized prospective studies by Vermesh et al.[31] and Murphy et al.[32] have demonstrated that laparoscopic therapy for the treatment of ectopic pregnancies has significantly reduced the hospital stay, cost, and delay to normal activity. In most cases, laparoscopy should replace laparotomy for the surgical treatment of ectopic pregnancies. MTX is noninvasive, effective, and less expensive than surgical interventions in selected patients and is a powerful tool in the armamentarium of the reproductive surgeon treating ectopic pregnancy.

References

1. Centers for Disease Control. Ectopic pregnancy: United States, 1987. *MMWR.* 1990;39: 2425.
2. Coste J, Job-Spira N, Aublet-Cuvlier B, et al. Incidence of ectopic pregnancy; first results of a population-based register in France. *Human Reprod (Oxf).* 1994;9:742–745.
3. Norman RJ, Buck RH, Rom L, Joubert S. Blood and urine measurement of human chorionic gonadotropin for detection of ectopic pregnancy? A comparative study of quantitative methods in both fluids. *Obstet Gynecol.* 1988; 71:315–318.
4. Romero R, Kadar N, Copel JA, Jeanty P, De Cherney AH, Hobbins JC. The effect of different human chorionic gonadotropin assay sensitivity on screening for ectopic pregnancy. *Am J Obstet Gynecol.* 1985;153:72–78.
5. Fossum GT, Davajan V, Kletzky OA. Early detection of pregnancy with transvaginal ultrasound. *Fertil Steril.* 1988;49:788–790.

6. Bateman BG, Nunley WC Jr, Kolp LA, Kitchen JD III, Felder R. Vaginal sonography findings and hCG dynamics of early intrauterine and tubal pregnancies. *Obstet Gynecol.* 1990;75: 421–426.

7. Bree RL, Edwards M, Bohm-Velez M, Beyler S, Roberts J, Mendelson EB. Transvaginal sonography in the evaluation of normal early pregnancy: correlation with hCG level. *Am J Radiol.* 1989;153:75–82.

8. Reich H, Johns DA, DeCaprio J, McGlynn F, Reich F. Laparoscopic treatment of 109 consecutive ectopic pregnancies. *J Reprod Med.* 1988; 33:885–889.

9. Nager CW, Murphy AA. Ectopic pregnancy. *Clin Obstet Gynecol.* 1991;34:403–411.

10. Murphy AA. Diagnostic and operative laparoscopy. In: Thompson JD, Rock JA, eds. *TeLinde's Operative Gynecology.* 7th ed. Philadelphia: Williams & Wilkins; 1991:361–384.

11. Sherman D, Langer R, Sadovsky G, et al. Improved fertility following ectopic pregnancy. *Fertil Steril.* 1982;37:497–502.

12. Tulandi T, Guralnick M. Treatment of tubal ectopic pregnancy by salpingotomy with or without tubal suturing and salpingectomy. *Fertil Steril.* 1991;51:53–58.

13. Pauerstein CJ, Croxatto HB, Eddy CA, Ramay I, Walters MD. Anatomy and pathology of tubal pregnancy. *Obstet Gynecol.* 1986;67:301–308.

14. Mecke H, Semm K, Lehmann-Weillenbrock E. Results of operative pelviscopy in 202 cases of ectopic pregnancy. *Int J Fertil.* 1989;34:93–100.

15. Henderson SR. Ectopic tubal pregnancy treated by operative laparoscopy. *Am J Obstet Gynecol.* 1989;160:1462–1464.

16. Stovall TG, Ling FW, Gray LA, Carson SA, Buster JE. Methotrexate treatment of unruptured ectopic pregnancy: a report of 100 cases. *Obstet Gynecol.* 1991;77:749–753.

17. Stovall TG, Ling FW, Gray LA. Single dose methotrexate for treatment of ectopic pregnancy. *Obstet Gynecol.* 1991;77:754–757.

18. Horne LA, Younger JB. Low-dose oral methotrexate therapy of presumed ectopic pregnancy. 45th Annual Meeting of the American Fertility Society, 1989, San Francisco, CA. Abstract #0-02.

19. Buster JE, Carson SA. Ectopic pregnancy: new advances in diagnosis and treatment. *Curr Opin Obstet Gynecol.* 1995;7:168–176.

20. Wolf GC, Witt BR. Outpatient laparoscopic management of ectopic pregnancy with local methotrexate injection. *J Reprod Med.* 1991; 36:489–491.

21. Tulandi T, Atri M, Bret P, Falcone T, Khalife S. Transvaginal intratubal methotrexate treatment of ectopic pregnancy. *Fertil Steril.* 1992; 58:98–100.

22. Stovall TG, Ling FW. Single-dose methotrexate as expanded clinical trial. *Am J Obstet Gynecol.* 1993;168:1759–1772.

23. Glock JL, Johnson JV, Brumsted JR. Efficacy and safety of single-dose systemic methotrexate in the treatment of ectopic pregnancy. *Fertil Steril.* 1994;62:716–721.

24. Stovall TG, Ling FW. Ectopic pregnancy diagnostic and therapeutic algorithms minimizing surgical intervention. *J Reprod Med.* 1993; 38:807–812.

25. Crenin MD, Washington AE. Cost of ectopic pregnancy management: surgery versus methotrexate. *Fertil Steril.* 1993;60:963–968.

26. Seifer DB, Silva PD, Grainger DA, Barber SR, Grant WD, Gutmann JN. Reproductive potential after treatment for persistent ectopic pregnancy. *Fertil Steril.* 1994;62:194–196.

27. Shapiro HI, Adler DH. Excision of an ectopic pregnancy through the laparoscope. *Am J Obstet Gynecol.* 1973;117:290–293.

28. Pouly MA, Mahnes H, Mage G, Canis M, Bruhat MA. Conservative laparoscopic treatment of 321 ectopic pregnancies. *Fertil Steril.* 1988;46: 1093–1097.

29. DiMarchi JM, Kosasa TS, Kobara TY, Hale RW. Persistent ectopic pregnancy. *Obstet Gynecol.* 1987;70:555–561.

30. Brumsted J, Kessler C, Gibson M. A comparison of laparoscopy and laparotomy for the treatment of ectopic pregnancy. *Obstet Gynecol.* 1988; 71:889–893.

31. Vermesh M, Silva PD, Rosen GF, Stein AL, Fossum GT, Sauer MV. Management of unruptured ectopic gestation by linear salpingostomy: a prospective randomized clinical trial of laparoscopy vs. laparotomy. *Obstet Gynecol.* 1989; 73:400–408.

32. Murphy AA, Nager CW, Wujek JJ, Kettel LM, Chin HG. Operative laparoscopy vs. laparotomy in the management of ectopic pregnancy: a prospective trial. *Fertil Steril.* 1992;57: 1180–1185.

13

Laparoscopic Tubal Surgery and Adhesiolysis

John S. Hesla and John A. Rock

Introduction and Background

Major advances in instrument design during the past two decades have allowed the development of endoscopic techniques for correction of pelvic pathology. These reconstructive procedures are in many circumstances supplanting traditional open abdominal microsurgery because of equivalence in outcomes and lower patient morbidity and expense. Operative laparoscopy provides excellent visualization and, when performed properly, fulfills the major tenets of microsurgery. These principles include the precise dissection and approxima-

tion of planes with minimal damage to adjacent tissue, use of atraumatic instruments, frequent irrigation to maintain serosal surface moisture, meticulous hemostasis, and minimal introduction of foreign bodies such as glove powder and lint into the peritoneal cavity.

Nevertheless, if the tissue planes cannot be clearly identified, the appropriate instruments are not available, or the surgeon lacks the experience and skill to safely and effectively perform the procedure, the endoscopic approach should be abandoned and a laparotomy performed. The surgeon must consider his or her abilities, the risk of complications of laparoscopy versus laparotomy, and the time required to complete the procedure with either approach to identify the most appropriate procedure for the patient. Major endoscopic fertility-promoting procedures for the treatment of tubal disease are described in this chapter.

Preoperative Preparation

Laparoscopy is an integral step in the investigation of the infertile couple. With the advent of endoscopic reconstructive techniques, both infertility diagnosis and therapy can be performed in a single operative procedure. Although not mandatory, hysterosalpingography performed in the initial stages of the infertility evaluation can provide information that will facilitate the planning for surgery, particularly if the study reveals salpingitis isthmica nodosa, distal tubal obstruction, or collections of contrast suggestive of periadnexal adhesions. The prognosis is worsened by an absence of ampullary mucosal folds or by the presence of a "honeycomb" pattern or other irregular reticular images of the ampulla that suggest intraluminal adhesions (Table 13.1). Conversely, increased pregnancy rates are seen when rugae are present on the preoperative hysterosalpingogram, even when the tubal obstruction is complete. With these radiological findings, the physician can begin to counsel the couple regarding the potential need for reconstructive

surgical procedures or in vitro fertilization (IVF) so as to achieve a pregnancy.

There may be some utility in performing a primary endoscopic reconstructive procedure before IVF even when prognostic factors for a successful surgical outcome are poor. Recent data suggest that embryo implantation rates may be higher in women with a history of tubal factor infertility whose hydrosalpinges have been excised or surgically opened before undergoing IVF as compared with those with intact hydrosalpinges. This may be caused by reduction in drainage of hydrosalpingeal fluid into the uterine cavity in the surgically treated patient group, resulting in an improved endometrial environment for nidation.

The surgeon should obtain cervical cultures or DNA screens for gonorrhea and chlamydia on all patients preoperatively. Because tissue trauma predisposes the patient to the development of postoperative infections, any woman with a history of postinflammatory pelvic adhesive disease, including fimbrial phimosis and hydrosalpinx formation, is routinely prescribed prophylactic antibiotics. A typical regimen includes intake of doxycycline on the day before surgery and for 3 days postoperatively along with parenteral administration of a broad-spectrum cephalosporin immediately before surgery.

Because an intestinal injury can occur during enterolysis, patients who have a history of previous laparotomies, pelvic inflammatory disease, or severe endometriosis should un-

TABLE 13.1. Classification of the extent of tubal disease with distal fimbrial obstruction.

Extent of disease	Findings
Mild	1. Absent or small hydrosalpinx (≤15-mm diameter)
	2. Inverted fimbria easily recognized when patency achieved
	3. No significant peritubal or periovarian adhesions
	4. Preoperative hysterosalpingogram reveals a rugal pattern
Moderate	1. Hydrosalpinx 13–30 mm diameter
	2. Fragments of fimbria not readily identified
	3. Periovarian or peritubal adhesions without fixation; minimal cul-de-sac adhesions
	4. Absence of a rugal pattern on preoperative hysterosalpingogram
Severe	1. Large hydrosalpinx (≥30-mm diameter)
	2. No fimbria
	3. Dense pelvic or adnexal adhesions with fixation of the ovary and tube to either the broad ligament, pelvic side wall, omentum, or bowel
	4. Obliteration of the cul-de-sac
	5. Frozen pelvis (adhesion formation so dense that limits of organs are difficult to define)

Adapted with permission from Rock JA, Katayama P, Martin EJ, et al. Factors influencing the success of salpingostomy techniques for distal fimbrial obstruction. *Obstet Gynecol.* 1978;52:591–596.

dergo a mechanical bowel preparation with an oral lavage solution such as GoLYTELY® 1 day before surgery. In addition, if there is a high possibility that the large intestine may be entered, neomycin 1 g and erythromycin base 1 g are administered orally three or four times on the day before the procedure to reduce the bacterial count in the colon.

The laparoscopic surgeon must compensate for a lack of tactile appreciation of the pelvic anatomy with detailed identification of the landmarks of structures. This inspection is enhanced by correct positioning of the patient's buttocks at the end of the surgical table to allow full range of motion of the rigid, curved uterine manipulator. Chromopertubation can also be performed with this cannula. When the posterior cul-de-sac is distorted by adhesions, a rectal probe facilitates dissection of the rectosigmoid from the posterior uterus or the adnexa. Surgical competence in the performance of cystoscopy can be extremely useful to the gynecologist, for laparoscopic identification of the ureter is greatly enhanced by placement of a ureteral stent. This is particularly noteworthy when the ovary is densely adherent to the lateral pelvic side wall as a consequence of endometriosis.

If extensive adnexal adhesions, marked ampullary dilatation, or thickening of the tubal wall are noted intraoperatively, salpingoscopy is useful to identify intratubal synechiae and mucosal denudation. Salpingostomy may also provide important prognostic information in patients who have relatively normal fimbria at the neostomy site, for the gross findings do not always correlate with the status of the ampullary mucosal folds. If luminal damage is extensive and IVF is an option for the couple, prolonged efforts to reconstruct the tubes are unwarranted.

Salpingo-ovariolysis

Indications and Patient Selection

Pelvic adhesions are frequently detected at the time of diagnostic laparoscopy, although their prevalence in the general population is not known. Of all operative laparoscopy procedures performed in the United States during the last decade, approximately 40% were for the evaluation and treatment of pelvic pain. Although 26%–48% of patients with chronic pelvic pain do have adhesions at the time of exploratory surgery, their presence does not necessarily connote a causative relationship. Peritoneal damage leading to adhesion formation may be initiated by pelvic inflammatory disease, surgical trauma, and endometriosis.

Adnexal adhesions may lead to infertility by preventing ovum capture by the fimbria and inhibiting normal tubal motility. Common patterns of adhesion development include immobilization of the ovary against the posterior leaf of the broad ligament or pelvic side wall, fixation of the distal oviduct to the ovary and broad ligament, envelopment of the ovarian cortex by avascular adhesions, scarring of the fimbria ovarica and encapsulation of the distal end of the fallopian tube, and obliteration of the posterior cul-de-sac.

The relationship between the grade of adhesions and conception rate is inverse and independent of the condition of the adnexae. The surgical prognosis depends on the type, location, and extent of adhesions. Both fine, avascular adhesions and thick, poorly vascularized adhesions are amenable to laparoscopic dissection. Patients with filmy adhesions that cover less than half of the ovary are the most benefited. Intimate adherence of one organ to another may arise from prior pelvic surgery and recurrent, severe infection. Such confluent adhesions and thick, highly vascularized fibrous bands may require laparotomy for effective therapy, although surgical separation of these tissue planes is itself likely to lead to denudation of the peritoneal surface and extensive adhesion reformation. Hence, prognosis is poor for this category of disease, regardless of the surgical technique employed. In vitro fertilization may be more appropriate for these patients.

Instrumentation and Procedure Specifics

Because pelvic diseases and the operative procedures that are used to correct anatomic disorders often produce adhesions, the laparoscopic surgeon must have a high index of suspicion that adhesions may exist between bowel and anterior abdominal wall in any patient with infertility or pelvic pain. Hence, one must exercise caution from the very start in placement of the Veress needle and laparoscopic trocar. Open laparoscopy may reduce the risk of viscus damage in the patient who is likely to have extensive adhesions; nevertheless, the bowel serosa may adhere to the anterior parietal peritoneum just underneath the umbilicus. It is possible to directly enter the lumen of the intestine during open laparoscopy while never appreciating any tissue plane other than the scar.

Lifting the abdominal wall after Veress needle insertion should result in a negative pressure reading on the insufflator. An increase in intraabdominal pressure during the insufflation process may be a sign of bowel or omental adhesions. After placement of the laparoscope, the anterior parietal peritoneum is inspected and ancillary trocars are placed under direct visualization. Omental or bowel adhesions of the lower abdomen that prevent safe insertion of accessory trocars may be separated by use of laser or scissors introduced through the operating channel of the laparoscope. Vascular adhesions should be coagulated with bipolar or endothermic crocodile forceps before division. Persistent bleeding of the omental pedicle may be secured by repeat electrocoagulation, by thermocoagulation, or by placement of an loop ligature or clip. To avoid thermal damage, use sharp dissection rather than laser or needle cautery to separate bowel from bowel and to divide dense adhesions of bowel to adjacent structures.

Careful inspection of the anatomic landmarks of the oviduct and ovary is necessary before undertaking adhesiolysis to prevent inadvertent incision of the fimbria ovarica, ovarian vasculature, and tubal serosa. Extensive dissection requires the introduction of two or three suprapubic trocar sheaths. Adhesion bands are stretched by one or two 5-mm grasping forceps or blunt probes to demarcate the adhesion from the adjoining organ.

Initial sharp dissection of filmy adhesions may facilitate subsequent separation of denser bands. Separation of more medial adhesions should be attempted before approaching sidewall disease. Multilayer adhesions should be divided one layer at a time to prevent trauma to underlying structures that may not be immediately recognizable. The microscissors or endoshears, needle electrode, or laser must be used at an angle perpendicular to the adhesion being lysed. Large vessels along the line of transection may be desiccated with cautery before division. Careless rupture of organized adhesion bands with a blunt probe produces areas of deperitonealization, which may promote adhesion recurrence and de novo adhesion formation.

In commencing salpingo-ovariolysis, adhesions of bowel to adnexal structures should be separated first to allow progressively greater exposure. Broad tubo-ovarian adhesions are initially incised near the point of their attachment to the tubal serosa (Fig. 13.1). The adhesion may then be tented with a pointed atraumatic forceps to allow complete excision from

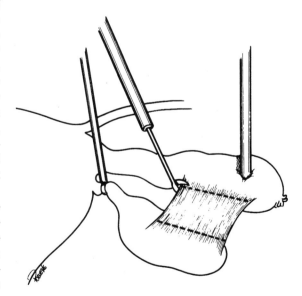

FIGURE 13.1. Lysis of avascular adnexal adhesions. Structures are manipulated with an aspiration cannula and atraumatic forceps, placing the adhesive band on traction. It is important to attempt to excise the adhesive band at its insertions, rather than performing a simple incision.

the ovarian surface. Avoid grasping the ovarian cortex so as to minimize trauma. When there are adhesions to the posterior leaf of the broad ligament, ovariolysis is aided by applying traction to the utero-ovarian ligament and rotating the ovary with grasping forceps. Residual filmy adhesions of the ovary and fallopian tube may be identified by instilling lactated Ringer's solution in the posterior cul-de-sac to float the adnexa. After applying traction with forceps, microscissors are used to remove these avascular bands (Fig 13.2).

Posterior cul-de-sac adhesions must also be excised because of the possibility that ovum capture may occur in this region. Use of the uterine manipulator facilitates placing the stretching and dissecting of such adhesions. Inspection of the peritoneal surfaces lying under the irrigation solution will reveal any small bleeding vessels that require coagulation. Precise hemostasis is achieved by microbipolar cautery. In cases of more widespread oozing, thermocoagulation may also be used.

The postoperative inflammatory response and extent of tissue destruction are lessened by sharp dissection with the scissors or scalpel as compared to laser or electrosurgery. Nevertheless, laser laparoscopy is associated with a low rate of postoperative adhesion recurrence and may avoid the formation of de novo adhesions. The laser beam with a small spot size in the enhanced superpulse mode is applied to the edge of the adherent surface in a sweeping motion to vaporize the tissue fibers. Care must be taken to avoid tearing the adhesion at its attachment by applying too much traction; bleeding leads to a reduction of absorption of the laser beam. The tip of a nonreflective titanium suction aspiration cannula, a manipulation wand, the platform of the waveguide sheath, or a pool of irrigant may serve as the backstop to the carbon dioxide (CO_2) laser beam. Because the laser provides a precise energy source and moderate hemostasis when used in the focused mode, it may be particularly helpful for the separation of dense adnexal adhesions that extend near or to the bowel and ureter. Copious irrigation of the site of vaporization with warm, heparinized Ringer's lactate will remove carbonized debris and blood.

An alternative technique for adhesiolysis involves the application of irrigant at pressures as high as 800 mmHg to develop cleavage planes between the pelvic side walls, fallopian tube, ovary, and bowel.[1] This hydrodissection is particularly effective when the scarring is filmy or

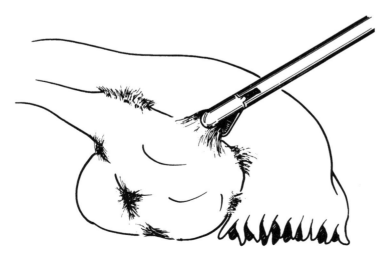

FIGURE 13.2. Removal of superficial ovarian adhesions. The adhesions are grasped with a biopsy forceps and gently removed, taking care to apply traction against the direction of the fibers, not peeling the ovarian cortex.

gelatinous in nature. Adhesions are frequently seen in this state during the early resolution phase of infection or shortly after a primary surgical procedure. The suction tip of the aspiration-irrigation system also may be used to grasp and manipulate the pelvic organs during adnexal surgery.

Dense adhesions of the distal fallopian tube and the ovary and of the ovary and the pelvic side wall are difficult to approach endoscopically and are often better treated by means of microsurgery. The objective of endoscopic adhesiolysis in such circumstances is to preserve as much peritoneum as possible while freeing the ovarian surface. Hydrodissection may be helpful to develop potential spaces among the adhesions that may, in turn, be dissected with endoshears or laser. A fragment of ovarian cortex or stroma left on the peritoneum of the ovarian fossa may predispose the patient to later pelvic pain as part of the ovarian remnant syndrome.

Ureteral injury may be caused by careless dissection or cauterization of the ovarian fossa, when nodularity or thickening is present in the region of the uterosacral ligament, or when there are unrecognized anomalies in the location of the ureter. The ureter enters the pelvis beneath the semitransparent peritoneum at the bifurcation of the common iliac artery on the left and the right external iliac artery on the right. It courses down the pelvic side wall along the medial leaf of the broad ligament usually just anterior to the hypogastric artery. The ureter passes beneath the uterine artery approximately 1.5 cm lateral to the cervix and at this point disappears into a condensation of endopelvic fascia. Once it enters this web, the ureter is no longer visible and cannot be palpated laparoscopically.

The ureter is most easily identified at the pelvic brim; its path into the pelvis can be confirmed by observing its peristaltic motion. Adhesions of the ovary to ovarian fossa or the sigmoid colon to the area of the bifurcation of the common iliac artery may prevent visualization of the ureter. Dissection of the retroperitoneum to identify its entire course is not usually justified because of the time involved and the morbidity associated with this procedure. A

better alternative is cystoscopy with ureteral catheterization. If the ureteral catheter is taped to a Foley catheter upon its emergence from the bladder, it may be moved during the laparoscopy to identify the ureter. Alternatively, placement of quartz fiber illuminated catheters may make ureteral identification easier. Dissection of the pelvic side wall should commence from the utero-ovarian ligament in a cephalad direction or from the infundibulopelvic ligament in a caudal direction, as opposed to dissecting directly underneath the ovary, to reduce the risk of blind injury to the ureter.

Fimbrioplasty

Indications and Patient Selection

Postinflammatory fimbrial damage may take the form of fimbrial agglutination, fimbrial encapsulation by fibrous tissue, or stenosis of the apex of the tubal infundibulum (prefimbrial phimosis). These conditions are amenable to laparoscopic treatment using techniques that have been derived from laparotomy procedures. The magnification of the operative field provided with the use of the video monitor facilitates the laparoscopic approach.

The efficacy of laparoscopic tubal reconstructive procedures has been established over the past decade. Nevertheless, treatment of extensive adnexal disease requires meticulous technique and should not be attempted by the inexperienced endoscopist. Laparoscopic interventions under such circumstances may result in further, irreversible damage to the fallopian tubes. Patients with significant fimbrial agglutination and phimosis but little tubal distention achieve excellent outcomes with microsurgery. It may be preferable to proceed directly to laparotomy in such cases rather than achieve a suboptimal repair through endoscopy.

Instrumentation and Procedure Specifics

The fallopian tube is distended via transcervical instillation of indigo carmine dye. Periadnexal adhesions are lysed and removed (see prior section) before fimbrial reconstruction is undertaken. The serosa of the fallopian tube is easily traumatized if not handled delicately. Any fibrous tissue covering the terminal end of the tube is excised with fine scissors, a unipolar needle-tip electrode, or the laser. The fallopian tube is stabilized by grasping the antimesenteric serosa of the distal ampulla with atraumatic forceps or the suction-irrigator. To correct minor fimbrial agglutination, closed 3-mm alligator forceps may be introduced through the small tubal ostium. The jaws of this instrument are opened within the lumen and are gently withdrawn to stretch the infundibulum.[2] This use of the alligator forceps may be repeated several times in different directions to achieve maximal dilation of the fimbriated end. The tubal ostium also may be entered with a conical tube probe to achieve the desired separation. However, these blunt dissection techniques may actually cause further damage to the tubal mucosa.

Fimbrial bridges can be freed with the needle-tip unipolar electrode or with a laser (Fig. 13.3). Avascular adhesions should be cut with microscissors. Identification of these adhesions may be enhanced by floating the fimbrial folds in irrigation fluid or with use of the salpingoscope. Microbipolar cautery may be necessary for hemostasis, although most bleeding will stop spontaneously.

Particular care must be taken in cases of severe agglutination, because forced insertion of the forceps into the stenosed tubal lumen may traumatize the fragile mucosa. Such damage may lead to complete fimbrial occlusion postoperatively, which would reduce the chance of successful repair in any repeat surgical procedure. Severe agglutination is better corrected by a salpingostomy procedure or through open microsurgery.

Prefimbrial phimosis is overcome by salpingostomy in which peritubal fibrous bands that constrict the infundibulum are divided with the laser or a pointed electrode and blended current. The ampullary serosa is grasped with atraumatic forceps and may be immobilized against the uterine fundus. A shallow linear incision should be made along avascular points, commencing at the fimbriated end and extending beyond the region of the phimosis. Any fibrous tissue surrounding the tubal ostium should be cut; bleeding points may be cauterized with the needle or microbipolar electrode.

A greater degree of eversion of the tubal mucosa may be achieved by placement of 4-0 to 6-0 interrupted synthetic absorbable suture(s) or by application of defocused laser or low-power cautery to the infundibular serosal surface. This latter technique lightly desiccates and constricts the superficial tissue layer, although the resultant thermal damage may promote adhesion formation or phimosis. Wrapping the distal fallopian tube with Interceed® may reduce this risk.

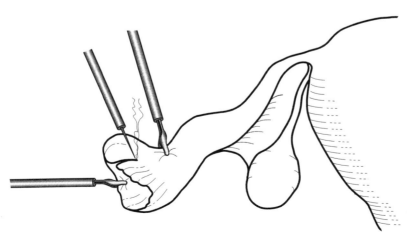

FIGURE 13.3. Fimbrioplasty. Fimbrial bridges can be freed with the needle-tip unipolar electrode or with laser.

Salpingoneostomy

Indications and Patient Selection

The introduction of microsurgical techniques has resulted in great improvements in pregnancy rates for many infertility surgical procedures. Although the application of these principles to the repair of distal tubal occlusion has resulted in a significant increase in postoperative tubal patency over conventional macrosurgery, the pregnancy rates after microsurgical salpingoneostomy remain poor as the result of irreversible damage of ciliary function and muscular peristalsis or inadequate restoration of normal tubo-ovarian anatomic relationships. Tubal function subsequent to salpingoneostomy depends primarily on the status of the fallopian tube at the time of surgical intervention rather than the surgical technique employed. Because of this, minimally invasive endoscopic techniques have been proposed as a reasonable alternative to open abdominal microsurgery.

Several classification systems have been proposed to characterize prognosis after surgical repair of the hydrosalpinx.[3] These systems incorporate the findings of hysterosalpingography and diagnostic laparoscopy, including the size of the hydrosalpinx, condition of fimbria and tubal mucosa, associated adnexal adhesions, and rugal pattern seen at the time of hysterosalpingography. Postoperative pregnancy rates are typically less than 10% in cases of severe disease. The hydrosalpinx with a rigid, thickened wall may show little evidence of dilation, but has an exceedingly poor prognosis because fibrosis of the muscularis layer interferes with tubal transport. Multiloculated cystic changes in the endosalpinx and severe associated peritubal and periovarian adhesive disease also adversely affect surgical outcome. Thin-walled hydrosalpinges allow better surgical dissection of the fimbria and eversion of the mucosa. Partial or complete destruction of the endosalpinx and multifocal luminal occlusion are usually the consequence of chlamydial and gonococcal salpingitis, whereas extrinsic tubal damage in association with fimbrial occlusion may arise from appendicitis, previous adnexal surgery, and rarely endometriosis. The sequelae of nongynecologic pelvic infection represent the best response category for tubal repair because of the lack of extensive involvement of the tubal mucosa.

Instrumentation and Procedure Specifics

The traditional microsurgical technique of salpingoneostomy requires meticulous attention to details that must not be sacrificed when operating with laparoscopic instruments. Visualization may be augmented by video camera monitoring. An intraumbilical and two or three suprapubic/lower abdominal incisions are necessary for placement of instruments. The fallopian tube is immobilized with atraumatic grasping forceps placed through the operating channel of the laparoscope or through a midline or lateral suprapubic sheath. Some surgeons insert the laser or scissors through a 5- to 7-mm trocar sleeve located at a medial site 3 to 5 mm superior to the suprapubic line. The shorter focal length of a laser introduced through an ancillary port provides greater power density than can be obtained through the operating channel of the laparoscope.

Infundibular tubal occlusion is frequently accompanied by perisalpingeal and periovarian adhesions. These must be freed before proceeding with the salpingoneostomy. Transcervical installation of dilute indigo carmine dye distends the hydrosalpinx and aides in the identification of the scarred ostium, fimbria ovarica, and adjacent structures. Inspection of the distal tube may demonstrate a central dimple with streaks of radial scarring, which should be used as guides for incising the tube with laser, scissors, or needle electrode (Fig. 13.4).

If the CO_2 laser is employed, a superpulse beam of 25 W or a continuous mode beam of 30 to 40 W with a 1.0-mm spot size is applied to the stellate scar of the occluded infundibulum after immobilizing the tube approximately 2 cm from its end with atraumatic forceps. Rather than perforating the full thickness of the wall and thereby promoting immediate collapse of the hydrosalpinx, the tube is superficially scored with the laser from the ostium to-

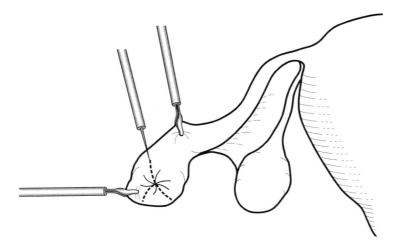

FIGURE 13.4. Salpingoneostomy. Inspection of the distal tube may demonstrate a central dimple with streaks of radial scarring, which should be used as guides for incising the tube with laser, scissors, or needle electrode. The tube is stabilized with atraumatic forceps.

ward the ovary and fimbria ovarica following the old scar line. The incision is then carried down until dye is encountered. The atraumatic forceps may then be repositioned to stabilize the margins of the incision, carefully avoiding all delicate mucosa that have been everted by outrushing indigo carmine dye.

Two or three radial incisions are usually necessary to achieve sufficient exposure of the residual fimbria; this results in a "Y"- or "X"-shaped incision of the terminal tube (Fig. 13.4). The platform of the waveguide sheath may be used as a backstop so that the beam does not penetrate the tubal wall and damage the endothelium of the other side of the oviduct. Ringer's lactate irrigant placed in the posterior cul-de-sac may also be used as a backstop for the laser beam. Grasping forceps may be inserted into the ostium to gently stretch and separate fine intraampullary and fimbrial adhesions. Microbipolar cautery is employed for hemostasis. If the tube is very vascular, 1 to 2 cc of a dilute vasopressin solution (20 U in 20 ml normal saline) may be injected directly into the tube with a laparoscopic needle to minimize bleeding. Finally, it is important to ensure maximum exposure of the tubal ostia to the ovarian surface by extending the tubal incision ventrally (Fig. 13.5). Placing a probe within the newly opened ostia is often helpful.

On completion of the incision(s), the serosal edge of the distal tube may be everted with the defocused, 2- to 5-W CO_2 laser (Fig. 13.6). This

desiccation causes contraction of the serosa. The degree of eversion should be exaggerated to prevent postoperative closure. Many expert laparoscopic surgeons prefer to place inter-

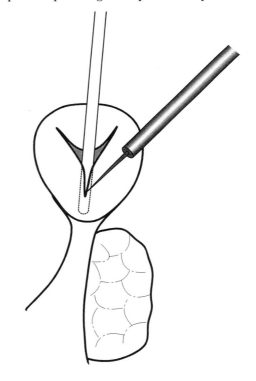

FIGURE 13.5. Salpingoneostomy. It is important to ensure maximum exposure of the tubal ostia to the ovarian surface by extending the tubal incision ventrally. Placing a probe within the newly opened ostia is often helpful.

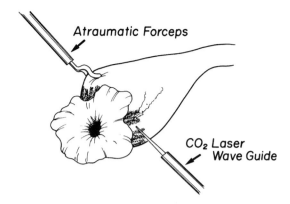

FIGURE 13.6. Salpingoneostomy. Eversion of fimbria via desiccation of serosal edge. The CO_2 laser beam is defocused and set at 2 to 5 W.

rupted 4-0 to 6-0 synthetic, delayed absorbable sutures via an intraabdominal instrument tie or an extracorporeal tie as described in Chapter 9 to secure the fimbrial margin to the ampullary serosa. This suture technique is particularly indicated in those cases in which the chance for reobstruction appears high, such as when the wall of the fallopian tube is thickened and the eversion created by laser is suboptimal.

An alternative technique for accomplishing salpingoneostomy involves the application of mechanical and electrocautery dissection.

Adhesiolysis is performed as described to mobilize the distal tube. After distending the hydrosalpinx by chromopertubation, the avascular lines are traced with fine monopolar needle-tip cautery or point thermocoagulation. The tube is then opened with laparoscopic microscissors or the needle-tip electrode. After the initial incision is made to allow access to the tubal lumen, additional dissection of the tubal wall may be approached from the interior, following the pattern of the fimbria and luminal folds. The mucosal flaps are mobilized with atraumatic forceps. Hemostasis is secured with microbipolar cautery. The neostomy edges are everted with suture, light electrocoagulation, or thermocoagulation; low current must be used to avoid damage to the muscularis. An alternative approach involves application of one or two Hulka clips or newly developed absorbable clips to everted edges of the tube.[4] The Hulka clips are removed 2 to 3 months later by second-look laparoscopy.

McComb and Paleologou[5] have described a technique of intussusception of the tubal epithelium to maintain tubal patency after salpingostomy (Fig. 13.7). A relatively short incision is made along the axis of the fimbria ovarica toward the antimesenteric border of the tube. The closed, blunt-tipped scissors and grasping forceps are introduced into the lumen and manipulated to dilate the infundibulum. The lat-

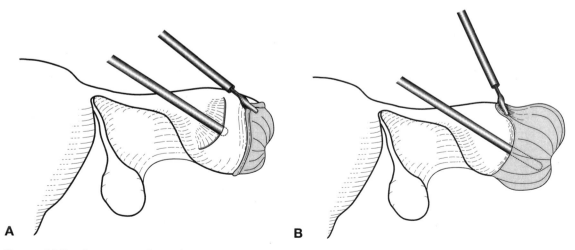

A   **B**

FIGURE 13.7. Intussusception salpingostomy. **A:** The point of a blunt probe or scissors is used to prolapse the ampullary mucosa through the neostium. **B:** The borders of the incision then act as a restrictive collar to maintain mucosal eversion.

eral margin of the ostium is then grasped with the forceps, and the end of the scissors or a similar blunt instrument is used to prolapse the ampullary epithelium and serosa through the ostium. The borders of the incision act as a restrictive collar to maintain the endothelium in an everted configuration.

The peritoneal cavity is copiously irrigated with Ringer's lactate solution containing heparin (5000 U/liter) throughout the tuboplasty procedure. Meticulous hemostasis is necessary to optimize outcome. Ancillary methods of impeding adhesion formation include placement of an absorbable adhesion barrier (Interceed®) between the fallopian tube and pelvic side wall or intraperitoneal instillation of 200 ml of 32% dextran-70 (Hyskon®) or Ringer's lactate (1–2 liters) at the conclusion of the procedure to achieve hydroflotation.

Results

Salpingo-ovariolysis

Reconstructive pelvic surgeries through laparoscopy or laparotomy are associated with both adhesion reformation and de novo scarring of peritoneal surfaces previously uninvolved with adhesions, despite appropriate surgical technique and the use of adjuvant therapy. Nevertheless, the majority of animal and clinical trials have reported that operative laparoscopy results in an improvement in adhesion scores from the preoperative state and fewer reformed and new adhesions as compared with open microsurgery.

Intrauterine pregnancy rates after salpingo-ovariolysis via laparotomy range from 32% to 66% in the literature.[2] The range of rates (29.5%–81%) reported in several laparoscopic series are similar.[1,2,4] In Gomel's report of 92 patients with moderate to severe adnexal adhesions, 46% of all intrauterine pregnancies occurred within 6 months of operative intervention.[2] Favorable prognostic features include the presence of filmy rather than primarily dense adhesions, normal tubal fimbria, and less than one-half of the ovarian surface affected by disease. Pregnancy rates are generally lower when adhesions involve both the fallo-

pian tube and ovary, presumably as the result of a greater likelihood of concurrent fimbrial involvement and impairment of oocyte recovery. The ectopic pregnancy rate following laparoscopic adhesiolysis averages 10%. Patients with extensive, confluent ovarian adhesions are best treated with IVF because functional surgical outcome is poor.

In general, there is poor correlation between the severity of pain and the extent and location of adhesions unless their presence is associated with active endometriotic implants. Adhesiolysis for the management of pelvic pain may improve the symptoms of a portion of patients; nevertheless, it is difficult to exclude a placebo effect. Adhesions encapsulating the ovary may be a source of pain from ovarian dysfunction. In addition, intestinal adhesions may cause pain through partial viscus occlusion or torsion.

Fimbrioplasty

Recent series of microsurgical fimbrioplasty via laparotomy report intrauterine pregnancy rates of 49% and 68%. The success rate achieved by laparoscopic fimbrioplasty has ranged from 21.5% to 50% in the literature,[2,6] and the ectopic pregnancy rate from this procedure is approximately 5% whether it is performed through the endoscope or via laparotomy. The cure rate depends on whether one or both tubes are damaged. In one recent report, the cumulative pregnancy curve was substantially lower in patients with moderate to severe fimbrial phimosis who required bilateral salpingostomy compared to those who underwent unilateral salpingostomy with or without contralateral lysis of fimbrial adhesions; nevertheless, the cure rate was not statistically different between the two groups in this study because of the inadequate sample size.[6]

Salpingoneostomy

The number of published reports on endoscopic salpingostomy and the sample size per series are rather small. Although the success rates have ranged from 0% to 44%,[1,4,6–8] the mean outcome of these series generally approximates the overall intrauterine pregnancy rate of 19% to 35% achieved via laparotomy.[3]

In a series of 90 consecutive cases of laparo-scopic salpingoneostomy, Dubuisson et al.[8] re-ported a pregnancy rate of 44% among those patients who had hydrosalpinges with normal mucosa or moderate attenuation of mucosal folds; this contrasted with a pregnancy rate of 0% among women with no folds or severe in-traluminal adhesions. Furthermore, the con-ception rate is lower when the hydrosalpinx is accompanied by dense adhesions as compared to a lesser degree of adhesions. This confirms the premise that the results of tubal surgery are mainly related to the severity of tubal dam-age and type and extent of adhesions rather than to the surgical technique employed. Nev-ertheless, the lower success rate noted in some reports illustrates that successful endoscopic repair of the hydrosalpinx is a tedious and technically difficult undertaking.

Salpingoneostomy or salpingostomy via lapa-roscopy is not contraindicated when the pa-tient has poor prognostic variables for a suc-cessful conception. However, unless the surgeon has demonstrated mastery of the en-doscopic approach, microsurgical reconstruc-tion via laparotomy is recommended for pa-tients whose prognosis for conception is good (i.e., if the tubal wall is thin, if distal dilatation is 2.5 cm or less, if the endosalpinx appears normal, and if there are few fixed adhesions). A poorly performed laparoscopic procedure does not benefit this category of disease.

Alternative Techniques

Endoscopic reconstructive procedures fulfill the principles of microsurgery and result in minimal physical impairment. There appear to be no significant differences in pregnancy rates among patients undergoing adhesiolysis and possibly fimbrioplasty procedures via mi-crosurgery, macrosurgery, or laparoscopy. Nev-ertheless, the main goal of reparative surgery of the fallopian tubes should be to provide the best possible chance for pregnancy. Although success is related more to the extent of disease than to the operative technique selected, the surgeon must be proficient in advanced endo-scopic procedures for one to reasonably expect an equivalent functional outcome with this ap-proach as compared with open operative tech-niques. Hence, there remains an important role for microsurgery in the patient with distal tubal disease, particularly in the small percent-age of patients whose prognostic features for future pregnancy following correctly per-formed tuboplasty are good.

Given the relatively poor outcome of most salpingostomy procedures, it is prudent to ad-vise patients with known bilateral partial or to-tal tubal occlusion and poor prognostic fea-tures against tuboplasty in favor of IVF therapy. Moreover, women over 37 years of age with sig-nificant adnexal adhesive disease should be counseled to proceed directly to IVF. Because one large series has reported that 86.7% of all intrauterine pregnancies occurred within the first year following salpingostomy, IVF should not be further delayed in patients who elect to receive primary surgical therapy and who do not conceive during this time period.[7]

Because of lack of insurance coverage for IVF therapy, many patients with pelvic adhesive disease are forced into accepting an operative procedure that has little chance of success. Nevertheless, with recent advances in preg-nancy rates achieved by programs of assisted reproduction, the relative costs of IVF to soci-ety may be equivalent to or less than that of surgery. In a comparative analysis of surgical versus IVF therapy among patients with tubal factor infertility in Norway, a highly significant increased rate of deliveries was achieved after three IVF treatment cycles (72.3% per patient) as compared with tubal surgery (23.7%, $P <$ .001).[9] Tan et al.[10] have reported a 51.5% cu-mulative pregnancy rate following five cycles of IVF in a group of 1161 patients with tubal dam-age. Judicious consideration of the woman's age, degree of adnexal damage, other infertil-ity risk factors, and financial resources will re-sult in the most appropriate individualized treatment plan to achieve parenthood.[9]

Adjunctive Procedures

Uterine Suspension

Endoscopic plication of the round ligaments may be performed in those circumstances in which a greater degree of uterine anteflexion is desired to impede postoperative adhesion formation of the adnexal structures and posterior cul-de-sac. The round ligament is grasped with atraumatic forceps, and an loop ligature, Silastic band, or laparoscopic clip is applied to the looped ligament to shorten it. (For more details, see Chapter 20.) This operation is rarely needed or performed.

Second-Look Laparoscopy

The term "second-look laparoscopy" generally refers to laparoscopy after a primary reconstructive procedure via laparotomy. The interval between the initial reproductive surgery and the laparoscopy may vary from 3 days to 2 or more years. Fibrosis of unlysed fibrin begins 3 days after serosal trauma and is completed by 21 days. Endoscopic adhesiolysis is performed in an attempt to restore a greater degree of normality to the pelvic structures and thus to improve intrauterine pregnancy rates. The success of such procedures is widely debated. A few studies have suggested that second-look laparoscopies effectively reduce peritoneal adhesions. The impact on conception rates is less certain, however, whether the second-look laparoscopy was performed within 8 days of the initial laparotomy or after 1 year. The interval from surgery to conception and the occurrence of ectopic pregnancy both appear to be reduced, although the cumulative pregnancy rate may not be significantly improved. Hence, the value of a second-look laparoscopy after a primary endoscopic reconstructive procedure appears to be modest.

References

1. Reich H. Laparoscopic treatment of extensive pelvic adhesions, including hydrosalpinx. *J Reprod Med.* 1987;32:736–742.
2. Gomel V. Salpingo-ovariolysis by laparoscopy in infertility. *Fertil Steril.* 1983;40:607–611.
3. Rock JA, Katayama P, Martin EJ, et al. Factors influencing the success of salpingostomy techniques for distal fimbrial obstruction. *Obstet Gynecol.* 1978;52:591–596.
4. Nezhat C, Winer WK, Cooper JD, et al. Endoscopic infertility surgery. *J Reprod Med.* 1989; 34:127–134.
5. McComb PF, Paleologou A. The intussusception salpingostomy technique for the therapy of distal oviductal occlusion at laparoscopy. *Obstet Gynecol.* 1991;78:443–447.
6. Dlugi AM, Reddy S, Saleh WA, et al. Pregnancy rates after operative endoscopic treatment of total (neosalpingostomy) or near total (salpingostomy) distal tubal occlusion. *Fertil Steril.* 1994;62:913–920.
7. Canis M, Mage G, Pouly JL, Manhes H, et al. Laparoscopic distal tuboplasty: report of 87 cases and a 4-year experience. *Fertil Steril.* 1991;56: 616–621.
8. Dubuisson JB, Chapron C, Morice P, et al. Laparoscopic salpingostomy: fertility results according to the tubal mucosal appearance. *Hum Reprod.* 1994;9:334–339.
9. Holst N, Maltau JM, Forsdahl F, Hansen LJ. Handling of tubal infertility after introduction of in vitro fertilization: changes and consequences. *Fertil Steril.* 1991;55:140–143.
10. Tan SL, Royston P, Campbell S, et al. Cumulative conception and live birth rates after in-vitro fertilization. *Lancet.* 1992;339:1390–1394.

14

Laparoscopic Tubal Anastomosis

Eugene Katz

Introduction

Despite the advent of newer methods of contraception and reformulated oral contraceptives, female voluntary sterilization remains popular. Although this is presented as a permanent method of sterilization, traditional microsurgical techniques have allowed more than 60% of women requesting reversal of sterilization to carry an intrauterine pregnancy.[1,2] Like most of the gynecologic procedures, tubal reanastomosis can also be performed laparoscopically.

Although the laparoscope may provide adequate magnification, the loss of precision inherent to the use of long instruments and the difficulty in handling microsuture material present a challenge to the successful performance of the reanastomosis. In the first such case, reported in 1989,[3] a catheter was pushed through the fimbria into the proximal portion of the tube. The tubes were attached with a biological glue made of human coagulation products, and the catheter was exteriorized through the abdominal wall in the iliac region for 48 hr. Four months later, the tube was patent on hysterosalpingogram but no pregnancy had been established.

Another surgeon reported a patient in whom the tube was reapproximated with two 2-0 polyglactin sutures thorough the muscularis layer and another suture in the serosa.[4] The same year, Tsin reported four women in whom the tubes were cannulated hysteroscopically; two 5-0 or 6-0 sutures were placed through the seromuscular layer of the tube and a third in the mesosalpinx.[5] The cannulas were removed 2 weeks postoperatively; however, no results were reported.

We describe herein our technique and results for performing minimally invasive tubal reanastomosis.[6]

Patient Selection

Patients are selected according to the same criteria used for reanastomosis via laparotomy. A higher success rate is expected among patients with tubes exceeding 4 cm in length and in whom an isthmic–isthmic reanastomosis is possible. Patients with an extremely short proximal segment may not benefit from the laparoscopic approach because of the difficulty in placing the rather straight needle through a tube almost flush with the uterus.

Technique

The patient is placed in the lithotomy position
with her thighs not elevated above the body.
Prophylactic antibiotics are given intraoperatively. A 0° angle laparoscope is introduced infraumbilically, and three 5-mm trocars are
placed suprapubically under direct visualization. A trocar is placed in the midline, and one
trocar is introduced slightly above and about 5
cm lateral to it on each side. The mesosalpinx
adjacent to the distal and proximal tubal
stumps is infiltrated with 5 ml of a solution
containing 1 U of Pitressin in 10 ml of normal
saline or lactated Ringer's solution. The tips
are pulled with any graspers, and the occluded
segments are cut with sharp scissors (Fig. 14.1).
Hemostasis can be achieved with bipolar coagulators, but they must be used judiciously because small bleeding points usually subside
with observation alone.

Patency of the proximal segment is documented by chromotubation through a cannula
previously introduced into the uterus. To facilitate the alignment of the tubes, the cannula is
removed and the proximal segment of one

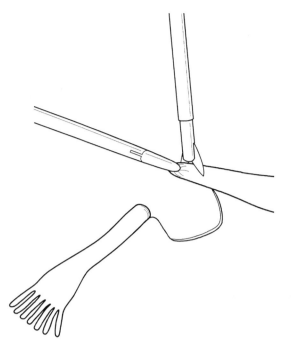

FIGURE 14.1. After the mesosalpinx is infiltrated
adjacent to the proximal and distal tubal stumps, it
is infiltrated with Pitressin; the tip of the stumps are
grasped and transected with sharp scissors.

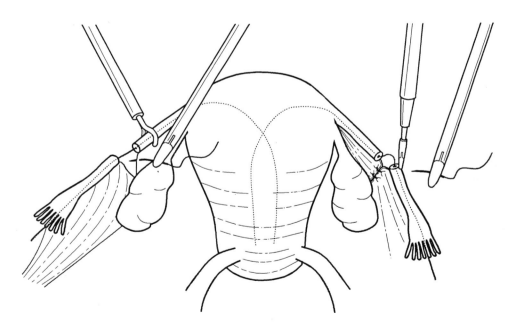

FIGURE 14.2. After transection, the proximal and distal tubal stumps are cannulated with a wireguide of a
3-Fc. catheter placed hysteroscopically. The mesosalpinx and the tubal wall are approximated.

FIGURE 14.3. The mesosalpinx is approximated using 4-0 or 5-0 polydioxanone suture (PDS II, Ethicon, Inc.) tied intraabdominally.

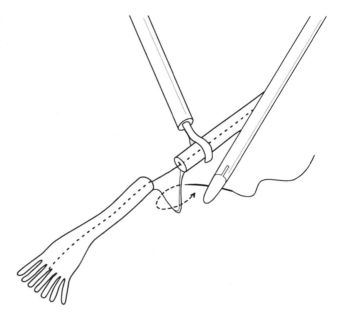

tube is cannulated under hysteroscopic guidance. A 5.5 French (5.5-Fr.) Novy catheter is introduced through the operative channel of the hysteroscope and placed in the uterotubal junction[7] (see Chapter 31). A 3-Fr. catheter, with a wireguide through its lumen, is introduced coaxially through the 5.5-Fr. catheter until the tip is seen laparoscopically exiting the proximal tubal stump (Fig. 14.2). The serosa of the distal segment is then grasped and manipulated until its lumen can be cannulated with the 3-Fr. catheter guidewire. The catheter is advanced until the tip is seen exiting the fimbriated portion of the fallopian tube.

The mesosalpinx is approximated with a 4-0 or 5-0 polydioxanone suture (Figs. 14.2 and 14.3) tied intraabdominally (see Chapter 9). The tubes are then approximated over the catheter with three sutures of 4-0, 5-0, or 6-0 polydioxanone (PDS II, Ethicon, Inc.) or polyglactin (Vicryl, Ethicon, Inc.), incorporating the entire tubal wall if the segment is ampullary or only the muscularis if the segment is isthmic (Fig. 14.2 and 14.4). The 4-0 polydioxanone suture on a ST-4 needle is particularly easy to handle. Again, all sutures are tied intraabdominally. If possible a second layer of three sutures incorporating the serosa can be placed. The 3-Fr. catheter is then removed and

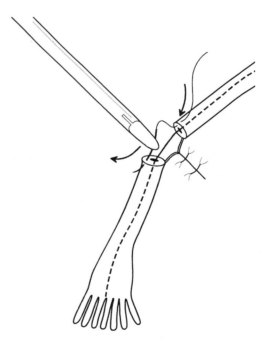

FIGURE 14.4. After the mesosalpinx has been sutured, the tubes are approximated over the wireguide using three sutures with either 4-0, 5-0, or 6-0 polydioxanone (PDS II, Ethicon, Inc.) or polyglactin (Vicryl, Ethicon, Inc.). The entire tubal wall is incorporated if the segment is ampullary; if the segment is isthmic, only the muscularis is sutured.

TABLE 14.1. Characteristics of the study group and outcome.

Patient	Age	Type of sterilization	Segment anastomosed	Hysterosalpingogram	Pregnancy
1	39	Bipolar coagulation	R: Isthmic-ampullary	Patent	No
			L: Isthmic-ampullary	Occluded	
2	26	Bipolar coagulation	R: Isthmic-isthmic	Not done	Yes
			L: Isthmic-isthmic	Not done	
3	29	Postpartum Pomeroy	R: Isthmic-ampullary	Occluded	No
			L: Isthmic-ampullary	Occluded	
4	39	Hulka clip	R: Isthmic-ampullary	Patent	Yes
			L: Isthmic-ampullary	Patent	
5	30	Postpartum Pomeroy	R: Isthmic-ampullary	Patent	Not exposed
			L: Isthmic-ampullary	Occluded	
6	30	Postpartum Pomeroy	R: Isthmic-ampullary	Patent	Yes
			L: Isthmic-ampullary	Occluded	

the contralateral tube cannulated. Although cannulating the tubes helps with alignment of the tubes and placement of the sutures, it is at times not possible to properly position the guidewire. Nonetheless, this has not impeded completing our procedure satisfactorily.

Results

Our initial experience is summarized in Table 14.1. Two patients who were lost to follow-up shortly after surgery were excluded. Patency was documented by hysterosalpingogram 2 to 6 months after surgery if the patient was not pregnant. Operating time varied from 4.5 hr for the first two cases to less than 3 h for all subsequent cases.

Half the operated tubes remained patent after surgery, and three of six patients became pregnant. Two patients delivered at term. Patient 6 suffered two early pregnancy losses in which human chorionic gonadotropin (hCG) titers declined before a gestational sac could be identified.

Our experience demonstrates the feasibility of performing tubal reanastomosis by laparoscopic guidance. The technique requires a proximal stump of sufficient length for easy placement of the suture needle. Clearly, this method is more difficult to learn than the more traditional approach by laparotomy. Results may improve with the introduction of instrumentation specifically designed to handle smaller suture needles and finer threads.

References

1. Gomel V. Microsurgical reversal of sterilization: a reappraisal. *Fertil Steril.* 1980;33:587–597.
2. Grunert GM, Drake TS, Takaki NK. Microsurgical reanastomosis of the fallopian tube for reversal of sterilization. *Obstet Gynecol.* 1981;58:148–151.
3. Sedbon E, Bouquet D, Boudouris O, Madelenat P. Tubal desterilization through exclusive laparoscopy. *Hum Reprod.* 1989;4:158–159.
4. Ostre O, Olsboe F, Trolle B. Laparoscopic tubal anastomosis: reversal of sterilization. *Acta Obstet Gynecol Scand.* 1993;72:680–681.
5. Tsin DA, Mahmood D. Laparoscopic and hysteroscopic approach for tubal anastomosis. *J Laparoendosc Surg.* 1993;3:63–66.
6. Katz E, Doneski BW. Laparoscopic tubal anastomosis. A pilot study. *J Reprod Med.* 1994;39:497–498.
7. Novy ML, Thurmond AS, Patton P, et al. Diagnosis of cornual obstruction by transcervical fallopian tube cannulation. *Fertil Steril.* 1988;50:434–440.

15

Laparoscopic Treatment of Endometriosis

Dan C. Martin

Introduction and Background

Laparoscopy has increased the gynecologist's ability to diagnosis endometriosis. In addition, laparoscopy is increasingly important as a treatment modality. No longer is laparoscopy used only to treat minimal and mild disease; advanced disease can be treated safely and effectively.[1] The laparoscopic approach to the treatment of endometriosis has many advantages over laparotomy. The decrease in morbidity and cost is established.[2] Additionally, laparoscopy may decrease the incidence of de novo adhesion formation when compared to laparotomy.[3]

The surgical approach to the treatment of endometriosis is determined in part by the goals of treatment. When a tissue diagnosis is needed, biopsy or excisional technique is used. When fertility is to be preserved, the techniques require a balance that removes as much tissue as possible but minimizes residual tissue trauma. An aggressive excisional approach may result in excessive adhesions that will be more a factor in infertility than the endometriosis itself. On the other hand, pain secondary to fibrotic endometriosis, particularly in the bowel, requires aggressive resection of all palpable and visible abnormalities. Although laparoscopy appears excellent for visually diagnosed disease, it is limited when palpation and excision of deep infiltrating lesions is required.

Morphologically different forms of endometriosis have been described. Recognition of lesions may be more important than the technique used. Near-contact laparoscopy and CO_2 laser excisional techniques have been used to identify and confirm lesions as small as 180 μ.[4] However, all lesions are not readily recognized at laparoscopy or laparotomy. Endometriosis found at second operations may be persistence rather than recurrence.[5,6] Small lesions can be missed because of their size,[7,8] larger lesions may be missed because of their position,[9,10] and any lesion can be hidden in or behind adhesions.[11] Deep lesions may be more palpable than visual.[9,12] However, some lesions are neither clinically active nor progressive; treatment to prevent progression is balanced against the possibility of causing adhesions.[3]

Video monitoring provides increased magnification and resolution through the use of large monitors[13] that increase the ability of personnel to assist at surgery. However, video imaging can decrease detection, resolution, depth of field, and palpation.

Indications and Patient Selection

Patients with endometriosis generally present with abdominopelvic pain, dysmenorrhea, dyspareunia, infertility, or pelvic mass. Some may already carry the diagnosis of endometriosis, based on previous surgery. Alternatively, some patients are diagnosed at the time of the initial operative laparoscopy.

Pelvic Pain

Patients undergoing diagnostic laparoscopy for pelvic pain generally have failed therapy with nonsteroidal antiinflammatory agents or oral contraceptives. Before surgery, a careful history should be obtained exploring other causes of pelvic pain such as chronic pelvic infection, bowel disease such as irritable bowel, or urinary tract disorders including bladder dysfunction or nephrolithiasis. Gastrointestinal or urologic evaluation and consultation may be considered. The clinical presentation depends to a certain degree on the location and the extent of disease, although the severity of symptoms does not correlate directly with the extent of disease.

As a general rule, patients with focal pain and tenderness commonly have a surgically treatable disease. On the other hand, those with diffuse or changing pain do not respond to surgery as well. Patients with lateral dysmenorrhea may be more likely to have endometriosis than those with central dysmenorrhea.

Infertility

Infertile patients undergoing diagnostic laparoscopy should have completed a basic evaluation, including semen analysis, documentation of ovulation (e.g., basal body temperature plotting with a luteal phase progesterone serum level or endometrial biopsy), hysterosalpingography, and a timed postcoital (Sims–Huhner) test. In these patients, laparoscopy should be both diagnostic and operative. At the time the consent is obtained, the patients should be counseled regarding the possibility of operative laparoscopy if endometriosis or other pathology is found.

Laparoscopy may not be indicated in all patients. Those with a benign history, benign physical exam, normal hysterosalpingogram, and a negative chlamydia trachomatis immunoglobulin (IgG) may benefit from intrauterine insemination or other reproductive technologies before proceeding to laparoscopy.

Pelvic Mass

Pelvic masses secondary to endometriosis are usually symptomatic, although not invariably. If bowel symptoms are present, sigmoid/

colonoscopy should be performed before or at the time of laparoscopy. When there is concern regarding pelvic cancer or bowel anastomosis, a gynecologic oncology or general surgery consultation is used. Moreover, all these patients should undergo bowel preparation before surgery. (See following.)

Preoperative Preparation

Preoperative medical suppression using gonadotropin-releasing hormone (GnRH) analogs has been useful in decreasing the size of lesions and in avoiding corpus lutea. Corpus lutea can frequently be confused as endometriosis. This appears to be most important in patients with large ovaries and with infiltrating endometriosis. On the other hand, medical suppression may obscure subtle lesions and can be associated with side effects in some patients. The majority of advantages of suppression occur in the first 2 months although some patients will continue to have decreased volume over the next 1 to 4 months.

Bowel prep is used in all patients who are prepared for elective laparotomy. A common reason for laparotomy is bowel adhesions or bowel involvement. The type of bowel prep used is generally determined by the general surgeon who is present at the time. Mechanical prep (enemas, magnesium citrate, Go-Lytely) and/or antibiotics have been used. Although many general surgeons were trained to do a colostomy on a laceration in unprepped bowel, many now believe that this is not needed. The experience in the Vietnamese War is said to have been that immediate closure of lacerated bowel was preferable to colostomy and delayed closure. Thus, when unprepped bowel is entered, it is repaired at that time and a colostomy avoided.

Although some authors have suggested that ureters should be stented with significant disease, my experience is that these can be dissected out. Stents may perforate the ureter, and there are reports of the ureter being clamped and cut with the stent in place. Furthermore, few patients with endometriosis have ureters attached. The ureter can usually be pushed away from the endometriotic areas.

Instrumentation and Techniques

Instrumentation

The laparoscopic techniques used to destroy endometriosis are coagulation (desiccation), vaporization, and excision. Coagulation as a term is used to encompass concepts that include but are not limited to heating, desiccation, denaturation, protein coagulation, cauterization, and carbonization of tissue. The effects of coagulation have been produced by bipolar electrosurgery, unipolar electrosurgery, thermal pelviscopy, and fiber-propagated lasers. Vaporization is accomplished by converting high power density laser or electrical energy into heat sufficient to vaporize intracellular water. Excision can utilize any of these techniques in addition to scissors. These methods may be accompanied by mechanical hemostatic devices such as loops, sutures, or clips.

Although coagulation and vaporization are adequate for most cases, the CO_2 laser has been used to resect deep lesions and to dissect the ureter and bowel away from endometriosis and adhesions. However, scissors, bipolar coagulation, thermal coagulation, and unipolar knives are pieces of equipment that are more generally available and appear adequate for most, if not all, dissections.[14] Furthermore, surgeons should master the use of scissors and electrocoagulation before learning to use lasers.

Treatment of Peritoneal and Retroperitoneal Endometriosis

Concepts regarding peritoneal and preperitoneal endometriosis have been a part of the concerns of endometriosis since early publications. Small areas of ovarian endometriosis were originally thought to be a sometimes self-limited disease. On the other hand, even small lesions were considered capable of dissemination. Large endometriomas appeared to be a more important clinical problem. Recent publications have characterized superficial and infiltrating disease by many characteristics including size, volume, appearance, mitotic activity, vascularization, depth of infiltration, volume of infiltration, characteristics of infiltration, biochemical fluid contents, and histologic differentiation. It seems reasonable to conclude that no one of these characteristics defines the behavior of endometriosis.

Small implants (≤2 mm) can be treated in any fashion. However, for diagnosis, these are sampled by biopsy or total excision before vaporization or coagulation. Bipolar or thermal coagulation is effective on lesions that are small or which can be held in the grasping jaws. Initial dissection may be needed so that the lesions can be grasped and controlled. Argon, potassium-titanylphosphate (KTP), and neodyium:yttrium-aluminum-garnet (Nd:YAG) lasers are useful for the destruction of these small lesions. However, all forms of coagulation can distort tissue because of thermal transfer and heating, which may interfere with lesion recognition and dissection.

Vaporization or excision can be useful for larger lesions, although deep lesions are more accurately excised than vaporized (Table 15.1;

TABLE 15.1. Advantages of lesion excision compared to vaporization for the treatment of endometriosis.

Results in less thermal distortion
Creates less smoke
Reduces carbon deposition
Provides tissue for diagnosis

Fig. 15.1). Destruction or excision of these lesions is carried down to the level of healthy tissue. Excision is started by cutting through the peritoneum and into the loose connective tissue surrounding the lesion, using either scissors, knife, or laser. The lesion is outlined and the incision continued into the loose connective tissue until fat is seen. A probe, irrigating solution, knife, or laser is then used to dissect these layers. Once the tissue is excised, it is removed. Specimens that are too large to be removed through the trocar can be removed by colpotomy, minilaparotomy, or morcellation.

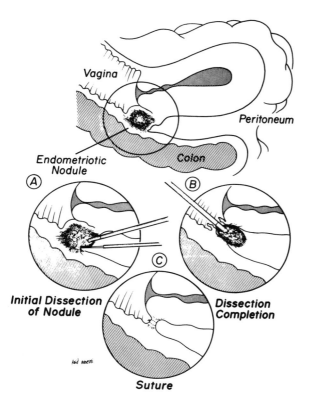

FIGURE 15.1. Deep laparoscopic dissection of the rectovaginal space, in combination with colpotomy, for the treatment of a large endometriotic nodule of the rectovaginal septum. **A:** Initial laparoscopic dissection of nodule. **B:** Completion of dissection via colpotomy incision. **C:** Suturing the rectovaginal septum.

Solutions can be used to push the peritoneum away from vessels, bowel, bladder, or ureter to keep these away from the area of vaporization.[13] These solutions appear most useful in situations where the purpose is to hide structures. On the other hand, when direct visualization and dissection of the ureter and bladder appear advantageous, these solutions are avoided as they may interfere with the surgery.

When carbon accumulates from electrosurgical or laser carbonization of tissue, the field is obscured both at the time of initial surgery and at subsequent procedures. Intraperitoneal carbon can be confused with or can hide endometriosis. The only way to confirm what is associated with carbon is to excise the area. In addition, carbon sublimates at 3652°C and creates a secondary thermal burn. High power density superpulse techniques avoid carbonization and unintended thermal damage by facilitating rapid vaporization. Carbon is usually removed by lavage; rubbing the carbon is avoided or limited.

Treatment of Ovarian Endometriosis

Ovarian endometriomas are managed according to their size. Those less than 5 mm are biopsied and coagulated, vaporized, or excised. The infiltration of these small lesions can be very irregular, and vaporization is taken 2 to 4 mm into healthy-appearing stroma. When these are between 5 mm and 2 cm, they are handled according to the general characteristics at the time of surgery.

At 2 to 5 cm in size, the ovary is opened and drained and the inner wall inspected. The ovary is opened at the dependent portion or on the lateral (broad ligament) side to avoid bowel adhesions. Old blood is drained and the inside lining wall irrigated. A relaxing incision is made cutting through the cortex and down to the level of the cyst wall. The cyst wall is preserved at this level to facilitate definition of the plane of the pseudocapsule (Fig. 15.2). The cyst wall is then stripped out of the ovary. When the capsule is adherent to the hilar vessels, coagulation is used instead of stripping to avoid tearing these vessels. Sutures are not used. For a further description of techniques for endometrioma removal, see Chapter 16.

When endometriomas exceed 5 cm, stripping techniques have an increased risk of requiring 2 to 5 hr at laparoscopy with a realization that laparotomy may be necessary 3 to 5 hr into the operation. In addition, removing these large cysts may increase the chance of sacrificing the ovary when compared to performing a "staged procedure." A staged procedure involves draining, biopsy, and coagulating the inner lining of large cysts at an initial laparoscopy. This is followed by serial sonography with or without medical suppression. A subsequent laparoscopy is per-

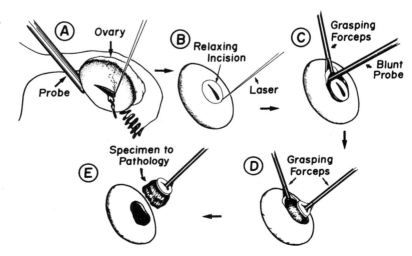

FIGURE 15.2. Resection of an endometrioma. A: An incision is made in the most dependent portion of the ovary. B: A relaxing incision is made circumferentially through the thinned and damaged cortex overlying the endometrioma, after drainage and irrigation of the cyst wall lining. C: A plane of dissection is established with either a blunt probe or forceps. D: Dissection is carried out bluntly or sharply. E: The entire cyst wall is sent to pathology.

formed if the cyst recurs. Staging the procedures appears to increase preservation of healthy ovary (see following.)

Ovarian endometriomas can be difficult to diagnose with certainty either visually or histopathologically. Brosens subdivided ovarian chocolate and hemorrhagic cysts into various appearances and confirmed endometriosis in 89% and 42% of what he termed "typical" and "atypical" cases.[15] Both Brosens and Martin found that red lesions on the inside lining were generally confirmed as endometriosis.[15,16] The appearance most commonly associated with positive histology was irregular brown or red mottling on the surface of a white capsule. On the other hand, a uniform brown appearance was as likely to be an old hemorrhagic corpus luteum as it was to be endometriosis. An interesting observation is that histologic examination of ovarian specimens presumed to be endometriomas actually resulted in a decrease in the rate of diagnosis of these lesions. This decrease in diagnosis was opposite to the increased prevalence of disease noted when analyzing peritoneal lesions.[4]

Treatment of Bowel Endometriosis

Bowel involvement is suggested by palpable tumor near the bowel, rectovaginal tenderness, a rectovaginal shelf, rectal bleeding at the time of menses, or persistent pain following laparoscopic removal of recognized lesions. Recognition requires careful palpation as lesions smaller than 1 cm can be easier to feel than to see. Palpation can be manual for low rectal lesions and for lesions in the rectovaginal septum. Mechanical techniques using laparoscopic or rectal probes may be useful for sigmoid and small bowel lesions. However, many lesions can be palpated adequately only at laparotomy. The majority of my cases have been treated at laparotomy.

Large lesions may present with the majority of the mass of the lesion pushing into the lumen. The superficial manifestation represents only the tip of an iceberg (Fig. 15.3). Approximately 50% of appendiceal lesions are more readily recognized by palpation than visualization. In addition, few lesions are found by barium enema, colonoscopy, sonography, computed tomography (CT), or magnetic resonance imaging (MRI) scan. The main advantage to colonoscopy in the presence of a bowel mass is to rule out adenocarcinoma of the bowel.

Tumor in the rectovaginal septum generally requires a gynecologist or general surgeon familiar with bowel surgery in this area. Deep rectosigmoid resection and anastomosis is a

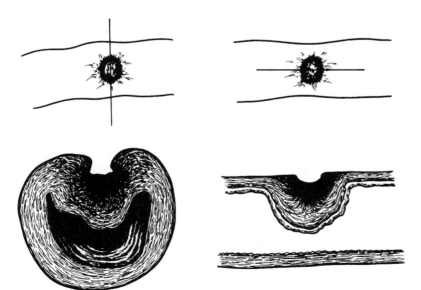

FIGURE 15.3. Endometriosis lesions of the bowel may present with the majority of the mass protruding into the bowel lumen, while superficially the lesion appears small. *Left,* transverse view; *right,* longitudinal view.

distinct possibility at this level, and laparotomy may be indicated. Furthermore, the uterosacral ligaments can be infiltrated with disease extending toward the sacrum or pelvic floor. At this level, the uterosacral ligaments and perirectal tissue are easier to palpate through the rectosigmoid than through the vagina. If disease at this location is not noted preoperatively, it is easy to miss at surgery. If the mucosa is fixed, full-thickness penetration is often present. With any concern regarding bowel muscularis involvement, a general surgery consult, barium enema, sigmoid-oscopy, and colonoscopy should be considered to rule out bowel cancer. Although laparo-scopic treatment in this area can be intention-ally superficial, unanticipated deep damage with delayed perforation may occur. Deep bowel procedures are generally avoided in in-fertility patients who do not have symptoms at-tributable to bowel infiltration. For a further discussion of resection of bowel endometriosis, see Chapter 23.

Attempts at partial resection of infiltration with bowel distortion have met with inconsis-tent results. Some authors believe that they can do this successfully, while others have had uni-form failure. The depth of infiltration into the bowel can be difficult to perceive while operat-ing laparoscopically. Although palpation has been useful at laparotomy in guiding superfi-cial muscularis resection, this has not been use-ful at laparoscopy.

Patients prepared for laparotomy are gener-ally bowel prepped because the most common indication for laparotomy is suspected bowel involvement. In addition, blood banking is dis-cussed with these patients as these procedures frequently last 3 to 5 hr and can be associated with significant blood loss and a need for sub-sequent transfusion.

Treatment of Bladder Endometriosis

Bladder implants up to 5 mm are handled as the peritoneal lesions discussed earlier. Larger lesions approach and may invade the bladder muscularis. Deep muscularis penetration should be anticipated as the lesions become larger. Lesions 2 cm and greater have required

resection of the bladder at laparotomy, when the indication was pelvic pain or when there was tubal distortion.

Treatment of Ureteral Endometriosis

When endometriosis lies over the ureter, two techniques are used to minimize damage to this organ during resection of the disease. A so-lution can be injected to push the ureter away and to provide a barrier between the ureter and the surgical area.[13] An alternate technique is to make an incision in the peritoneum above and away from the ureter. The peritoneum is then grasped and pulled toward the midline. A blunt probe is used to push the ureter away, or the laser is used to incise periureteral loose connective tissue; the laser is not aimed at the ureter. The lesion is resected in its entirety us-ing this technique.

When the ureter will not push away from the peritoneum, the chance that endometriosis has infiltrated the ureter is increased. Peri-ureteral vessels can also bleed, and attempts at hemostasis may harm the ureter. If the ureter is transected or damaged in the process of re-secting disease, some urologists believe that anastomosis in a diseased area should not be performed and that a ureterocystotomy im-plantation is indicated. If you are not prepared for ureteral implantation, avoid cutting near the ureter, especially when it is adherent to en-dometriosis.

Staged Procedures

Staged treatment is generally aimed at patients with extensive disease or large endometriomas. The initial surgery destroys or removes as much endometriosis as reasonable at the initial surgery while avoiding tubes, bowel, ureter, bladder, or other delicate structures. Patients are then observed or placed on 3 to 9 months of hormonal suppression. Endometriosis, par-ticularly around the ureter, bowel, or major blood vessels, is often left behind intentionally. Observation may prove that partial treatment provides sufficient relief so that laparotomy or medical therapy is not necessary. When the pain is persistent, medical therapy, a second laparoscopy, or laparotomy are considered. Repeat laparoscopy for recurrent endometriosis is particularly useful in younger patients.

P. Koninckx of the University of Leuven in Belgium, (personal communication) has suggested a staged procedure for ovarian endometriomas that involves drainage, irrigation, examination, biopsy, and coagulation the inner lining of large cysts at an initial laparoscopy. Serial sonography with or without medical suppression is used to monitor persistence or recurrence. A subsequent laparoscopy is performed if the cyst recurs. This may decrease the extent of removal of a healthy ovary.

Laparotomy may reveal palpable lesions that are not seen at laparoscopy. Because of the increased incidence of palpable bowel disease in this group, bowel prep is routinely performed on all patients who are prepared for laparotomy.

Results

Resolution of Infertility

The 92% pregnancy rate following laparoscopic resection of ovarian endometriomas reported by Reich and the 80% pregnancy rate following laparoscopic treatment of extensive endometriosis are among the higher pregnancy rates reported for this type disease.[17] The collected pregnancy rates were similar using either CO_2 or Nd:YAG laser[18,19,20] (Table 15.2). The argon and CO_2 lasers had similar decreases in success rates as a function of increased years of infertility (Table 15.3). These findings suggest that young patients delaying their family and patients who have short-term infertility have approximately a 65% chance of conceiving. On the other hand, patients with long-term infertility or male factor have lower fertility rates and should be given a realistic prognosis.

Life table analysis indicates that laparoscopic resection of endometriosis is equal to medication or to laparotomy for mild to moderate diseases and equal to or better than laparotomy for severe cases.[13] This outcome may be related to limiting the amount of surgery, to limiting the trauma from retraction, to avoiding suture placement, to encouraging early ambulation, or to using laparoscopy.

The long-term effectiveness of laparoscopic resection of endometriosis for infertility is unclear. In spite of what appears to be an initial increased fecundity, there may be no differences between treated and nontreated patient groups at 3 years. However, for those patients who become pregnant quickly, this avoids potential exposure to another laparoscopy, expensive medical suppression, or in vitro fertilization. In addition to potential decrease of cost, time, and morbidity using these techniques, there is an emotional advantage to early pregnancies.

TABLE 15.2. CO_2 and Nd:YAG laser laparoscopy for endometriosis.

Laser	Isolated/factor		Multiple factors	
	Patients (n)	Pregnant	Patients (n)	Pregnant
CO_2	754	513(86%)	782	351(45%)
Nd:YAG	16	11(69%)	13	4(31%)

Adapted from Martin[19] and from Kojima et al.[20]

TABLE 15.3.   Argon and CO_2 laser laparoscopy for endometriosis.

Laser	0–2 years of infertility		3 or more years of infertility	
	Patients	Pregnant	Patients	Pregnant
CO_2	44	30(68%)	71	26(37%)
Argon	8	5(63%)	48	14(29%)

Adapted from Martin[18] and from Keye et al.[21]

Resolution of Pain

Pain relief is much harder to quantitate than pregnancy rates or resolution of focal tenderness. Pain may be caused by endometriosis, by a combination of endometriosis and other factors, or only by other factors with endometriosis as a coincidental finding. Focal tenderness associated with scarred lesions resolves when these lesions are resected. Diffuse pain is much harder to predict, and pain associated with positive chlamydia IgG titers or with previous sexual abuse can be the hardest to relieve.

Postoperative Adhesions

Postoperative adhesions appear to occur less often with laparoscopy than with laparotomy. Whether this is related to reduced tissue desiccation, decreasing the amount of surgery, avoiding sutures, early ambulation, increased bowel peristalsis, or other factors is a matter of conjecture. Portuondo[22] demonstrated that 92% of ovaries had adhesions following wedge resection at laparotomy compared with a 0% adhesion rate following ovarian wedge resection by multiple ovarian biopsies at laparoscopy. Moreover, he noted the bed of the ovary was dry at the end of the laparoscopic surgery in contrast to the laparotomy procedure. He concluded that hemostasis was necessary to maintain this low adhesion rate. This decrease in adhesions is confirmed by a de novo adhesion rate that was 51% following laparotomy[23] compared to 12% at laparoscopy.[3] However, the adhesion reformation rate was similar following either laparoscopy or laparotomy. Clinically, laparoscopy and laparotomy appear equal in their ability to remove adhesions while laparoscopy appears to cause fewer new adhesions.

Alternative Techniques

Medical Suppression

Long-term medical suppression is used in specific clinical circumstances. Danazol and GnRH analogs have produced the most rapid and predictable relief of pain and have been

TABLE 15.4. Indications for gonadotropin-releasing hormone (GnRH) suppression in the treatment of endometriosis.

Preoperative preparation to decrease ovarian size and functional cysts
Failure to respond to oral contraceptives or progestin suppression
Cornual tubal occlusion
Planned joint myomectomy

preferred for short-term (6 months or less) use, while oral contraceptives or progestins are less expensive and are generally used for long-term (more than 6 months) purposes. Table 15.4 indicates those clinical circumstances in which clinical suppression appears useful.

Laparotomy Surgery

Laparotomy has been the standard for surgical therapy of endometriosis. Palpation, examination of retroperitoneal spaces, examination of bowel, and delicate handling of deep lesions are enhanced at laparotomy when compared with laparoscopy. Laparoscopic excision of deep bowel lesions has been associated with a high persistence. Laparotomy is most useful in patients with persistent pelvic pain following initial laparoscopic surgery and in those with a tumor that appears more involved than can be appropriately handled at laparoscopy.

Endometriosis: A Disease of Coping

Endometriosis requires coping with pelvic pain, dyspareunia, dysmenorrhea, infertility, marital discord, medical expenses, unsuccessful medical therapy, unsuccessful operations, and the inability of multiple physicians to correct the problem. Even the most skilled surgeon may be unable to properly treat the patient without utilizing multiple modalities and consulting with other health care providers.

Self-help and support groups can be helpful to many patients and their families. Group and individual counseling have also been useful. Some physicians have sponsored group counseling sessions in their office.

Conclusions

Bipolar coagulators, unipolar knives, thermal coagulators, lasers, and endoscopic scissors have been used to ablate (coagulate, vaporize, or excise) endometriosis. A combination of these techniques is superior to concentrating on any one of them. Careful attention to the nature and presentation of endometriosis can assist in choosing the technique most useful in a specific clinical situation. However, further study is needed to determine the most appropriate technique or the technique that will be the easiest to teach and to apply for a given clinical situation.

References

1. Adamson GD, Subak LL, Pasta DJ, Hurd SJ, Von Franque O, Rodriguez BD. Comparison of CO_2 laser laparoscopy with laparotomy for treatment of endometriomata. *Fertil Steril.* 1992;57: 965–973.
2. Luciano AA, Lowney J, Jacobs SL. Endoscopic treatment of endometriosis-associated infertility: therapeutic, economic and social benefit. *J Reprod Med.* 1992;37:573–576.
3. Diamond MP, Operative LSG, Daniell JF, et al. Postoperative adhesion development after operative laparoscopy: evaluation at early second-look procedures. *Fertil Steril.* 1991;55:700–704.
4. Martin DC, Hubert GD, Van der Zwaag R, El-Zeky FA. Laparoscopic appearances of peritoneal endometriosis. *Fertil Steril.* 1989;51: 63–67.
5. Wheeler JM, Malinak LR. Computer graphic pelvic mapping, second look laparoscopy, and the distinction of recurrent versus persistent endometriosis. Fertility and Sterility Program, 43rd Annual Meeting Suppl. 1987, Reno. Abstract 194.
6. Davis GD, Brooks RA. Excision of pelvic endometriosis with the carbon dioxide laser laparoscope. *Obstet Gynecol.* 1988;72:816–819.
7. Russell WW. Aberrant portions of the mullerian duct found in an ovary. *Johns Hopkins Hosp Bull.* 1899;94-96:8–10.
8. Murphy AA, Green WR, Bobbie D, Dela Cruz ZC, Rock JA. Unsuspected endometriosis documented by scanning electron microscopy in visually normal peritoneum. *Fertil Steril.* 1986; 46:522–524.
9. Nesbitt RE, Rizk PT. Uterosacral ligament syndrome. *Obstet Gynecol.* 1971;37:730–733.
10. Moore JG, Binstock MA, Growdon WA. The clinical implications of retroperitoneal endometriosis. *Am J Obstet Gynecol.* 1988;158: 1291–1298.
11. Sampson JA. Perforating hemorrhagic (chocolate) cysts of the ovary. Their importance and especially their relation to pelvic adenomas of the endometrial type ('adenomyoma' of the uterus, rectovaginal septum, sigmoid, etc.). *Arch Surg.* 1921;3:245–323.
12. Ripps BA, Martin DC. Correlation of focal pelvic tenderness with implant dimension and stage of endometriosis. *J Reprod Med.* 1992;37: 620–624.
13. Nezhat C, Crowgey SR, Nezhat F. Videolaseroscopy for the treatment of endometriosis associated with infertility. *Fertil Steril.* 1989; 51:237–240.
14. Redwine DB. Conservative laparoscopic excision of endometriosis by sharp dissection: life table analysis of reoperation and persistent or recurrent disease. *Fertil Steril.* 1991;56:628–634.
15. Brosens IA, Puttemans PJ, Deprest J. The endoscopic localization of endometrial implants in the ovarian chocolate cyst. *Fertil Steril.* 1994;61: 1034–1038.
16. Martin DC, Berry JD. Histology of chocolate cysts. *J Gynecol Surg.* 1990;6:43–46.
17. Reich H, McGlynn F. Treatment of ovarian endometriomas using laparoscopic surgical techniques. *J Reprod Med.* 1986;31:577–584.
18. Martin DC. CO_2 laser laparoscopy for endometriosis associated with infertility. *J Reprod Med.* 1986;31:1089–1094.
19. Martin DC. Therapeutic laparoscopy. In: Martin DC, ed. *Laparoscopic Appearance of Endometriosis.* Vol. I. Memphis: Resurge Press; 1990:21–29.
20. Kojima E, Yanagibori A, Yuda K, Hirakawa S. Nd:YAG laser endoscopy. *J Reprod Med.* 1988;33: 907–911.
21. Keye WR, Hansen LW, Astin M, Poulson AM. Argon laser therapy of endometriosis: a review of 92 consecutive patients. *Fertil Steril.* 1987; 47:208–212.
22. Portuondo JA, Melchor JC, Neyro JL, Alegre A. Periovarian adhesions following ovarian wedge resection or laparoscopic biopsy. *Endoscopy* 1984;16:143–145.
23. Diamond MP, Daniell JF, Feste J, et al. Adhesion reformation and de novo adhesion formation after reproductive pelvic surgery. *Fertil Steril.* 1987;47:864–866.

16

Laparoscopic Ovarian and Parovarian Surgery

Michael P. Steinkampf and Ricardo Azziz

Laparoscopic Oophorectomy and Ovarian Cystectomy

Indications

Indications for laparoscopic removal of the ovary include pelvic pain from ovarian adhesions not amenable to simple adhesiolysis, chronic inflammation, severe endometriosis, nonmalignant ovarian neoplasms in which preservation of ovarian function is not desired, or rarely castration for the treatment of breast cancer and other estrogen-sensitive disorders.

In general, ovarian cystectomy is preferable to oophorectomy in women who desire future fertility, particularly when only a single ovary is present. Oophorectomy is preferable in postmenopausal women so as to remove the entire tumor for pathologic examination and minimize spillage. Nonmalignant ovarian tumors amenable to laparoscopic treatment include endometriomas, dermoids, serous and mucinous cystadenomas, and parovarian cysts.

Patient Selection and Preoperative Evaluation

A thorough history and physical generally suggest the etiology of the mass. Worsening dysmenorrhea and infertility are characteristic of pelvic endometriosis, while a history of sexually transmitted diseases and pelvic pain suggests an inflammatory mass. Laboratory testing should be individualized depending on the patient's clinical presentation. Pelvic sonography, particularly using a transvaginal probe, is quite useful in guiding therapy.

Masses that are bilateral, predominantly solid, have significant papillations or excrescences, or are more than 10 cm in diameter are more likely to be malignant, and these patients should be prepared for radical surgery if ovarian malignancy is detected at laparoscopy. If ascites is detected preoperatively, in association with an ovarian mass(es) and in the absence of prior ovarian stimulation, the patient should proceed directly to a laparotomy because the likelihood of a cancerous process is great. However, it should be kept in mind that small amounts of free peritoneal fluid can frequently be detected in normal reproductive-age women using transvaginal sonography.[1]

Patients of reproductive age whose adnexal tumor is predominantly cystic should be followed expectantly for at least six weeks because functional ovarian cysts will spontaneously regress over this period. The use of oral contraceptives to hasten resolution of functional ovarian cysts has been recommended, but we have abandoned this treatment after failing to confirm efficacy in a controlled study.[2] Furthermore, preoperative estrogen/progestin treatment may increase the risk of pulmonary embolism.[3]

Although the risk of a malignancy in the presence of an adnexal mass is higher among postmenopausal patients, these women are also candidates for laparoscopic treatment, if they meet strict criteria. Parker and Berek predicted a benign adnexal mass in 25 postmenopausal women by (a) ultrasound findings of a cystic adnexal mass of less than 10 cm with distinct borders and no evidence of irregular solid parts, thick septa, ascites, or matted bowel; and (b) a normal serum CA-125 value (<35 U/ml).[4] All patients had benign lesions, and laparoscopic treatment was successfully performed in 22 (88%).

Table 16.1 summarizes the factors to consider in deciding which patients should undergo an attempt at laparoscopic treatment of their adnexal mass. In general, women with be-

nign adnexal pathology should be considered for laparoscopic treatment, while patients at high risk of adnexal malignancy should be prepared for treatment by laparotomy, although diagnostic laparoscopy to assess the possibility of malignancy should be considered in at least some of these women as well. We suggest that a frank and thorough discussion of the potential benefits and complications of laparoscopic ovarian surgery be carried out with the patient before the procedure. We have found that most patients are willing to accept the small risk of inadvertent disruption of a malignancy in return for the obvious benefits that laparoscopic surgery offers.

Significance of Intraoperative Cyst Rupture

A major advantage of laparoscopy, the use of small incisions, necessarily increases the risk of cyst rupture. This has been suggested to increase morbidity in patients with both benign and malignant tumors. Occasionally mucinous cystadenomas spontaneously perforate, resulting in seeding of the peritoneum and extensive intraabdominal production of mucin (pseudomyxoma peritonei). In these patients removal of the cyst and evacuation of the mucin does not prevent intraabdominal reaccumulation. Nonetheless, pseudomyxoma peritonei is almost invariably found at the initial operation and does not appear to be a complication of

TABLE 16.1. Considerations in deciding on laparoscopy versus laparotomy in patients with an adnexal mass.

Laparotomy is favored for the following reasons:
 Postmenopausal patients
 Family history of ovarian cancer
 Systemic symptoms (weight loss, bowel obstruction, etc.)
 Endocrine functionality (e.g., excess androgen or estrogen production)
Ascites
Sonographic evidence of papillations, thick septae, or solid mass; bilaterality in postmenopausal
 Size >10 cm
 Serum CA-125 >35 U/ml in the postmenopausal patient

cyst rupture at surgery by either laparotomy or laparoscopy.

Although spontaneous or iatrogenic rupture of ovarian teratomas can induce peritoneal granuloma formation and adhesions, these complications have not been reported with intraoperative rupture. Mage and colleagues removed 91 cystic teratomas laparoscopically without complication.[5] Nezhat and associates performed second-look laparoscopy on four patients in whom dermoid cysts had been excised laparoscopically and found no evidence of granuloma formation.[6] Thus, it would appear that the risk of complications from rupture of benign cysts during laparoscopy is small. Minimizing spillage at the time of tumor excision is beneficial nevertheless, because the oily contents of some teratomas are not easily removed by aqueous irrigants. Extensive irrigation and aspiration of the pelvis should follow the drainage (either spontaneous or intentional) of cyst contents.

The adverse effects of spill from a malignant cyst at the time of laparoscopic removal are less certain. Ovarian cancer generally spreads by peritoneal dissemination, and it seems reasonable that the dissemination of malignant cells into the abdominal cavity would increase the risk of tumor recurrence. On the other hand, it is likely that the manipulation of tumors during *any* attempt at removal results in the sloughing of some cancerous cells into the peritoneal cavity. Early studies on the prognostic effect of ovarian tumor rupture at laparotomy were inconclusive. Parker and colleagues noted that rupture of the ovarian tumor capsule had no effect on survival,[7] while a retrospective study of data from the Mayo Clinic indicated that survival was decreased for these patients.[8] These studies are difficult to interpret because of small patient numbers, inadequate staging, and the failure to account for confounding factors that might affect the risk of recurrence. More sophisticated analyses[9,10] have failed to identify intraoperative cyst rupture as an independent risk factor for tumor recurrence.

Nevertheless, some caveats still apply to the management of potentially malignant ovarian cysts. While most studies indicate that intraoperative rupture of malignant cysts does not in-

crease the risk of tumor recurrence, these data come from patients undergoing immediate staging and hysterectomy at the time of tumor excision; the prognostic implications of tumor spill at laparoscopy followed by hysterectomy some weeks later is unknown. Even if staging and hysterectomy are performed at the initial surgery, some oncologists still prefer to treat women with stage IA ovarian cancer more aggressively if intraoperative spill has occurred. Furthermore, patients with tumor spill at laparoscopy may not be considered to be adequately staged if peritoneal washings were not obtained before cyst rupture; these patients may not be eligible for those therapies managed under the auspices of the Gynecologic Oncology Group (GOG). Thus, to preserve the staging process it is extremely important to obtain pelvic washings at the time of the original surgery, prior to ovarian manipulation.

Principles of the Laparoscopic Management of Adnexal Masses

Table 16.2 denotes the principles for handling an adnexal mass laparoscopically. If a malignancy is encountered at the time of laparoscopy or is determined by histopathology in the immediate postoperative period, a prompt

TABLE 16.2. Principles of laparoscopic management of adnexal masses.

Select properly patients by history, age, menopausal status, sonographic appearance, and tumor markers.
Thoroughly counsel patients regarding risks and complications, surgical experience and skill, and possible need for laparotomy.
Consider mechanical/antibiotic bowel prep if gastrointestinal tract (GI) involvement is suspected.
At surgery:
1. Examine pelvis and abdomen for tumor implants, excessive bowel adhesions at mass, or peritoneal excrescences.
2. Obtain washings before commencing resection, particularly in postmenopausal patients.
3. Minimize spillage and attempt to remove cyst intact.
4. If cyst is opened, examine lining.
5. If the cyst appears functional, or cannot be removed, always obtain a biopsy of cyst wall.
6. Enucleate or excise; do not drain.
7. When in doubt, obtain a frozen section.

staging laparotomy should be performed by a qualified surgeon. While the laparoscopic treatment of a stage I ovarian cancer has been reported,[11] long-term outcomes of women treated by this approach have not been reported.

Technique: Oophorectomy or Salpingo-oophorectomy

The technique of oophorectomy or salpingo-oophorectomy employs the same principles as for removal by laparotomy: lysis of periovarian adhesions, control of the blood supply, and excision. It is most important to identify the course of the ureter and the iliac vessels before dissection. The left ureter will often be more difficult to locate because of its proximity to the root of the sigmoid mesentery. If necessary, the retroperitoneal space can be opened lateral to the infundibulopelvic (I-P) ligaments to facilitate identification. It is also very important to fully mobilize the ovary and tube from surrounding structures before their removal to minimize the chance of damaging bowel or

ureter or of leaving a portion of ovarian cortex attached to the pelvic sidewall.

A simple oophorectomy can be accomplished using a simple loop ligature, as follows (Fig. 16.1):

1. A loop ligature (e.g., 0-chromic) is placed into the abdominal cavity and over the ovary after determining the course of the ureter.
2. The ovary is grasped with a 5- or 10-mm claw forceps and placed through a contralateral suprapubic incision and through the suture loop.
3. The ovary is pulled through the loop ligature, toward the midline, and the meso-ovarium is ligated.
4. In this fashion, a total of three loop ligatures are placed. A reinspection of the course of the ureter is made before excision of the ovary. Care must be taken not to draw or kink the ureter into the ligatures.
5. The meso-ovarium is incised with scissors, leaving at least a 3mm pedicle. Minimal bipolar coagulation of the stump may be needed.

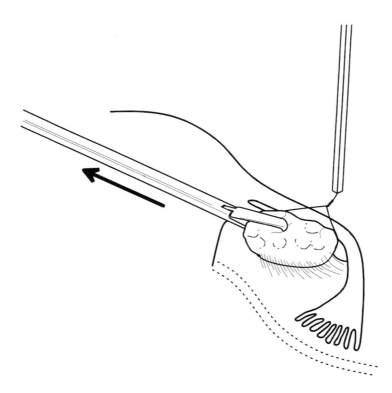

FIGURE 16.1. Oophorectomy using a loop ligature. A small or normal-sized ovary can be resected by placing two loop ligatures (e.g., 0-chromic) around the hilum of the ovary, after fully identifying the course of the infundibulopelvic ligament and ureter (dotted lines). Medial traction on the ovary can be applied using a 5- or 10-mm claw forceps, inserted contralaterally. The utero-ovarian ligament may be coagulating with bipolar before or after ligature.

While the method described just makes use of the suture ligature, equally satisfactory results can be obtained with bipolar cauterization. Furthermore, loop ligature excision is appropriate only for relatively normal-sized ovaries, while the bipolar technique depicted may also be used for enlarged ovaries. Removal of the ovarian tissue is described next.

When needed, a complete adnexectomy can be performed, as follows (Fig. 16.2).

1. The adnexa is freed from surrounding adhesions.
2. Because the ovary, side wall, and cul-de-sac are often involved with adhesions, we generally prefer to begin our dissection at the

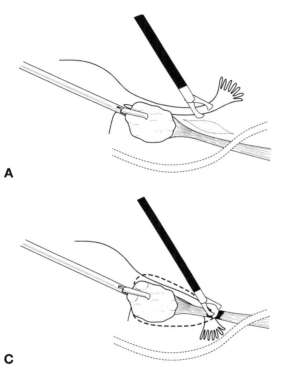

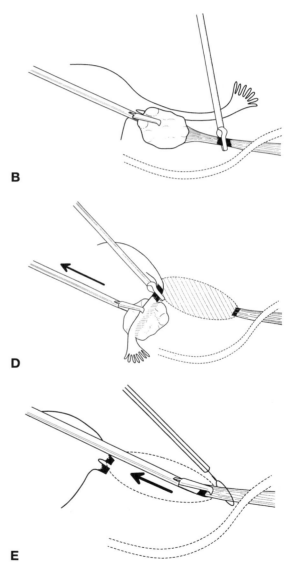

FIGURE 16.2.   Complete adnexectomy. After freeing the adnexa from surrounding adhesions, the infundibulopelvic (I-P) ligament and overlying ureter are identified at the pelvic brim. **A:** An incision is made lateral and parallel to the ligament and vessels. **B:** The I-P ligament is isolated from the pelvic sidewall and thoroughly coagulated with bipolar forceps in at least a 5-mm-wide strip. The ureter *(dotted lines)* and underlying iliac vessels must be clearly identified before desiccation. **C:** After incising the coagulated I-P ligament, the intervening peritoneum is progressively incised *(heavy dashed line)* toward the uterus, placing gentle traction medially on the adnexa. **D:** The utero-ovarian ligament and tubal isthmus are then coagulated and transected. **E:** A loop ligature can be placed over the remaining stumps either before or after transection.

pelvic brim. At that site, the I-P ligament and overlying ureter are identified. An incision is made lateral and parallel to the ligament and vessels, and the I-P ligament is isolated from the pelvic side wall, away from the ureter.

3. The isolated I-P ligament is then grasped with bipolar forceps and thoroughly coagulated. It is most important to first completely occlude the vessels with the bipolar paddles before coagulation and to desiccate at least a 5-mm-wide strip. As indicated previously, the ureter and underlying iliac vessels must be clearly identified before desiccation.

4. The coagulated tissue is incised with scissors, taking care to transect through the middle of the dissected band. For added protection, particularly if the vessels are prominent, the cut infundibulopelvic ligament can be further ligated with one or two loop ligatures.

5. Placing gentle traction medially on the adnexa, the intervening peritoneum, below the ovary and lateral to the fallopian tube, is progressively incised toward the uterus. Electrocoagulation is rarely required for this dissection because this tissue is relatively avascular. After the adnexa is completely excised, any bleeding points on the pelvic side wall can be controlled with the bipolar cautery.

6. The utero-ovarian (U-O) ligament and tubal isthmus are then coagulated and transected. A loop ligature can be placed over the remaining stump either before or after transection.

7. Resected tissue is removed from the pelvis as described next.

Technique: Ovarian Cystectomy

As for laparotomy, laparoscopic removal of an ovarian cyst should be preceded by careful inspection of the pelvic peritoneum, contralateral ovary, and the abdominal contents. If signs of malignancy such as peritoneal implants, ascites, or capsular excrescences are noted, laparoscopic removal of the cyst should not be attempted. With larger cysts, generally those

greater than 3 cm, even if they appear functional (i.e., a follicular or corpus luteum cyst), a biopsy of the cyst wall should be obtained and sent for pathologic examination.

It should be remembered that the greatest risk of laparoscopic misdiagnosis is not confusing a malignancy with a benign process but rather mistaking a serous or mucinous cystadenoma for a functional cyst.[4,12] We generally do not encourage simple aspiration, unless the cysts are quite small. The approach to laparoscopic cystectomy differs somewhat depending on whether the tumor is an endometrioma, particularly if ruptured, or whether it is a benign neoplasm.

Resection of Ruptured Endometriomas

Endometriomas generally are involved in dense adhesions to the pelvic side wall or sigmoid (Fig. 16.3) while other tumors are not. Furthermore, endometrioma will often drain

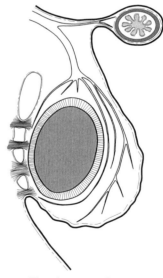

Endometrioma

FIGURE 16.3. Transverse anatomy of an endometrioma. Note that there are extensive adhesions on the posterior aspect of the ovary to the side wall, usually at the site of most cortical fibrosis and thinning. The cyst wall is usually also fused to the cortex at this site. Note also that the hilar ovarian vessels do not penetrate the cyst wall.

freely ("rupture") during dissection of the ovary from surrounding structures, and the enucleation site will be dictated by the drainage site. Finally, while the ovarian cortex covering most of the endometrioma is healthy, the area where the cyst was attached to the pelvic side wall is generally thinned out, fibrotic, and infiltrated with endometriosis. Furthermore, the cyst wall is usually also fused to the cortex at this site. Endometriomas can be enucleated as follows (Fig. 16.4):

1. The ovary is freed from surrounding adhesions, and the ureter and pelvic side-wall vessels are clearly identified (Fig. 16.4A).
2. Enucleation should generally begin at the site of rupture or at the site of maximum cortical damage. To establish the correct

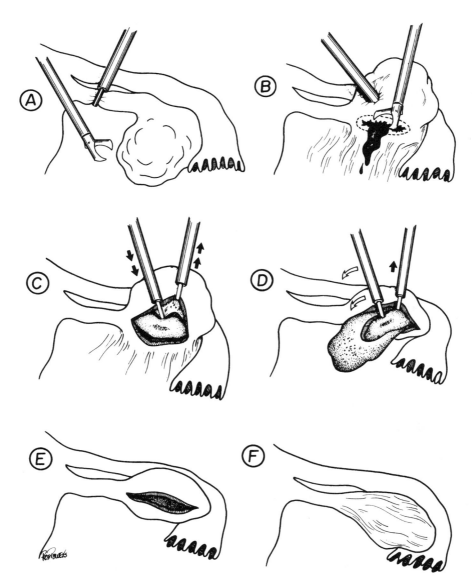

FIGURE 16.4. Laparoscopic ovarian cystectomy. The dissection planes are easiest to attain if the cyst remains distended during the initial phase of enucleation. This may not always be possible because many ovarian endometriomas will leak during their initial dissection from the pelvic side-wall.

dissection plane between cyst wall and normal ovarian cortex, it is extremely important to circumferentially excise the fused abnormal ovarian cortex and cyst wall surrounding the rupture site (Fig. 16.4B and 16.5).

3. After the edges of the normal ovarian cortex and cyst wall are clearly seen at the border of the circumferential incision, they are gently teased apart using two biopsy forceps with a central fixing pin. Manipulation and grasping of the ovarian cortex, however, is minimized (Fig. 16.4C).

4. Continued dissection of the cyst wall from the ovarian bed is performed circumferentially, by continuously regrasping the tissue. To minimize tearing of the normal ovarian cortex, the tips of the forceps are kept in close proximity when pulling the layers apart. Rarely, fibrous strands are cut using the scissors (Fig. 16.4D).

5. Twisting the cyst wall over a biopsy forceps, while applying gentle traction, has been reported to facilitate removal (Fig. 16.6), although it may increase the risk of tearing the ovarian cortex.

6. After cyst enucleation, the cyst bed should be inspected and any remaining fragments removed (Fig. 16.4E).

7. Hemostasis of the ovarian bed can be obtained with a bipolar fulguration. Contrary to what has often been assumed, hilar vessels do not penetrate into the cyst wall (see Fig. 16.3), and significant bleeding is not often encountered if a proper dissection plane was initially created.

8. As for any laparoscopic procedure, thorough lavage of the pelvis is performed with lactated Ringer's solution.

9. The ovarian incision may be covered with Interceed® Adhesion Barrier (Johnson & Johnson Medical, Inc., Arlington, TX) to minimize adhesion formation. Suturing of the ovary is rarely needed, and only in circumstances in which the normal ovarian cortical anatomy has been severely disrupted (Fig. 16.4F). More frequently, redundant thinned-out ovarian cortex is circumferentially resected.

10. The cyst tissue is removed from the pelvis, as described next.

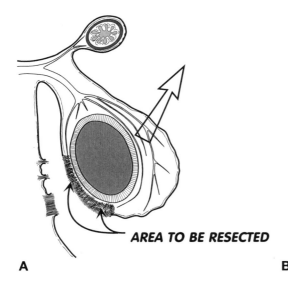

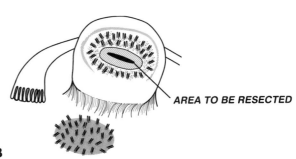

A   **B**

FIGURE 16.5. Two views (**A,B**) of resection of the ovarian cortex surrounding the endometrioma rupture site. While the ovarian cortex covering most of the endometrioma is healthy, the area where the cyst was attached to the pelvic side wall is generally thinned out, fibrotic, and infiltrated with endometriosis. To establish the correct dissection plane between cyst wall and normal ovarian cortex, it is extremely important to circumferentially excise the abnormal ovarian cortex surrounding the rupture site.

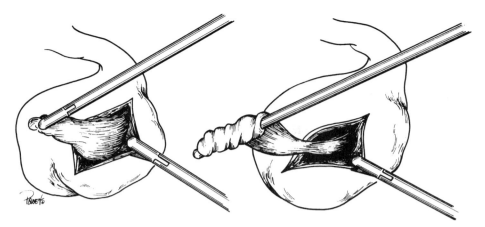

FIGURE 16.6. To facilitate cyst enucleation, the cyst wall can be grasped with biopsy forceps and twisted while applying gentle traction, peeling the cyst wall from the underlying ovarian bed. This maneuver however may increase the risk of tearing the ovarian cortex.

Resection of a Presumed Benign Neoplasm

The ovarian cortex overlying benign neoplasms is generally healthy. Nonetheless, it may be very thinned out, depending on the size of the tumor. The procedure is as follows.

1. If a tumor other than an endometrioma is suspected, peritoneal washings should always be obtained before commencing cystectomy. The specimen can be discarded if the cyst, once removed, is thought to be definitively benign.
2. As previously, the ovary is freed from surrounding adhesions, and the ureter and pelvic side-wall vessels are clearly identified.
3. For cyst dissection, if needed the ovary can be rotated upward with the use of a blunt probe. While a grasper placed at the U-O ligament can also be used, this ligament generally will tear, particularly if the cyst is larger than 3 cm.
4. For ovarian tumors that lie within the body of the ovary and minimally distort the ovarian cortex, an incision should be made directly over the cyst with scissors (Fig. 16.7). The incision should preferably be made parallel to the long axis of the ovary, and as far posterior as possible, taking care to incise only ovarian cortex and not cyst wall. The placement of the incision posteriorly will minimize the possibility of adhesions to the bowel, uterus, or tube, in contrast to the classic antimesenteric incisions.
5. If ovarian cortex overlying the cyst is exceedingly thin or the cyst is very large, a circumferential incision is made with scissors around the base of the cyst (Fig. 16.7). The incision should be made at the limit between healthy full-thickness cortex and the thinned-out encapsulation of the cyst.
6. A plane is created between cyst wall and ovarian cortex by using a blunt probe or by gently spreading the tips of the scissors. For countertraction, the edge of the cortex can be grasped using a biopsy forceps or adhesion grasper.
7. While some laparoscopic surgeons routinely empty the cyst before removal, we find that an intact cyst facilitates dissection. Once an adequate dissection plane is created circumferentially around the cyst, the cyst can be either aspirated and opened or enucleated intact for removal. If possible, we prefer to enucleate the cyst intact, removing it from the abdomen either by placing into a retaining sac or through a colpotomy incision (see following).
8. If exceedingly large, the cyst may need to be aspirated before enucleation and removal. We try to minimize spillage of cyst contents by first aspirating through a

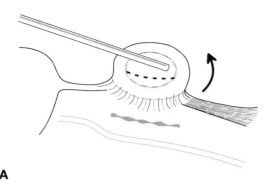

A

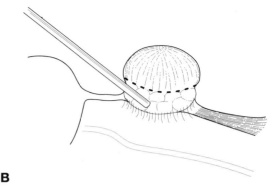

B

FIGURE 16.7.   Cortical incisions for the resection of benign ovarian neoplasms. Only the ovarian cortex, and not the underlying cyst wall, should be incised. **A:** For ovarian tumors that lie within the body of the ovary and minimally distort the ovarian cortex, an incision *(dotted line)* should be made directly over the cyst with scissors, parallel to the long axis of the ovary and as far posterior as possible. **B:** If the cyst is very large or the ovarian cortex overlying the cyst is exceedingly thin, a circumferential incision *(dotted line)* is made with scissors around the base of the cyst, at the limit between healthy full-thickness cortex and the thinned-out encapsulation of the cyst.

large-bore (18- or 16-gauge) spinal needle placed transabdominally. Placing a suction cannula near the drain site also helps minimize spill. However, drainage of dermoids or mucinous cystadenomas generally requires fenestration, followed by extensive irrigation and aspiration.

9. Once the cyst is drained, it is opened for inspection. Using the laparoscope, the inner aspect of the cyst wall is examined closely to detect the presence of excrescences or papillations suggestive of ovarian malignancy. If solid areas are found within the cyst wall at laparoscopy or following removal, a frozen section is obtained. If malignancy is detected, a staging laparotomy is performed.

10. After the cyst is opened and inspected, the cyst wall is pealed away from the ovarian bed, as discussed for the removal of endometriomas (see Fig. 16.4).

11. Whether the cyst is enucleated intact or after drainage, hemostasis of the ovarian bed can be obtained with a bipolar fulguration. The pelvis is thoroughly lavaged with lactated Ringer's solution, and the ovarian incision may be covered with Interceed® Adhesion Barrier. The cyst tissue is then removed from the pelvis, as described next.

Removal of Resected Tissue from the Pelvic Cavity

Removal of resected tissue from the abdominal cavity, particularly an intact ovary or cyst, is often the most difficult part of the laparoscopic treatment of adnexal masses. If there is the minimum suspicion of malignancy, we prefer to place the ovaries or intact cysts within a plastic bag. We prefer the Pleatman sac (Cabot Medical, Inc., Langhorne, PA), which does not have a pursestring and is sturdier, although other makes are also useful (e.g., Endobag, Dexide, Fort Worth, TX). We generally remove the bag through the umbilical incision, pulling it out together with the umbilical sleeve.

If there is no risk of malignancy and the tissue is small, the entire organ can be removed through the midline suprapubic port, perhaps after some degree of morcellation with scissors. Nonetheless, this may hinder the pathologic examination. If the amount of tissue is larger, the midline suprapubic incision may be enlarged; then, after grasping the excised tissue or bag, the grasper and port sleeve are removed together in one smooth movement.

If the ovary or cyst is larger, generally more than 5 cm, we prefer to remove it through a colpotomy incision. This method seems to be associated with less postoperative pain than a minilap incision. It is, however, restricted to those patients with relatively normal cul-de-sac anatomy. It is imperative to confirm that the rectum is well away from the site of the planned incision, and dissection of the colon from the cul-de-sac may be necessary. Generally, we first wedge the ovary or cyst into the cul-de-sac using a suprapubic grasper (Fig. 16.8). We then make a posterior colpotomy incision, much like the initial incision of a vaginal hysterectomy. Once the peritoneal cavity is breached, a single-tooth or similar tenaculum is used to grasp the tissue, pulling it toward the vagina. The cyst(s) may be aspirated transvaginally before removal, as needed to reduce its size. The colpotomy incision can also be extended, using lateral digital traction. The ovarian tissue is progressively pulled ("walked") out of the peritoneum by successively grasping the mass with two alternating graspers.

An alternative approach to the colpotomy may be to perform the incision transperitoneally, by placing a sponge stick into the posterior vaginal fornix and incising the vagina laparoscopically, with either a laser or needle cautery. This method is however associated with the rapid loss of pneumoperitoneum and subsequent difficulty in finding and grasping the ovarian tissue transvaginally, with an increased risk of damage to surrounding structures.

Results of Laparoscopic Management of Adnexal Masses

Many authors have demonstrated the success of laparoscopic ovarian surgery. Reich reported 116 laparoscopic oophorectomies without complication.[13] Perry and Upchurch reported 12 patients undergoing a unilateral and 5 a bilateral salpingo-oophorectomy.[14] Only 1 patient required a laparotomy for postoperative bleeding. We have performed more than 40 oophorectomies or adnexectomies without significant complications.

Mage and colleagues reported that of 481 patients undergoing a laparoscopy for a presumed benign cyst, 42 (8.7%) underwent a laparotomy as it was not possible to perform the surgery endoscopically because of dense adhesions or excessively large tumors (>10 cm).[4] In 19 of 481 (3.9%) patients a laparotomy was performed, following the laparoscopy, for the presence or suspicion of a malignancy. Among the 420 patients treated laparoscopically for ovarian cysts, only 3 (0.7%) suffered significant complications (pelvic infection in 2 and acute pain in 1). Hauuy and colleagues reported that of 165 attempts at laparoscopic treatment of ovarian cysts,[12] the operation was successful in 158 (93%).[12] The failure rate was highest for endometriomas (18.1%) and dermoids (5.7%). We have had to proceed to a laparotomy in 3 of 30 (10%) patients with endometriomas secondary to the density of periovarian adhesions.

The fertility rate following laparoscopic treatment of endometriomas is unclear. Reich and McGlynn reported a pregnancy rate of 60% (12/20) among patients treated with laparoscopy only.[15] Kojima and colleagues reported a 37.5% (6/16) pregnancy rate following surgery.[16] Daniell and associates noted that 12 of 32 (38%) patients treated by laparoscopy

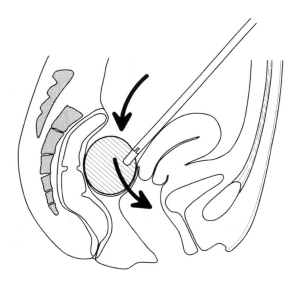

FIGURE 16.8. Removal of resected ovarian tissue through a colpotomy incision. The resected ovary, or cyst, is wedged into the cul-de-sac. The cyst can be drained transvaginally, after the colopotomy incision is made, as needed to reduce its size sufficiently to allow removal.

achieved pregnancy following their initial surgery.[17] In our practice, among 20 infertile patients with laparoscopically treated endometriomas, 6 (30%) became pregnant, with one miscarriage. We suspect that the success of laparoscopic ovarian surgery will depend not only on the skill of the surgeon but, more importantly, on proper preoperative evaluation and patient selection.

Laparoscopic Treatment of Anovulation

Polycystic ovary syndrome (PCOS) is a disorder of chronic anovulation and infertility. The ovaries typically are symmetrically enlarged, with a smooth, thickened capsule and multiple ovarian follicular cysts 4 to 8 mm in diameter. Wedge resection of the ovaries has been known to result in temporary normalization of ovarian function, with pregnancy resulting in 60% to 70% of infertile women.[18,19] The mechanism for this effect is unclear, but may involve reduction in ovarian androgen production through decrease in stromal mass or disruption of parenchymal blood flow. A number of alternatives to wedge resection by laparotomy have been proposed to decrease the morbidity and the associated postoperative adhesion formation.

Indications and Preoperative Evaluation

Because of the risk of postoperative adhesions, we believe that only infertile patients who have failed to ovulate with clomiphene citrate or human menopausal gonadotropins (HMG) should be considered candidates for the laparoscopic treatment of PCOS. Furthermore, patients failing to ovulate on clomiphene should be counseled regarding the option of proceeding to ovulation induction with HMG before surgery is performed. Unfortunately, because ovarian drilling is technically easy to perform while gonadotropin therapy requires a greater degree of expertise, many patients are being steered toward the laparoscopic procedure without proper counseling or preoperative selection.

Patients with PCOS usually have a history of infrequent, irregular menses from puberty; the sudden onset of amenorrhea, especially with progressive virilization, should alert one to the possibility of a hormonally active adrenal or ovarian tumor. Other causes of androgen excess should also have been excluded, including the hyperandrogenic-insulin resistant-acanthosis nigricans (HAIRAN) syndrome and 21-hydroxylase-deficient nonclassic adrenal hyperplasia. Because laparoscopic ovarian drilling is performed for the treatment of infertility, a basic infertility evaluation should have been completed, including a semen analysis and hysterosalpingography. Lack of ovulatory response to clomiphene or HMG should have been documented.

Technique of Laparoscopic Ovarian Cauterization for Polycystic Ovary Syndrome

Laparoscopy is performed in the standard manner. After careful inspection of the pelvis, the entire surface of the ovary is fulgurated at evenly spaced points (Fig. 16.9). The ovary

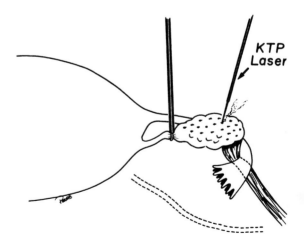

FIGURE 16.9. Laparoscopic cauterization for the treatment of polycystic ovarian syndrome (PCOS). The surface of the ovary is fulgurated at evenly spaced points. If unipolar cautery is used, 4 to 8 points per ovary are required. However, if the laser is utilized, the number of punctures required may be as high as 25 to 40 per ovary.

may need to be rotated upward with a blunt probe to expose its posterior aspect. If needle-point unipolar electrocautery is used, eight spots per ovary are satisfactory, with current maintained until both the ovarian capsule and cortex are penetrated. If the laser (CO_2 or potassium-titnyl-phosphate, KTP) is used, the number of punctures required may be higher, with 25 to 40 reportedly used by some surgeons.[20] After cauterization, the pelvis is irrigated and inspected for bleeding, although this is a rare complication. Although laparoscopic wedge resection is feasible, the results have not been shown to be superior to simple fulguration of the ovary.

Results of Laparoscopic Treatment for Polycystic Ovary Syndrome

Campo and co-workers performed multiple ovarian biopsies at laparoscopy in 12 patients with PCOS who had not responded to clomiphene; pregnancy subsequently occurred in 5 patients.[21] Gjonnaess performed systematic ovarian electrocautery in 62 women with PCOS.[22] Ovulation occurred within 3 months in 92% of patients, and regular menstrual cycles were established in 86%. More importantly, 7 of the 9 women who had been resistant to clomiphene therapy ovulated after electrocautery, and the remaining 2 then responded to clomiphene stimulation. Also, 28 (80%) of the 35 women with PCOS as their only infertility factor, and 3 of 9 of the clomiphene-resistant patients, became pregnant. The number of sites electrocauterized varied from 5 to 8 points per ovary. Only 66% of patients ovulated if fewer than 6 points were cauterized per ovary, compared to 97% if more than 10 points per ovary were used. Since then, a number of studies have demonstrated the efficacy of ovarian cautery for infertile women with clomiphene-resistant PCOS, with pregnancy rates ranging from 50% to 80%.[20,23–25]

The effectiveness of this technique on PCOS patients who ovulate on clomiphene or gonadotropins but fail to achieve conception has not been demonstrated. In addition it appears that the effects of electrocautery are of limited duration. Of 12 anovulatory women who did not become pregnant within 3 months of ovarian cautery, only 3 (25%) demonstrated persistent menstrual regularity for more than 2 years.[22]

A significant concern with ovarian cauterization in the treatment of PCOS relates to the possibility of postoperative periovarian adhesions. At unselected second-look procedures following ovarian electrocautery, approximately 25% of patients demonstrate mild to moderate adhesions.[26,27] In contrast, Gurgan et al. treated 17 patients, all of whom had an early second-look laparoscopy.[25] In 7 patients undergoing ovarian electrocautery and 10 undergoing laser vaporization, 6 (85%) and 8 (80%), respectively, demonstrated postoperative adhesions. In none of the patients were the adhesions severe, but in 2 (12%) the adhesions were of moderate extent. Subsequently, Gurgan and colleagues treated 40 women with clomiphene-resistant PCOS by laparoscopic neodymium:yttrium-aluminum-garnet (Nd:YAG) laser photocoagulation of the ovaries and assigned them randomly to either an early second-look laparoscopy and lysis of adhesions or expectant management.[28] Of the 19 patients undergoing second-look laparoscopy, 13 (68%) demonstrated periovarian adhesions, all of minimal or mild degree. Interestingly, in this randomized study, performance of an early second-look laparoscopy did not improve pregnancy rates.

In conclusion, it is yet unclear to what extent periovarian adhesions form following ovarian cautery. In studies in which early second-look laparoscopies were performed in all patients, approximately 70% to 90% of patients demonstrated adhesions, the majority being minimal to mild. Nevertheless, the extent of adhesions will probably relate to the extent of ovarian cortex damage achieved.

Laparoscopic Resection of Parovarian Cysts

Introduction

Parovarian cysts may present as an adnexal mass and are usually detected by pelvic examination or sonography, which reveals a simple uniloculated cystic structure in the adnexa. Genadry and colleagues reviewed 132 benign parovarian cysts and observed that 51% of tumors greater than 3 cm in diameter were of mesothelial (peritoneal inclusion) origin, 19% were paramesonephric, and none were of mesonephric (Wolffian) origin.[29] The majority of these cysts (79%) were encountered in women between the ages of 20 and 49 years. Mesothelial cysts in particular can reach more than 10 cm in size. These cysts are usually composed of a single layer of epithelium or mesothelium and are encapsulated in a thin fibrous connective tissue layer. The mesosalpingeal vasculature surrounds but does not penetrate this connective tissue layer encapsulating the cyst.

Indications and Patient Selection

Often a parovarian cyst will be diagnosed by pelvic examination or incidentally during pelvic ultrasonography or diagnostic laparoscopy. At the time of the laparoscopy it is most important to determine whether there are any solid components within the parovarian cyst, or peritoneal implants suggesting malignant transformation. Furthermore, it is important not to confuse a tumorous extension of an ovarian neoplasm into the mesosalpinx with a parovarian cyst. Benign parovarian cysts are rarely bilateral. If the appearance of the cyst on sonography and laparoscopic inspection of the adnexa suggests that the structure is benign, laparoscopic resection can proceed.

Technique

Semm and colleagues prefer to enucleate the cysts without prior drainage,[30] but Herbert and associates have described a technique that involves the initial aspiration of the cyst.[31] These authors prefer not to drain the cyst before enucleation, to facilitate dissection. However, exceedingly large tumors may require partial aspiration before resection. If indicated, an 18- or 20-gauge spinal needle is placed through the midline of the anterior abdominal wall and the cyst is partially aspirated.

Following is the authors' preferred method of removing parovarian cysts, using a standard three-puncture operative laparoscopy approach (Fig. 16.10):

1. Once the cyst has been clearly identified, the peritoneum overlying the mass, halfway between the tube and the ovary, is picked up with micrograspers and incised with hook or microscissors. The incision is performed parallel to the long axis of the tube. Care should be taken not to enter the cystic cavity at this time. Although the fallopian tube may often be stretched and distorted, the surgeon should avoid any manipulation that may endanger this structure because the fallopian tube returns to normal once the parovarian cyst is removed.

2. Hook scissors are now introduced through the incision, between the cyst wall and overlying peritoneum, and circumferential dissection is begun bluntly by spreading the tips of the scissors.

3. Once the cyst has been exposed, a biopsy forceps (with a central grasping pin) is used to firmly grasp the cyst. At this time it is important not to relax the forceps so as to avoid excessive leakage of cyst fluid and loss of the dissection planes. Enucleation of the parovarian cyst away from surrounding connective tissue and vasculature is accomplished more easily when it is distended.

4. Alternatively, if the cyst is quite large the biopsy forceps may be relaxed allowing fluid to drain into the cul-de-sac, reducing cyst size. If needed, the mesosalpingeal incision is extended parallel to the tube.

5. In general, small peritoneal vessels can be transected with the hook scissors with minimal bleeding, which clots promptly. Larger vessels should be cauterized before incision.

6. Continuous traction of the cyst toward the midline and progressive circumferential dissection with the scissor tips will free the cyst from the surrounding connective tissue and peritoneum.

7. If there remains a thicker pedicle of coalesced connective tissue attached between the bed and base of the cyst, it is cauterized slightly with bipolar and transected. Bleeding is generally minimal and does not re-

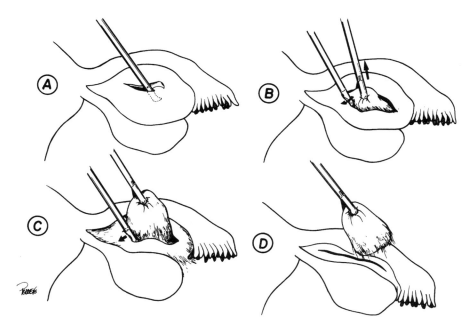

FIGURE 16.10. Laparoscopic resection of a parovarian cyst. Dissection is generally facilitated if the cyst is left intact. **A:** An incision is made through the serosa, taking care not to puncture cyst. **B:** Cyst is grasped, preferably with biopsy forceps, and the surrounding connective tissue dissected away using gentle traction and countertraction. **C:** Enucleation of the cyst continues. **D:** Cyst is removed intact. Bleeding is minimal and generally does not require electrocoagulation. The peritoneum should not be closed with sutures after resection of the cyst.

quire extensive electrocoagulation. If there is oozing from the parovarian cyst bed, it is preferable to apply pressure with a suprapubic blunt probe for approximately 5 min, followed by extensive irrigation. The placement of catgut loop ligatures at the base of the parovarian cyst is usually unnecessary and has the potential of creating significant postoperative adhesions. As stated previously, no vessels directly penetrate into the ovarian cyst wall, and careful dissection with a blunt-edge scissors should free the cyst in its entirety without the formation of an artificial "pedicle" of coalesced connective tissue.

8. Once the cyst has been enucleated from its mesosalpingeal location, it is allowed to drain and removed through a 5- or 10-mm suprapubic sleeve.

9. The peritoneal defect that is left behind does not require suturing. Furthermore, excessive cauterization of the area should be avoided.

Results

We have removed more than 20 parovarian cysts, ranging from 3 to 7 cm, in the manner described without difficulty. Minimal bleeding is encountered, which usually ceases spontaneously or following the application of pressure. Rarely is cauterization required. Cysts larger than 5 cm may require partial aspiration before dissection to reduce the size of the peritoneal incision.

References

1. Nichols JE, Steinkampf MP. Detection of free peritoneal fluid by transvaginal sonography. *J Clin Ultrasound*. 1993;21:171–174.
2. Steinkampf MP, Hammond KR, Blackwell RE. Hormonal treatment of functional ovarian cysts: a randomized, prospective study. *Fertil Steril*. 1990;54:775–777.
3. Vessey MP, Doll R, Fairbairn AS, et al. Postoperative thromboembolism and the use of oral contraceptives. *Br Med J*. 1970;3:123–126.

4. Parker WH, Berek JS. Management of selected cystic adnexal masses in postmenopausal women by operative laparoscopy: a pilot study. *Am J Obstet Gynecol.* 1990;163:1574–77.

5. Mage G, Canis M, Manhes H, et al. Laparoscopic management of adnexal cystic masses. *J Gynecol Surg.* 1990;6:71–79.

6. Nezhat C, Winer WK, Nezhat F. Laparoscopic removal of dermoid cysts. *Obstet Gynecol.* 1989; 73:278–280.

7. Parker RT, Parker CH, Wilbanks GD. Cancer of the ovary. *Am J Obstet Gynecol.* 1970;108: 878–888.

8. Webb MJ, Decker DG, Mussey E, et al. Factors influencing survival in stage I ovarian cancer. *Am J Obstet Gynecol.* 1973;116:222–228.

9. Dembo AJ, Davy M, Stenwig AE, et al. Prognostic factors in patients with stage I epithelial ovarian cancer. *Obstet Gynecol.* 1990;75:263–273.

10. Young RC, Walton LA, Ellenberg SS, et al. Adjuvant therapy in stage I and stage II epithelial ovarian cancer: results of two prospective randomized trials. *N Engl J Med.* 1990;322: 1021–1027.

11. Reich H, McGlynn F, Wilkie W. Laparoscopic management of stage I ovarian cancer. *J Reprod Med.* 1990;35:601–605.

12. Hauuy JP, Madelenat P, Bouquet de la Joliniere J, Dubuisson JB. Laparoscopic surgery of ovarian cysts. The indications and the limits as found in a series of 169 cysts. *J Gynecol Obstet Biol Reprod.* 1990;19:209–216.

13. Reich H. Laparoscopic oophorectomy without ligature or morcellation. *Contemp OB/GYN.* 1989;34(3):34–46.

14. Perry CP, Upchurch JC. Pelviscopic adnexectomy. *Am J Obstet Gynecol.* 1990;162:79–81.

15. Reich H, McGlynn F. Treatment of ovarian endometriomas using laparoscopic surgical techniques. *J Reprod Med.* 1986;31:577–584.

16. Kojima E, Morita M, Otaka K, et al. YAG laser laparoscopy for ovarian endometriomas. *J Reprod Med.* 1990;35:592–596.

17. Daniell JF, Kurtz BR, Gurley LD. Laser laparoscopic management of large endometriomas. *Fertil Steril.* 1991;55:692–695.

18. Adashi EY, Rock JA, Guzick D, et al. Fertility following bilateral ovarian wedge resection: a critical analysis of 90 consecutive cases of the polycystic ovary syndrome. *Fertil Steril.* 1981;36: 320–325.

19. McLaughlin DS. Evaluation of adhesion reformation by early second-look laparoscopy following microlaser ovarian wedge resection. *Fertil Steril.* 1984;42:531–537.

20. Daniell JF, Miller W. Polycystic ovaries treated by laparoscopic laser vaporization. *Fertil Steril.* 1989;51:232–236.

21. Campo S, Garcea N, Caruso A, et al. Effect of celioscopic ovarian resection in patients with polycystic ovaries. *Gynecol Obstet Invest.* 1983;15: 213–222.

22. Gjonnaess H. Polycystic ovarian syndrome treated by ovarian electrocautery through the laparoscope. *Fertil Steril.* 1984;41:20–25.

23. Armar NA, Lachelin GCL. Laparoscopic ovarian diathermy: an effective treatment for anti-oestrogen-resistant anovulatory infertility in women with the polycystic ovary syndrome. *Br J Obstet Gynaecol.* 1993;100:161–164.

24. Naether OGJ, Fisher R, Weise HC, Geiger-Kotzler L, Delfs T, Rudolf K. Laparoscopic electrocoagulation of the ovarian surface in infertile patients with polycystic ovarian disease. *Fertil Steril.* 1993;60:88–94.

25. Gurgan T, Urman B, Aksu T, Yarali H, Develioglu O, Kisnisci HA. The effect of short-interval laparoscopic lysis of adhesions on pregnancy rates following Nd-YAG laser photocoagulation of polycystic ovaries. *Obstet Gynecol.* 1992;80: 45–47.

26. Naether OGJ, Fischer R. Adhesion formation after laparoscopic electrocoagulation of the ovarian surface in polycystic ovary patients. *Fertil Steril.* 1993;60:95–98.

27. Dabirashrafi H, Mohamad K, Behjatnia Y, Moghadami-Tabrize N. Adhesion formation after ovarian electrocauterization on patients with polycystic ovarian syndrome. *Fertil Steril.* 1991;55:1200–1201.

28. Gurgan T, Kisnisci H, Yarali H, Develioglu O, Zeyneloglu H, Aksu T. Evaluation of adhesion formation after laparoscopic treatment of polycystic ovarian disease. *Fertil Steril.* 1991;56: 1176–1178.

29. Genadry R, Parmley T, Woodruff JD. The origin and clinical behavior of the parovarian tumor. *Am J Obstet Gynecol.* 1977;129:873–880.

30. Semm K. *Operative manual for endoscopic abdominal surgery.* Chicago: Year Book Medical Pub; 1987.

31. Herbert CM, Segars JH, Hill GA. A laparoscopic method for the excision of large retroperitoneal parovarian cysts. *Obstet Gynecol.* 1990;75: 139–141.

17

Laparoscopic Myomectomy

Bradley S. Hurst

Uterine fibroids are benign smooth muscle tumors that are found in at least 20% of women over the age of 30 years. The incidence of fibroids increases with age until the time of menopause. Fibroids may be identified in as many as 50% of nulliparous women at the age of 50.[1]

Most women with uterine leiomyomata are asymptomatic. However, symptoms attributed to myomas may include pelvic pain, pelvic pressure, urinary frequency caused by direct compression of the bladder, constipation or tenesmus from compression of the colon, abdominal bloating, or abnormal uterine bleeding. Submucous myomas or large intramural myomas may be associated with recurrent pregnancy loss and infertility.

Surgery is indicated when significant symptoms are directly attributed to the uterine fibroids. Additionally, surgery is recommended for rapidly growing myomas that may be malignant. Abdominal myomectomy has been the standard of care for a patient who desires to maintain her reproductive potential. Hysterectomy, either by abdominal or vaginal route, is the most common surgical procedure for symptomatic patients who do not wish to have children. With the development and improvement of endoscopic equipment and surgical techniques, however, laparoscopic myomectomy is now considered to be an alternative to major abdominal or vaginal surgery.

Preoperative Evaluation and Preparation

Preoperative Evaluation

The goal of the preoperative evaluation is to determine if surgery is required and, if so, what procedure is optimal. Causes for infertility and multiple pregnancy losses should be completely evaluated before surgery. Additional causes for the physical symptoms associated with fibroids should be explored. Abnormal uterine bleeding from cervical factors, ovulatory dysfunction, and endometrial abnormalities such as polyps, hyperplasia, or adenocarcinoma should be excluded before myomectomy. When no other correctable findings are identified, the patient must decide if her symptoms are sufficiently severe to warrant surgery.

Radiographic imaging may help to determine whether an endoscopic procedure is appropriate and advisable. Ultrasonography may provide information about the size, number, and location of fibroids. Fluid contrast ultrasound may be used to determine endometrial distortion caused by submucous or sessile myomas. Laparoscopic myomectomy is most likely to be successful when fibroids are single and pedunculated and do not distort the uterine cavity. Although laparoscopic myomectomy may be possible when fibroids are either large or quite numerous, one must question whether the endoscopic approach is safest for the patient and is least likely to result in operative complications.

Magnetic resonance imaging (MRI) can accurately provide specific information about the location of the myoma(s). MRI may be more precise than conventional ultrasound in defining whether the myoma is submucous, intramural, subserous, or pedunculated. However, the high cost and limited availability of MRI prohibit the routine use of this imaging technique.

Hysterosalpingography (HSG) is an extremely useful tool in the preoperative assessment of the patient suspected of having a submucous myoma. An HSG outlines the intrauterine portion of the myoma and may give a hint as to the site and extent of the myometrial attachment (see Fig. 28.1). Furthermore, an HSG will define the relationship of the myoma to the fallopian tube(s) and provide a preoperative assessment of tubal patency. If subserous, intramural, or pedunculated myomas are confirmed by either ultrasound or MRI, it may be possible to remove them laparoscopically. However, multiple deep intramural myomas may result in unac-

ceptable blood loss and myometrial damage if removed with the laparoscope and should probably be removed by laparotomy.

Preoperative Preparation

Laparoscopic myomectomy is one of the more difficult procedures that may be performed by the gynecologic laparoscopist, and should be attempted only by those with extensive experience in operative endoscopy. The potential morbidity associated with this procedure includes massive blood loss, infection, uterine rupture during pregnancy, and extensive postoperative adhesions. With these cautions in mind, several operative principles should be observed when laparoscopic myomectomy is performed.

The ability to perform a laparoscopic myomectomy is greatly limited by the size, position, and number of myomas. Preoperative gonadotropin-releasing hormone (GnRH) analogs may provide several potential benefits when laparoscopic surgery is proposed. First, GnRH analogs reduce cyclic or dysfunctional uterine bleeding and allow for a normalization of hemoglobin in patients who are anemic. Second, GnRH analogs decrease the uterine volume and the size of myomas, which may make them easier to remove.[2] Third, uterine blood flow and myometrial vascularity decrease with GnRH analog treatment. If preoperative ovarian suppression is elected, patients should be treated for 2 to 4 months before surgery to maximize the efficacy of this therapy.

The patient and surgeon should always be prepared for the possibility of an abdominal myomectomy. Laparotomy may be necessary because of bleeding or technical difficulty with the laparoscopic procedure. Furthermore, the patient should be informed that hysterectomy may be necessary if attempts at uterine repair are unsuccessful. Although hysterectomy is rarely necessary during abdominal myomectomy, there are no reports that address the incidence of emergency hysterectomy when laparoscopic myomectomy is attempted.

Autologous blood should be available before surgery whenever possible. If impossible, the patient should be cross-matched for a possible transfusion. Unlike most laparoscopic surgeries, the patient may require postoperative admission for close observation for bleeding, fever, infection, or other complications that arise from laparoscopic myomectomy. While fever is quite common after myomectomy, infection is unusual. Nevertheless, prophylactic antibiotics are frequently administered before laparoscopic myomectomy although there are no prospective trials evaluating their efficacy. Unless there is an immediate postoperative complication, there is no need to require a prolonged recuperation or to schedule an extended leave from work.

Techniques and Instrumentation

Instrumentation

Laparoscopic instruments necessary for myomectomy are similar to those required for other extensive laparoscopic procedures. An operating laparoscope or a straight laparoscope may be used. A video monitor system is necessary to allow visualization by the operator and assistants. Four incisions (three suprapubic and one umbilical) are generally required. A laparoscopic needle and syringe are necessary if the myometrium is to be injected with vasopressin. Alternately, this can be done transabdominally with a spinal needle under direct laparoscopic visualization.

A CO_2, potassium-titanyl-phosphate (KTP), argon, or neodymium:yttrium-aluminum-garnet (Nd:YAG) laser may be used to make the serosal incision, but lasers are not required. The incision may be made effectively with a monopolar microcautery tip, a laparoscopic knife, or common laparoscopic scissors. A grasper with teeth is essential and must be large enough to grasp the fibroid and provide adequate traction. Alternately, a laparoscopic myoma screw can be used for traction. Sharp scissors are necessary to dissect the myoma from the pseudocapsule. This can also be accomplished with lasers, particularly the sapphire tip of a Nd:YAG laser. An instrument for morcellation should be available.

Bipolar cautery, monopolar cautery, diathermy, or a laser with coagulation capabilities is essential to establish myometrial hemostasis. For a pedunculated myoma, large bipolar electrocautery paddles may be quite useful. A rapid irrigating and aspirating system is absolutely required. An automatic high-flow insufflator that provides a continuous pneumoperitoneum is now considered standard. Laparoscopic suturing equipment, such as the Auto Suture® EndoStitch® must be readily available, and the surgeon must be thoroughly experienced with their use.

Intracorporeal or vaginal ultrasound can be used in the operating room to define the position and size of an intramural fibroid and help determine the optimal incision site if intramural myomas are to be removed.[3] In addition, an adhesion barrier such as expanded polytetrafluoroethylene (E-PTFE, Preclude®, W.L. Gore, Inc.) should be available. Instruments to perform vaginal abdominal surgery should be accessible. If myomas are too large to be removed through the laparoscope and cannot be morcellated, they may be removed through a posterior colpotomy or a minilaparotomy incision.

Because operating time may be prolonged, a Foley catheter is placed to be sure that the pelvis will not be obscured by an enlarging bladder. A rigid instrument such as a Humi® (Unimar) cannula is used to allow for uterine manipulation.

Procedure Specifics

Basic operative laparoscopic techniques are used to prepare the patient for surgery. A sub- or intraumbilical incision is made for the laparoscope, and a midline suprapubic incision is used for suction, irrigation, or operative instruments. The placement site of the additional suprapubic operating ports will depend on the location of the myoma. A retracting instrument is generally placed through the port opposite the dissecting instrument, which can be placed either through the midline or a lateral port.

Removal of Pedunculated Subserosal Myomas

The following steps are recommended for removal of a pedunculated myoma. First, the fibroid is grasped and held in a position to allow bipolar cautery paddles to be placed across the pedicle. If the stalk is thin, a pretied loop of absorbable suture such as an Endoloop® can be placed and secured at the base (Fig. 17.1A). If the stalk is thick, a suture placed through the base of the stalk and tied fore and aft will ensure hemostasis. The bipolar instrument is then passed through the incision opposite the retracting instrument. Whenever possible, the bipolar cautery should be placed across the entire pedicle, above the suture ligature and close to the myoma (Fig. 17.1B). If this is not possible, the stalk may be coagulated in two or more sections. The bipolar cautery is activated until coagulation has stopped and there is no current flow.

The surgeon should attempt to minimize electrocautery damage to normal myometrium. While continuing to gently hold the myoma with the grasper, the bipolar cautery is replaced with scissors. The stalk is then sharply resected (Fig. 17.1C). Monopolar cautery scissors may be used to resect the stalk instead of the bipolar cautery system. If this instrument is used, a cutting current should be applied between the suture ligature and the myoma. If required, the defect produced by excision of the myoma may then be cauterized with bipolar or monopolar cautery until hemostasis has been accomplished.

A fibroid less than 1 cm in diameter can be pulled directly through the 10-mm trocar with grasping forceps or a myoma screw. For a

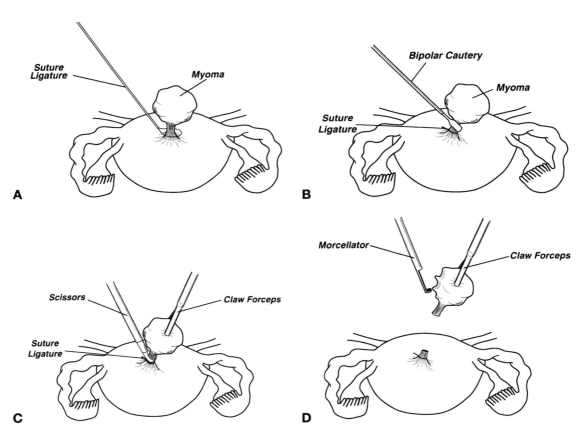

FIGURE 17.1.   Techniques for removal of a pedunculated myoma. **A:** A pretied loop of absorbable suture is secured at the base of the stalk. **B:** The fibroid is grasped and held to allow a bipolar cautery to be placed across the entire pedicle above the su- ture ligature. **C:** Scissors are used to resect the stalk at the bipolar cautery site. **D:** Large claw forceps are used to grasp the myoma. The morcellator is used to decrease the size of the myoma.

larger myoma, sharp morcellation can be attempted (Fig. 17.1D). If morcellation is not possible, the fibroid can sometimes be grasped with one instrument and progressively cut into smaller pieces with a monopolar cautery or scissors placed through the other operating channel. The myoma should be shaved in the anterior cul-de-sac to reduce the possibility of injury to the bowel. Fragments can be removed through the 10-mm laparoscope channel. If the myoma cannot be removed in this manner, it may be necessary to remove it through a colpotomy or abdominal incision, as is described later in this chapter.

Removal of Subserosal/Intramural Myomas

The laparoscopic removal of fibroids that are subserosal or intramural presents more of a challenge than does the resection of pedunculated fibroids. The operative principles followed should be the same as those used at laparotomy. Specifically, the incision should be in the anterior uterus when possible. Endoscopic or vaginal ultrasound may help identify the optimal incision site of an intramural myoma that would otherwise be difficult to visualize with the laparoscope.[3] On occasion, more than one myoma can be removed through the uterine incision. Care should be taken to avoid trauma to the surrounding normal myometrium. To reduce blood loss, the incision site may be injected with vasopressin. One ampule (20 U) of vasopressin is diluted with 20 ml of saline and injected directly into the incision site either transabdominally or via a laparoscopic needle. Blanching of the serosa should be observed.

An incision is then made over the fibroid with a CO_2, KTP, argon, or Nd:YAG laser, a fine-tip monopolar cautery or knife, or scissors (Fig. 17.2A). The choice of instrument is made at the discretion of the surgeon, as there are no data that suggest that any one method is superior to another. The incision is carried into the body of the myoma. A blunt probe is used to differentiate and expose the superficial aspect of the myoma from the myometrial pseudocapsule (Fig. 17.2B). The myoma is then grasped with forceps with teeth or a my-

oma screw. Dissecting scissors are inserted through the contralateral lower abdominal incision. Countertraction is applied with the holding instrument while the myoma is sharply dissected from the pseudocapsule with scissors (Fig. 17.2C).

When dissection becomes difficult, the grasping forceps and scissors are reversed and placed through the opposite trocars, and dissection is continued in the opposite side of the myoma. The myoma should never be pulled or twisted from its base because this may disrupt the endometrium. Rather, the base of the myoma should be sharply excised. After the myoma has been removed, it is placed in the posterior cul-de-sac. Monopolar or laser coagulation of the base may be required to achieve hemostasis.

If additional myomas are found, they should be removed through the initial uterine incision if possible. The myometrium is grasped and retracted to provide maximal exposure of the second myoma through the prior incision. The incision is made deeper into the myometrium and the additional myomas exposed. Again, the superficial aspect of the myoma is separated from the pseudocapsule by dissection with a blunt manipulator. The myoma is grasped and sharply cut from the pseudocapsule as previously described. All fibroids collected should be placed in the posterior cul-de-sac to avoid losing any tissue.

Once the myomectomy has been completed, the myometrium is coagulated until adequate hemostasis is achieved (Fig. 17.3A). An irrigator system is invaluable for maintaining a clear operative field and identifying small bleeding sites. Hemostasis may be achieved by either bipolar cautery, monopolar cautery, a thermal endocoagulator, an Nd:YAG laser, or a defocused CO_2 laser. Of these, the defocused CO_2 laser is probably the least efficient, while all the other options are acceptable. Both irrigation fluid and blood will dramatically reduce the effectiveness of any of these coagulation modalities, so the operative area should be kept as dry as possible to achieve hemostasis.

New instruments for laparoscopic suturing have greatly simplified closure of the myometrial defect. The AutoSuture Endo Stitch® al-

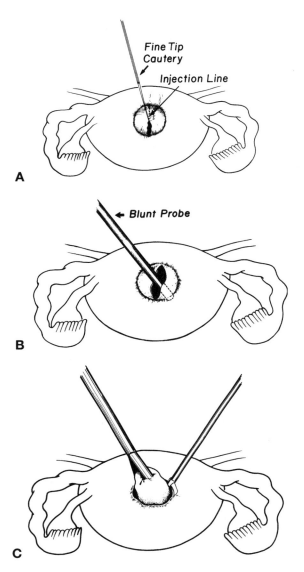

FIGURE 17.2. Technique for removal of a subserous or intramural myoma. **A:** Vasopressin is injected into the incision site *(dotted line)*. The incision is made down to the myoma. **B:** A blunt probe is used to expose the superficial aspect of the myoma. **C:** The myoma is grasped and countertraction is applied while the myoma is dissected from the pseudocapsule with scissors.

lows easy passage of the needle through tissue of limited thickness with controlled transfer of the needle. Because the device cannot be used for thick layers of myometrium, closure in multiple layers may be necessary. To facilitate closure of the base of the myomectomy incision, the myometrium should be grasped adjacent to the desired suture placement (Fig. 17.3B). The suture is tied intracorporeally with a surgeon's knot, and the myometrial layer is closed with a continuous interlocking suture. A grasper is necessary to hold and prevent slippage of the suture. Two or three layers may be required to close the myometrium and eliminate the dead space, depending on the depth of the defect. The serosa is closed with a continuous interlocking layer of 4-0 absorbable suture to give maximal hemostasis.

Recent studies have shown that microsurgical closure of myomectomy sites is associated with a high incidence of adhesions, and it is expected that a similarly high rate of adhesions will occur after a laparoscopic myomectomy.[4] Expanded polytetrafluoroethylene (E-PTFE, Preclude®) has been shown to reduce adhesions at myomectomy sites during laparotomy

FIGURE 17.3. Technique for removal of a subserous
or intramural myoma. **A:** After myomectomy, the
myometrium is coagulated with either endocoagulation *(depicted)* or electrocoagulation to achieve hemostasis. **B:** The myometrium is closed in layers with
absorbable suture. An automatic suturing device is
used for placement and transfer of the needle
through tissue *(Endo Stitch,* Ethicon, Inc., Cincinnati, OH). A grasper can be used to hold and expose adjacent myometrium to facilitate suture placement. **C:** A permanent adhesion barrier (e.g.,
Gore-Tex surgical membrane, W. L. Gore and Associates Medical Products, Phoenix, AZ) is placed over
the suture line, overlapping the edges of the incision by at least 1 cm. The barrier should be secured
with at least one permanent suture or staple.

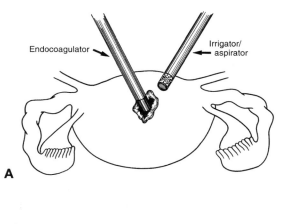

A

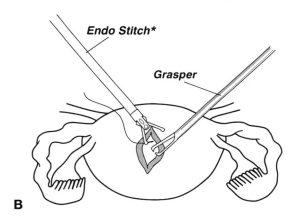

B

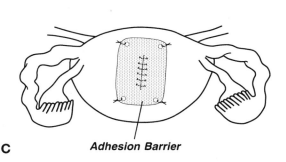

C

and can be used for laparoscopy. A piece large
enough to completely cover the defect and
overlap the new edge by at least 1 to 2 cm
should be used (Fig. 17.3C); Usually a 4 × 6
cm barrier is adequate. The barrier is rolled
and introduced through a 5- or 10-mm channel, then unrolled intracorporeally and placed
over the defect. The barrier must be permanently secured, with a fine (4-0 or smaller) permanent suture or by using a laparoscopic stapling device such as the AutoSuture Endo
Hernia Stapler® with a roticulating head. Although only one permanent fixture is required, the four edges should be secured by
fine absorbable or permanent suture or with
staples. As E-PTFE is FDA approved as a permanent implant, subsequent removal is not required.

Closure of the endometrium deserves special
attention. With careful dissection, creation of

an endometrial defect should be rare. However, despite the best technique, sometimes an
endometrial defect is created during dissection
and must be repaired. As with conventional
surgery, the edges of the endometrial defect
should be gently retracted with graspers. The
endometrium is repaired with fine (4-0) interrupted absorbable sutures, placed so that the
knots are positioned within the uterine cavity.
Use of the EndoStitch® device facilitates this
closure. The myometrium can be closed as previously described.

Removal of Myoma Tissue from the Pelvic Cavity

Fibroids may be removed through the trocar as
described previously, but two other methods
should be considered if a direct approach is
unsuccessful. First, a minilaparotomy may be

performed. Before a minilaparotomy is done, several preliminary steps must be completed because the laparotomy will likely result in loss of most or all of the pneumoperitoneum and will make further laparoscopic procedures virtually impossible. Hemostasis is obtained at all operative sites and all fluids are aspirated from the pelvis. That is, the laparoscopic procedure is effectively completed with the exception of removing the fibroids from the pelvis. The fibroid is then held with the laparoscopic grasper or hook and held up to the spot where the minilap incision will be made. The abdominal incision should be slightly larger than the myoma. Once the incision has been made and the peritoneum has been opened, the grasping instrument is passed through the incision and the myoma directly removed from the abdomen.

A third alternative is removal of the myomas through a colpotomy incision. Again, hemostasis should be established and the pelvis irrigated before colpotomy because the incision will cause loss of the pneumoperitoneum. The fibroid is held with the laparoscopic grasper or hook so that the fibroid may be directly passed through the colpotomy incision when it is made. The colpotomy is opened under laparoscopic guidance, and the myomas are removed. The incision is closed in the usual manner.

Need for Laparotomy

Laparotomy may be necessary in the face of difficulty or complications, and should never be considered a procedure of last resort. It is foolhardy to continue a procedure laparoscopically if serious morbidity is a distinct possibility. Significant bleeding that cannot be quickly controlled is an indication for immediate laparotomy. Major surgery is also necessary for small bleeders that cannot be completely controlled. Long or deep myometrial incisions that cannot be repaired laparoscopically should be handled via laparotomy, using microsurgical techniques to limit blood loss and to reduce adhesion formation. If multiple myomas are unexpectedly identified, or if the myomas are too large or too deep in the muscle of the uterus to remove safely, laparotomy should be performed. Laparotomy also should be performed if the endometrium is exposed or disrupted during the procedure and cannot be sufficiently repaired laparoscopically. In short, laparotomy should never be perceived as a defeat, but rather as a prudent step to ensure the safety and well-being of the patient in the case of a difficult procedure or significant complications.

Postoperative Care and Complications

Although same-day discharge can be expected after resection of a pedunculated myoma, a patient who has undergone a successful subserous or intramural laparoscopic myomectomy should be hospitalized as an inpatient for 24 hr. Serial hemoglobin levels should be obtained postoperatively, and the patient's vital signs should be monitored every 4 hr. There need be no physical restrictions on activity postoperatively if the patient's vital signs are stable.

Several delayed complications may be more likely following a laparoscopic myomectomy compared to abdominal myomectomy. Bleeding may occur from the intraabdominal operative sites, and the patient may become hemodynamically unstable. For a patient with a progressively declining hemoglobin or unstable vital signs, further diagnosis and probable reoperation will be necessary. Laparoscopy may be performed initially to determine whether or not there is bleeding from the incision. If bleeding is identified, laparoscopic coagulation is acceptable. However, if the site cannot be controlled laparoscopically, or if there are multiple bleeding sites or brisk bleeding, laparotomy should be performed.

Fever is quite common after abdominal myomectomy and can also occur after a laparoscopic myomectomy. Postoperative fever should be evaluated and managed just as it is for the patient undergoing an abdominal procedure. The additional danger, however, comes from an unsuspected bowel injury. If there is significant suspicion or evidence of bowel injury, or if fever does not respond to aggressive antibiotic therapy, laparotomy is warranted.

Extensive adhesion formation and the risk of bowel obstruction caused by adhesions may occur after laparoscopic myomectomy as a result of large defects in the uterus. For this reason, use of adhesion barrier such as E-PTFE is strongly recommended. Interceed® has not yet been tested on myomectomy incisions, but animal studies have shown an increase in adhesions when this product is used to cover a bleeding site.[5] Hyskon and other adjuvants are of limited use. An unexplored approach to reduce postoperative adhesions following laparoscopic myomectomy is the use of early second-look laparoscopy for adhesiolysis.

Uterine rupture during pregnancy is a potential concern with laparoscopic myomectomy. Uterine rupture has been reported after laparoscopic myomectomy, but the overall incidence of this complication is not known.[6] It is hoped that adequate closure of myometrial incisions will keep this a rare complication. Routine cesarean section is not advocated unless the procedure has been complicated by an infection or hematoma at the incision site, a deep defect of the myometrium has been made, or the endometrial cavity has been entered during the procedure. However, all patients should be informed of the potential risk of uterine rupture with pregnancy before considering laparoscopic myomectomy.

Alternative Techniques

Expectant management should be elected for patients with minimal symptoms unless there is rapid growth of fibroids or if the adnexae cannot be evaluated.[1] Symptoms caused by fibroids may improve after a course of GnRH analog therapy. Symptomatic relief may persist even after regrowth of fibroids after GnRH analog therapy.[2] Hysterectomy is the procedure of choice for patients with symptomatic fibroids who no longer desire fertility. Abdominal myomectomy remains the primary procedure for symptomatic patients who desire preservation of fertility.

Myoma coagulation is a new alternative to laparoscopic myomectomy. This procedure, sometimes referred to as "myolysis," is performed by coagulation and devascularization of the myoma base at multiple sites.[7] The size of large myomas may be reduced by more than 50%, and fibroids smaller than 3 cm may be completely lysed. The Nd:YAG laser was used initially for myolysis.[7] A special bipolar needle electrode has recently gained popularity for this procedure, although the benefits of this approach remain to be proven.

Unfortunately, there is little information about the long-term outcome of myolysis, and it is not certain that surgeons will be able to duplicate or exceed published results. Until more studies are available, it would be unwise to assume that fertility will be preserved or enhanced with laparoscopic myolysis. Furthermore, it is not known if the physical and functional integrity of the uterine wall will be preserved with this technique or if the risk of uterine rupture will be increased. Long-term assessment of uterine bleeding, uterine pain, and regrowth of fibroids must be addressed. Outcome analysis is needed to compare myolysis, laparoscopic myomectomy, and abdominal myomectomy.

Outcome and Results

Published results of laparoscopic myomectomy are encouraging. Although adhesions may be found during second-look laparoscopy in as many as two-thirds of patients after these procedures, other authors have described surprisingly low rates of postoperative adhesions and laparoscopic myomectomy.[8,9] Relief of pain and pressure symptoms following laparoscopic myomectomy is excellent.[8-10]

One must remember that many surgical series are biased and may go unreported if results are poor. Additionally, most reports describe the study of a very limited number of patients. Therefore, laparoscopic myomectomy should be limited until key questions as to the relative efficacy and safety of the procedure can be determined by appropriate studies. Until such data are available, abdominal myomectomy remains the procedure of choice, except for select patients.

Conclusions

Advanced instruments and surgical techniques have made increasingly difficult endoscopic procedures a possibility. Laparoscopic myomectomy requires highly advanced surgical skills. One must recognize that the availability of equipment and the technical ability to perform these procedures does not allow one to conclude that these procedures are optimal or even appropriate for uterine fibroids. Most fibroids that can easily be removed with the laparoscope probably do not require surgical resection at all.

The potential complications associated with laparoscopic myomectomy are serious enough that incidental or elective laparoscopic myomectomy is rarely, if ever, indicated. On the other hand, carefully selected patients may be good candidates for laparoscopic or hysteroscopic myomectomy in the hands of an experienced endoscopist. When an endoscopic myomectomy is performed, technique must be impeccable and hemostasis scrupulously confirmed. The surgeon should have a very low threshold for laparotomy should complications arise.

References

1. Entman SS. Uterine leiomyoma and adenomyosis. In: Jones HW, III, Wentz AC, Burnett LS, eds. *Novak's Textbook of Gynecology.* 11th ed. Baltimore: Williams & Wilkins; 1988:443–454.
2. Schlaff WD, Zerhouni EA, Huth JAM, et al. A placebo-controlled trial of depot gonadotropin-releasing hormone analog (leuprolide) in the treatment of uterine leiomyomata. *Obstet Gynecol.* 1989;74:856–862.
3. Hurst BS, Tucker KE, Awoniyi CA, et al. Endoscopic ultrasound: a new instrument for laparoscopic surgery. *J Reprod Med.* 1996;41:67–70.
4. The Myomectomy Adhesion Multicenter Study Group. An expanded polytetrafluoroethylene barrier (Gore-Tex Surgical Membrane) reduces post-myomectomy adhesion formation. *Fertil Steril.* 1995;63:491–493.
5. Linsky CB, Diamond MP, Cunningham T, et al. Effect of blood on the efficiency of barrier adhesion reduction in the rabbit uterine horn model. *Infertility.* 1988;11:273–280.
6. Harris WJ. Uterine dehiscence following laparoscopic myomectomy. *Obstet Gynecol.* 1992; 80:545–546.
7. Goldfarb HA. Nd:YAG laser laparoscopic coagulation of symptomatic myomas. *J Reprod Med.* 1992;37:636–638.
8. Hasson HM, Rotman C, Rana N, et al. Laparoscopic myomectomy. *Obstet Gynecol.* 1992;80: 884–888.
9. Nezhat C, Nezhat F, Bess O, et al. Laparoscopically assisted myomectomy: a report of a new technique in 57 cases. *Int J Fertil Menopause Stud.* 1994;39:39–44.
10. Mettler L, Semm K. Pelviscopic uterine surgery. *Surg Endosc.* 1992;6:23–31.

18

Laparoscopic Uterine Nerve Ablation, Presacral Neurectomy, and Uterovaginal Ganglion Excision

C. Paul Perry

A number of less frequently used laparoscopic procedures are discussed in this chapter. These techniques may be useful in the treatment of certain forms of pelvic pain. Nevertheless, experience with these procedures is still limited, patients should be selected very carefully, and the surgery should be performed only by experienced laparoscopists.

Laparoscopic Uterosacral Nerve Ablation or Resection

Introduction

In 1955 Doyle reported the vaginal interruption of the uterosacral ligaments for the relief of dysmenorrhea, as the majority of uterine sensory fibers traverse these ligaments. Various surgeons now interrupt these nerves laparoscopically.[1,2]

Indications and Patient Selection

Patients undergoing laparoscopic surgery and those who complain of significant central dysmenorrhea may be considered candidates for laparoscopic uterosacral nerve ablation (LUNA). No significant benefit will result from LUNA if the origin of the pain is extrauterine, including pelvic peritoneal surfaces, distal tubes, or ovaries. Patients with severe dysmenorrhea and minimal extrauterine pathology are the best candidates for this procedure.

At the time of laparoscopy, if distortion of the pelvic anatomy from scarring or endometriosis impedes clear identification of the uterosacral ligament, LUNA should not be attempted.

Technique

Laparoscopic ablation of the uterosacral nerve is relatively easy to perform. Potassium-titanyl-phosphate (KTP), argon, or contact-tip neodymium: yttrium-aluminum-garnet (Nd:YAG) fiber lasers can be used through the operative channel of the laparoscope or suprapubically. Alternatively, smoke production and lack of desiccation with the carbon dioxide (CO_2) laser make this instrument less than ideal for this purpose. Finally, LUNA can be performed with bipolar electrodesiccation and transection/resection with scissors. Bipolar desiccation before transection is advised.

The uterus should be displaced toward the anterior abdominal wall using an intrauterine manipulator. The ureter should be identified and atraumatically deviated laterally beforehand with a blunt probe. The uterosacral ligament is identified and followed to its insertion on the uterus. Laser energy is applied to the medial aspect of the ligament at its junction with the uterus until totally or partially ablated (Fig. 18.1). Total transection can be facilitated by grasping the unroofed uterosacral ligament with atraumatic forceps and stretching toward

the midline. A relaxing incision can be made in the peritoneum just lateral to the uterosacral ligament and medial to the ureter. This greatly facilitates the isolation and safe, complete transection of the nerve fibers (Fig. 18.2) Usually a 1.5- to 2-cm-long by 1.0-cm-deep area of vaporization through the ligament is required. There are some small vessels deep in the ligament that will require desiccation. A superficial "U"-shaped area of vaporization, connecting the two interrupted uterosacral ligament segments, may also be performed along the posterior aspect of the utero–cul-de-sac junction. This transects interconnecting fibers otherwise missed. Care must be used to avoid injury to the rectum during this step.

Incisions or ablation too far lateral to the ligament should be avoided because this may result in significant bleeding or ureteral injury. Any bleeding occurring after LUNA should be managed by bipolar and not unipolar electrodesiccation to decrease the possibility of ureteral injury.

Total uterosacral ligament excision occasionally may be preferable if endometriosis is deeply invasive in this area. This can be accomplished by first making the peritoneal relaxing incision just lateral and parallel to the ligament and medial to the ureter. The ureter must be clearly visible throughout its pelvic course be-

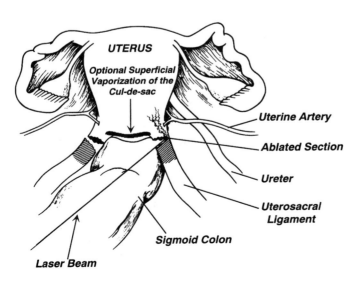

FIGURE 18.1. Laparoscopic uterosacral nerve ablation (LUNA). The uterus should be displaced toward the anterior abdominal wall by an intrauterine manipulator. The uterosacral ligament and the ureter are identified along their entire course in the pelvis. Laser energy is applied to the medial aspect of the ligament at its junction with the uterus until totally or partially ablated. Usually a 1.5- to 2-cm-long by 1.0-cm-deep area of vaporization through the ligament is required. A superficial "U"-shaped area of vaporization, connecting the two interrupted uterosacral ligament segments, may also be performed along the posterior aspect of the utero–cul-de-sac junction, which transects interconnecting fibers otherwise missed.

FIGURE 18.2. A relaxing incision is made medial to the ureter and lateral to the uterosacral ligament. This greatly enhances the safety of LUNA, and excision can be accomplished if necessary.

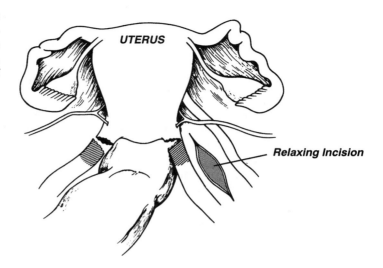

fore performing this maneuver. The uterosacral ligament may then be bluntly isolated, its origin and insertion coagulated with bipolar electrodesiccation, and the entire ligament safely excised. No data are yet available comparing pain relief with this technique to that with the standard LUNA procedure.

Results

The success of LUNA for relief of primary dysmenorrhea has ranged from 70% to 49% after 1 year of follow-up.[1,2] Relief of secondary dysmenorrhea caused by endometriosis by the LUNA procedure was reported to be 71%.[1] Unfortunately, no long-term follow-up studies are available, but it appears that the effectiveness of LUNA may decrease over time.[2] We have performed this procedure in more than 300 patients with endometriosis. A retrospective analysis of 91 patients found that one-half of our patients experienced at least 50% reduction in their pain during the first 2 years following surgery. By the third year, only 32% were experiencing at least 50% reduction in their pain level.

Early in our experience with LUNA, two patients required laparotomy for control of bleeding. Acquisition of bipolar electrodesiccation skills will decrease the need for open hemostasis. Further long-term studies are required to fully determine the efficacy and complication rate of this procedure.

Laparoscopic Presacral Neurectomy

Introduction

Since its introduction in 1898 by Jaboulay, presacral neurectomy for pelvic pain and dysmenorrhea has enjoyed periods of fluctuating enthusiasm. Cotte, the first surgeon to perform the procedure in the United States, reported some 1500 cases in 1938 with a 98% success rate. Presacral neurectomy was performed frequently throughout the 1940s and 1950s for both primary and secondary dysmenorrhea. Black compiled almost 10,000 cases from the literature, physician questionnaires, and personal experience and reported an overall success rate ranging from 75% to 80%.[3] The next 20 years were marked by the development of superior medical therapies for dysmenorrhea. Oral contraceptives, nonsteroidal antiinflammatory agents, and gonadotropin-releasing hormone agonists succeeded in pain control for most patients. However, even today some patients fail to respond to, or do not tolerate, conservative therapy.

Recent advances in operative laparoscopy offer the potential for relief of central dysmenorrhea by presacral neurectomy, without the need to resort to laparotomy. Laparoscopic presacral neurectomy (LPSN) may prove to be the treatment of choice in certain carefully selected patients. However, it must not be overutilized, for the fewer we do, the better results we will experience. Also, it should be undertaken only after proper training.

Indications and Patient Selection

Patients with central, not lateral, primary or secondary dysmenorrhea are considered the best candidates. They should have failed other conservative treatments, including LUNA if appropriate. Patients with endometriosis (other than minimal) might best be treated with laparoscopic resection of endometriosis and LPSN, because extrauterine pain responds poorly to LUNA. Nevertheless, low back pain, lateral pelvic pain, and dyspareunia may or may not respond to LPSN.

Patients should be fully informed regarding the potential risks and need for laparotomy. Vascular and ureteral injury along with possible incomplete pain relief or pain recurrence should be discussed. Constipation and vaginal dryness have been a problem for a few patients postoperatively. Painless first stage of labor and urinary retention should be mentioned, but these have been rare in our experience.

Technique

Laparoscopic presacral neurectomy (LPSN), unlike LUNA, requires a significant degree of surgical skill. It should be undertaken only by those surgeons familiar with the retroperitoneal anatomy. The presacral nerve is actually the superior hypogastric plexus, which is 1 of about 23 sympathetic collateral plexuses supplying efferent stimulation to the viscera. The superior portion is retroperitoneal and runs from the bifurcation of the aorta to the junction of the vertebral bodies of L5–S1. There it forms the middle hypogastric plexus, which divides at the level of the first sacral vertebral body into the right and left inferior hypogastric plexus. Somatic afferent fibers travel along with these sympathetic nerves, transmitting pain sensation to the spinal cord from the various target organs and peritoneal surfaces.

Most of the sensory fibers from the uterus and cervix traverse this plexus. Other afferent nerve fibers follow vascular supplies and cannot be interrupted by presacral neurectomy. Sacral parasympathetic fibers referring pain to the low back and low lateral suprapubic area usually are not affected. From their embryologic derivation, the distal third of the fallopian tubes and the ovaries receive their nerve supply from the aortic collateral plexus on the right and the renal collateral plexus on the left. Therefore, presacral neurectomy should not be expected to be consistently effective for lateral pelvic pain.[4]

Expert, meticulous dissection is required during LPSN. The boundaries for resection are exactly the same as those at laparotomy: superiorly, the bifurcation of the aorta; on the right, the right internal iliac artery and right ureter; on the left, the inferior mesenteric and superior hemorrhoidal arteries; and inferiorly, just below the division of the right and left inferior hypogastric plexus; and deep, the periosteum of the vertebral bodies (Fig 18.3).

This retroperitoneal area may be approached from above through the umbilical incision or from below with the suprapubic placement of the laparoscope as described by Perry and Perez.[5] Dissection is carried out via a four-puncture technique using atraumatic graspers and a blunt irrigation probe. To ensure hemostasis, bipolar desiccation should always be available. A Nd:YAG contact laser fiber (Surgical Laser Technologies, Malvern, PA) may be used through the operating channel of the laparoscope or one of the three suprapubic incisions. This instrument greatly facilitates isolation of the plexus by hemostatically interrupting fine vessels and nerve fibers that anastomose with the plexus from all directions. The fiber can be oriented so it enters the field of vision at 12 o'clock to minimize its interference with visibility. The CO_2–argon beam coagulator, laser, and electrosurgery should be used in this area with great caution because of the vulnerable left common iliac vein.

The patient is placed in exenteration stirrups with 30° Trendelenburg and a left lateral tilt to displace the bowel from the sacral promontory. If required, laparoscopic management of endometriosis is performed first. Following, all structures defining the anatomic extent of dissection are identified. The peri-

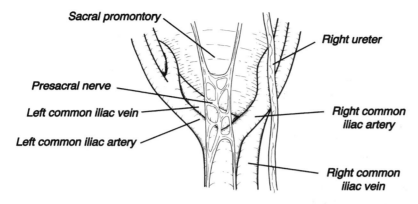

FIGURE 18.3. The anatomic landmarks for a laparoscopic presacral neurectomy (LPSN). Note the vulnerable left common iliac vein.

toneum overlying the sacral promontory is then grasped and elevated before incision. A superficial transverse peritoneal incision is made over the sacral promontory (body of the L5 vertebra) between the inferior mesenteric artery on the left and the right internal iliac artery, about 1 cm cephalad to the right ureteral crossing (Fig. 18.4). The peritoneal edges retract after being cut and require very little manipulation to maintain exposure. Blunt dissection, bipolar electrodissection, or laser energy can be used to separate the fine

nerves and vessels between the undersurface of the peritoneum and the loose connective tissue layer of the presacral space. This will help mobilize the presacral tissues.

The presacral nerve is isolated by developing the avascular space between the nerve and right internal iliac artery down to the periosteum (Fig. 18.5). The plexus usually runs to the left of the midline. Therefore, the next area of dissection should be carried out far enough on the left to ensure complete neural resection but without disturbing the inferior

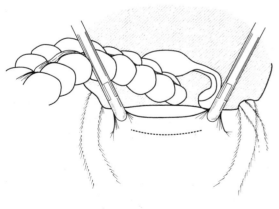

FIGURE 18.4. A transverse incision is made in the peritoneum over the presacral nerve at a level 1 to 2 cm rostral to the crossing of the ureter and the right common iliac artery.

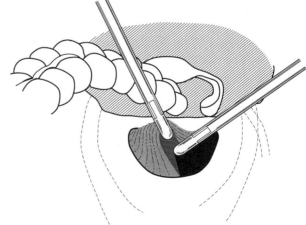

FIGURE 18.5. Isolation of the right border of the presacral nerve down to the periosteum of the L5 vertebral body.

mesenteric artery, the root of the sigmoid mesentery, or the left ureter. This space between the inferior mesenteric artery and the presacral nerve should be dissected bluntly down to the periosteum as well. Care should be taken not to injure the left common iliac vein, which is frequently found in the deep connective tissue of this area (Fig. 18.6).

When both the right and left borders of the superior hypogastric portion of the presacral nerve have been developed, the nerve is grasped and elevated off the sacral periosteum. The middle sacral artery and vein are closely adherent to the periosteum and can usually be avoided by careful elevation of the nerve before desiccation. The cephalad portion of the nerve is then desiccated and transected either by contact-tip laser energy or scissors. Gentle traction is applied to the remaining nerve trunk while isolating the middle plexus and right and left inferior hypogastric branches (Fig. 18.7). This dissection should proceed no more than 3 to 4 cm caudal from the point where the nerve has been transected so as not to invite troublesome bleeding from the sacral venous plexus. The inferior nerve trunks are then isolated, elevated, and coagulated. Tran-

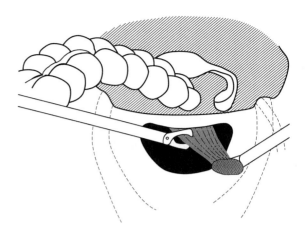

FIGURE 18.7. Traction is applied to the severed presacral nerve, and the right and left inferior hypogastric branches can be visualized, desiccated, and excised.

section is accomplished proximal to the coagulated neural and fatty tissue. The resected tissue should measure about 3 cm in length and can be easily drawn out of the abdomen via one of the suprapubic sites. Pathologic examination is useful to determine the presence of the nerve.

If bleeding from the middle sacral vessels is encountered, this usually responds to bipolar desiccation. Hemostasis may rarely require the application of stainless steel tacks on bone wax. In case of brisk bleeding, left common iliac vein laceration, or other major vessel injury, laparotomy should not be delayed.

Results

The success rate of LPSN seems to be comparable to the open procedure. A combined series of 87 patients undergoing presacral neurectomy reported a success rate of 91% with 24 months maximum follow-up.[5] We have personally performed more than 100 LPSNs at our institution. Most patients had endometriosis and had not responded to other conservative measures. At this writing we have 6 failures, with 5 patients lost to follow-up, for an overall success rate of 94% with as long as 4 years of follow-up. One patient experienced late thrombosis of the left common iliac vein from trauma sus-

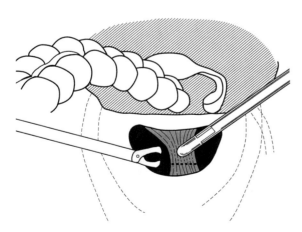

FIGURE 18.6. Isolation of the left border of the presacral nerve is demonstrated. This dissection can be difficult because of unclear dissection planes between the mesentery of the sigmoid colon and the presacral fat with the danger of left common iliac vein injury.

tained by efforts of hemostasis. No laparotomies have been necessary.

The most common reasons for failure are expected to be poor patient selection and incomplete removal of the ganglion. Incomplete removal of the plexus may result from anatomic variance or lack of presacral neurectomy experience. A 10-year follow-up will be necessary before LPSN can be properly compared with traditional presacral neurectomy.

Laparoscopic Uterovaginal Ganglion Excision (LUVE)

Introduction

In 1990, Gillespie[6] performed the first procedure to selectively ablate a portion of the uterovaginal ganglia. Destruction of the vesicoureteric plexus was used in the treatment of pain from hypersensitive bladder disorders. Of 175 patients who underwent bilateral plexus ablation, 64% reported significant relief, 33% had moderate improvement, and 7% failed to benefit.

The vesicoureteric plexus is closely associated with the uterovaginal ganglion. As the uterovaginal ganglion may be blocked with paracervically administered anesthetic, attempt to treat chronic pelvic pain based upon responses to preoperative nerve block was begun in 1993.

Indications and Patient Selection

Those patients complaining of persistent unilateral or bilateral lower pelvic pain unresponsive to other medical or surgical therapy can be considered for laparoscopic uterovaginal ganglion excision (LUVE).

After completing a visual analog pain scale, patients are administered a bilateral paracervical block (10 ml of 0.5% plain bupivacaine is used) and are asked to assess their pain 1 hr after the block. If all other therapeutic options have been exhausted, those patients noting a decrease in their pain score may be offered LUVE.

Technique

The uterovaginal ganglion is composed of parasympathetic fibers derived from nervi erigentes (S2–S4) and sympathetic fibers from the inferior hypogastric plexus (T10–L2). This coalescence of both parasympathetic and sympathetic visceral afferents offers an unusual opportunity to interrupt pain transmission from both types of autonomic fibers.

The uterovaginal ganglion is located on each side of the cervix. This nervous plexus lies in the loose connective tissue bordered by the cervix medially, the uterine artery ventrally, the vaginal or inferior vesicle artery dorsally, and the pelvic side wall laterally. The ureter lies approximately in the center of this triangle as it traverses the ureteric tunnel (Fig. 18.8).

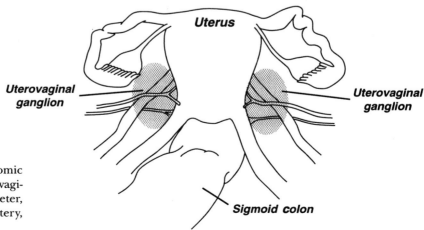

FIGURE 18.8. The anatomic relationship of the uterovaginal ganglion to the ureter, uterine artery, vaginal artery, and cervix.

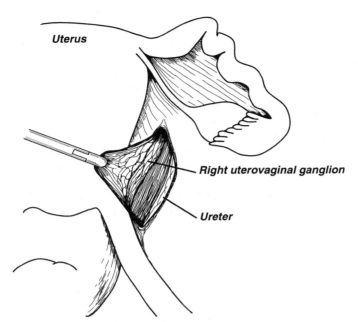

FIGURE 18.9. The right uterovaginal ganglion is being excised.

Ureteric catheters are placed to facilitate dissection of the ganglion and to safeguard the ureter. The peritoneum is incised over the ureter, and blunt dissection isolates the loose connective tissue and retroperitoneal fat containing the ganglion. Hemostatic clips are preferred over bipolar desiccation to diminish periureteral fibrosis. A segment of tissue is removed from the area bordered by the ureter above, the uterosacral ligament below, the ureteric tunnel caudally, and the midportion of the uterosacral ligament rostrally. The dissection extends laterally to the loose connective tissue of the side wall (Fig. 18.9). This tissue is submitted to pathology for confirmation of ganglion and peripheral nerves. The procedure may be performed bilaterally or unilaterally as dictated by the patient's symptoms. The peritoneum is left open.

Results

Our preliminary results include 27 patients with unilateral and bilateral LUVE procedures; 10 patients received excellent relief, 7 patients received good relief, and 2 patients were lost to follow-up with 8 failures for an overall success rate of 71%. The longest follow-up has been 2 years with good relief.

There have been no complications, and one laparotomy was required to complete the surgery because of extensive bowel adhesions in the pelvis. Four other patients required lysis of adhesions before dissection of the pelvic side wall. Three patients required oophorectomy, and one patient required bilateral salpingo-oophorectomy to complete the surgery.

No recommendations can yet be made regarding specifics of patient selection or long-term benefit. However, unlike the LUNA and LPSN, the LUVE procedure may offer selected patients relief from low lateral pelvic pain.

References

1. Feste JR. Laser laparoscopy, a new modality. *J Reprod Med.* 1985;30:413–417.
2. Lichten EM, Bombard J. Surgical treatment of primary dysmenorrhea with laparoscopic uterine nerve ablation. *J Reprod Med.* 1987;32:37–41.
3. Black WT. Use of presacral sympathectomy in the treatment of dysmenorrhea. *Am J Obstet Gynecol.* 1964;89:16–22.
4. Curtis AH, Anson BJ, Ashley FL, et al. The anatomy of the pelvic autonomic nerves in relation to gynecology. *Surg Gynecol Obstet.* 1942;75:743–750.
5. Perry CP, Perez JJ. The role of laparoscopic presacral neurectomy. *J Gynecol Surg.* 1993;9:165–168.
6. Gillespie L. Destruction of vesicoureteric plexus for the treatment of hypersensitive bladder disorders. *Br J Urol.* 1994;74:40–43.

19

Laparoscopic Treatment of Tubo-ovarian and Pelvic Abscess

Harry Reich

A pelvic abscess is a localized collection of a large number of organisms, inflammatory exudate, and necrotic debris often separated from surrounding tissue by a fibrous pseudocapsule. A tubo-ovarian complex is a tubo-ovarian abscess (TOA) that lacks a classic pseudocapsule and is made up of the agglutination of tube and ovary to adjacent pelvic and abdominal structures following reaction to purulent exudate from the inflamed tube. A true pelvic abscess with a classic pseudocapsule can occur in the ovary and after rupture of a diverticulum. Whatever the terminology, purulent material exists in a collection within the pelvis.

Abscess is the end result of an acute or subacute infection, often beginning with an initial stage of peritonitis in which aerobic bacteria predominate, followed by the development of an intraabdominal abscess with emergence of anaerobic bacteria as the predominant flora. Abscesses contain a large number of organisms in high concentration but not in a rapid growth phase, making them less susceptible to antimicrobial agents that require actively growing organisms for efficacy. In addition, the fibrous pseudocapsule, which the host makes in an attempt to control the infection, may inhibit adequate levels of antimicrobial agents from entering the abscess. The anaerobic milieu itself may hinder host defense mechanisms, reducing the ability of neutrophils to phagocytize and kill bacteria. Thus, therapy for abscesses must include some technique to drain the pus, along with appropriate antimicrobial therapy.

Until the early 1970s, clinicians who suspected a pelvic or tubo-ovarian abscess considered extirpative surgery, a total abdominal hysterectomy, and bilateral salpingo-oophorectomy (TAH/BSO). More recently, unruptured abscesses have been treated with intravenous antibiotics, with surgery reserved for poor responders to medical therapy. Although this approach avoids immediate operation, prolonged contact between necrotic and inflamed tissue often causes dense fibrous adhesions that impair reproductive potential. In an effort to avoid this problem, some gynecologists have advocated the use of laparoscopy with early lysis of acute adhesions as an alternative.

The commonly accepted belief that surgical intervention during acute pelvic infection results in greater injury than waiting for the infection to subside was initiated with the report of Simpson[1] in 1909. This opinion prevailed until recently, even though the risks associated with surgical intervention had changed drastically since the early part of the twentieth century. In reality, it is much easier to operate on acute adhesions than on the dense adhesions that later form between structures, obliterate the normal anatomic relationships, and develop neovascularization. For example, second-look laparoscopic adhesiolysis soon after infertility surgery is much easier to perform than the original operation.[2]

Electrosurgery, laser surgery, and sharp scissor dissection, all of which are useful for chronic pelvic inflammatory disease, have no place in the treatment of acute inflammatory adhesions. Simply stated, the laparoscopic treatment of acute adhesions, with or without abscess, does not require the high level of technical skill necessary to excise an endometrioma, open a hydrosalpinx, or remove an ectopic pregnancy under laparoscopic control. It is essentially an exercise in careful blunt dissection using a probe or aquadissection with a suction-irrigation device that can be performed by gynecologists experienced in operative laparoscopy using equipment available in most hospitals.

Why Laparoscopic Treatment Works

Peritoneal defense mechanisms that protect the host from invading bacteria include absorption of the microbes from the peritoneal cavity by the lymphatic system, phagocytosis by macrophages and polymorphonuclear leukocytes, complement effects, and fibrin trapping.[3] Fibrin trapping and sequestration of the bacterial inoculum by the omentum and intestine and the formation of a tubo-ovarian complex act to contain the infection initially, although abscesses may form eventually. Although the deposition of fibrin traps bacteria and decreases the frequency of septicemic death, thick fibrin deposits ultimately represent a barrier to in situ killing by neutrophils, with resultant abscess formation. Once formed, the abscess walls inhibit the effectiveness of antibiotics and the ability of the host to resolve the infection naturally.

Ahrenholz and Simmons[4] studied the role of purified fibrin in the pathogenesis of experimental intraperitoneal infection. Their conclusion was that fibrin delays the onset of systemic sepsis, but that the entrapped bacteria cannot be eliminated easily by the normal intraperitoneal bactericidal mechanisms and as a result an abscess can form. They also believed that radical peritoneal debridement or anticoagulation may reduce the septic complications of peritonitis. Stated another way, procedures that decrease fibrin deposition or facilitate fibrin removal, either enzymatically or surgically, decrease the frequency of intraperitoneal abscess formation. From this derives the rationale for extensive peritoneal lavage and radical excision of inflammatory exudate in patients with TOA. Success with the laparoscopic and laparotomy treatment of TOA by the author[5,6] and others[7–12] substantiates the laboratory work of Ahrenholz and Simmons. Laparoscopic drainage of a pelvic abscess, followed by lysis of all peritoneal cavity adhesions and excision of necrotic inflammatory exudate, allows host defenses to effectively control the infection.

Indications

Women with lower abdominal pain and a palpable or questionable pelvic mass should undergo laparoscopy to determine the true diagnosis because even "obvious TOAs" may prove to be endometriomas, hemorrhagic corpus luteum cysts, or an abscess surrounding a ruptured appendix. The worldwide average rate of misdiagnosis of pelvic inflammatory disease (PID) is 35% when laparoscopy has been used for confirmation.[13]

The diagnosis of TOA should be suspected in women with a recent or past history of PID who have persistent pain and pelvic tenderness on examination. Fever and leukocytosis may or may not be present.[14] Ultrasound frequently documents a tubo-ovarian complex or what appears to be an abscess. After the presumptive diagnosis of TOA is made, hospitalization should be arranged for laparoscopic diagnosis and treatment soon thereafter.

In patients suspected of having a TOA, intravenous antibiotics should be initiated on admission to the hospital, usually 2 to 24 hr before laparoscopy. Adequate and sustained blood levels of antibiotics are required to combat transperitoneal absorption of aerobic and anaerobic organisms during the operative procedure. This author prefers cefoxitin, 2 g intravenously, every 4 h from admission until discharge, which occurs usually on postoperative day 2 or 3.[15] The newer cephamycins, cefmetazole 2 g every 8 hr, or cefotetan 2 g every 12 hr can also be considered. Oral doxycycline is started on the first postoperative day and continued for 10 days. Although clindamycin and metronidazole both have demonstrated greater ability to enter abscess cavities and reduce bacterial counts therein, cefoxitin is used to simplify therapy to a single IV agent and assess further the efficacy of the laparoscopic surgical procedure; that is, the IV antibiotic alone should not be considered the reason for successful therapy. One pioneer in this area, Dr. Jeanine Henry-Suchet, starts antibiotics during the laparoscopic procedure only after cultures have been taken.

Instrumentation and Technique

The laparoscopic procedure is always performed under general anesthesia. A high-flow CO_2 insufflator is valuable to maintain the pneumoperitoneum and compensate for the rapid loss of CO_2 during suctioning. A Cohen or Rubin's cannula is then placed in the endocervical canal for uterine manipulation and tubal lavage. A 10-mm laparoscope is inserted through a vertical intraumbilical incision. Lower quadrant puncture sites are made above the pubic hairline and just lateral to the inferior epigastric vessels. The upper abdomen is examined and the patient is placed in a 20°

Trendelenburg's position before focusing attention on the pelvis. A Foley catheter is inserted. Through the right-sided ancillary puncture site, either a blunt probe or a grasping forcep is inserted and used for traction and retraction. Through the left-sided suprapubic sleeve, a suction-irrigation cannula (Aquapurator®, Wisap Co., Sauerlach, Germany, and Tomball, TX) or a suction probe attached to a 50-cc syringe is inserted and used to mobilize omentum, small bowel, rectosigmoid, and tubo-ovarian adhesions until the abscess cavity is entered. Purulent fluid is aspirated while the operating table is returned to a 10° Trendelenburg's position. Cultures should be taken from the aspirated fluid, from the inflammatory exudate excised with biopsy forceps, and from exudate near the tubal ostium using a bronchoscope cytology brush.

After the abscess cavity is aspirated, the dissection is continued, separating the bowel and omentum completely from the reproductive organs and lysing tubo-ovarian adhesions. Aquadissection is performed by placing the tip of the suction-irrigation cannula against the adhesive interface between bowel–adnexa, tube–ovary, or adnexa–pelvic side wall, then using both the cannula tip and the pressurized physiologic solution to develop a dissection plane (Fig. 19.1). The dissection can then be extended either bluntly or with continued fluid pressure. A 3- or 5-mm grasping forcep places the tissue to be dissected on tension so that the surgeon can identify the distorted tissue plane accurately before aquadissection. When the dissection is completed, the abscess cavity (necrotic inflammatory exudate) is excised in pieces using a 5-mm biopsy forceps.

It is important to remember that after ovulation purulent material from acute salpingitis may gain entrance to the inner ovary by inoculation of the corpus luteum, which may then become part of the abscess wall. Thus, after draining the abscess cavity and mobilizing the entire ovary, a gaping hole of varying size may be noted in the ovary that heretofore had been intimately involved in the abscess cavity. This area should be well irrigated; it will heal spontaneously, and significant bleeding is rarely encountered.

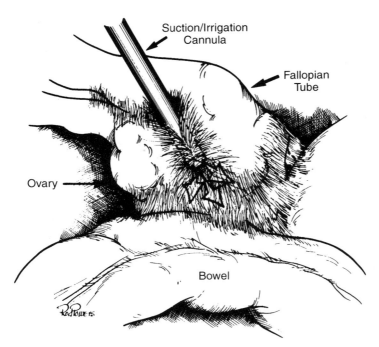

Suction/Irrigation
Cannula

Fallopian
Tube

Ovary

Bowel

FIGURE 19.1. Laparoscopic treatment of a pelvic abscess can be accomplished using an aspiration-irrigation cannula and a blunt probe. Under continuous irrigation with a physiologic solution (Ringer's lactate or normal saline), blunt dissection of the acutely adherent organs is performed.

Next, the grasping forceps are inserted into the fimbrial ostia and spread to free the agglutinated fimbriae. Irrigation of the tube through the fimbriated end should be performed to remove infected debris and diminish chances of recurrence. The fimbrial endosalpinx is visualized at this time and its quality assessed for future prognosis.

Tubal lavage with indigo carmine dye through the Cohen cannula in the uterus should be attempted. With early acute abscesses, the tubes are rarely patent because of interstitial edema. In contrast, when the abscess process has been present for longer than 1 week or the patient was previously treated with antibiotics, lavage frequently documents tubal patency. Rarely, necrotic material can be pushed from the tube during the lavage procedure.

The peritoneal cavity is extensively irrigated with Ringer's lactate solution until the effluent is clear. The total volume of irrigant often exceeds 20 liters. As part of this procedure, 2 liters of Ringer's lactate solution are flushed through the aquadissector into the upper abdomen, one on each side of the falciform ligament, to dilute any purulent material that may

have gained access to these areas during the 20° Trendelenburg's positioning. Reverse Trendelenburg's position is then used for the "underwater" exam. The laparoscope and the aquadissector are manipulated into the deep cul-de-sac beneath floating bowel and omentum, and this area is alternately irrigated and suctioned until the effluent is clear. An "underwater" examination is then performed to observe the completely separated tubes and ovaries and to document complete hemostasis. At the close of each procedure, at least 2 liters of Ringer's lactate is left in the peritoneal cavity to prevent fibrin adherences from forming between surfaces during the early healing phase and to dilute any bacteria present.

The umbilical incision is closed with 4-0 Vicryl. The lower quadrant 5-mm and 3-mm incisions are loosely approximated with a vascular clamp and covered with collodion to allow drainage of excess Ringer's lactate solution should increased intraabdominal pressure be present. No drains, antibiotic solutions, or heparin are used. A second-look laparoscopy is encouraged.

Without question, the more acute the abscess, the easier the dissection. Patient and physician delay often makes the laparoscopic procedure more difficult than it need be. However, even chronic abscesses can be successfully treated by careful blunt aquadissection.

Postoperative Care

Postoperatively, the patient is usually ambulatory and on a "diet as tolerated" after recovery from anesthesia. Temperature elevation rarely persists past the first postoperative day. We prefer to continue IV antibiotics until the patient is afebrile for at least 24 hr, and she is discharged on oral antibiotic coverage. The patient is usually discharged in 2 to 3 days if she remains afebrile, and is examined 1 week after discharge. All restrictions are removed at that time.

Alternative Techniques

Unruptured abscess are currently treated with intravenous antibiotics, with surgery reserved for poor responders to medical therapy. This approach often avoids immediate operation but commonly has reproductive consequences. Those that do not avoid surgery commonly undergo a TAH/BSO or at best a unilateral salpingo-oophorectomy. Most reports on operative technique for treatment of TOA by laparotomy emphasize that the tissues are edematous, congested, friable, and tear easily. Moreover, they note that capillary and venous oozing can be profuse. Hemostasis is often judged less than ideal in such cases, and blood loss requiring transfusion is common. These reports also suggest that meticulous dissection is virtually impossible and caution that the bowel is particularly vulnerable to injury when it is being separated from the pelvic viscera.

In contrast, laparoscopic adhesiolysis using aquadissection is rarely bloody. Capillary oozing does occur, but it ceases spontaneously as the procedure progresses. In my experience, blood loss is rarely greater than 100 ml, and blood transfusion has not been reported following laparoscopic treatment of a pelvic abscess.

Complications of treatment of pelvic abscess by laparotomy include superficial or deep wound infection, wound dehiscence, bowel injury including delayed perforation secondary to unrecognized injury, bowel obstruction, persistent undrained collections of pus, thrombophlebitis, pulmonary embolism, septic shock, and subdiaphragmatic abscesses. In contrast, neither wound disruption nor dehiscence is possible utilizing a laparoscopic approach, and the other possible complications have not been reported.

Results

The author has treated 40 pelvic abscesses using laparoscopic surgical techniques from 1976 to 1989.[6] One patient required TAH/BSO in 1977 for recurrence 1 month postoperatively; all other patients demonstrated long-term resolution of their TOA. Eight second-look laparoscopies documented minimal filmy adhesions. Similar results have been described by others,[7-12] with approximately 5% to 20% of patients requiring further surgery. It is possible that patients treated laparoscopically have fewer postoperative sequelae than those undergoing laparotomy. Between 1983 and 1988, Mecke and colleagues treated 25 patients with pelvic abscesses by laparotomy and 41 by pelviscopy.[12] Treatment was not randomized and was based on physician discretion. Conservative therapy was possible in 80% of patients treated laparoscopically. Furthermore, 27% of patients treated endoscopically complained of chronic abdominal pain at 1 to 2 years of follow-up, compared to 37% of patients treated by laparotomy, although this may have reflected selection bias. Nonetheless, it is clear that laparoscopic treatment of pelvic and tubo-ovarian abscesses is possible and may result in increased preservation of fertility.

Conclusions

The goal in the management of acute tubo-ovarian abscess is prevention of the chronic sequelae of infection, including pelvic adhesions, tubal occlusion, infertility, and pelvic pain, which often lead to further surgical intervention. Laparoscopic treatment in addition to antibiotic therapy is effective and economical. It offers the gynecologist 100% accuracy in diagnosis while simultaneously accomplishing definitive treatment with a low complication rate. Preventing infertility may be a possibility also, as an estimated 20% of infertility in the United States results from the sequelae of PID.

Laparoscopy allows for conservation of the tube and ovary with subsequent fertility potential. Additionally, laparoscopy has a high degree of patient acceptance because of minimal incision size, short hospital stay, and early return to full activity. The combination of laparoscopic treatment and effective IV antibiotics is a reasonable approach to the spectrum of PID from acute salpingitis to ruptured tubo-ovarian abscess.

Presently, many physicians are reluctant to advocate the routine use of laparoscopy for the diagnosis and treatment of acute pelvic adhesions and pelvic abscess. Whether the combination of laparoscopic surgery and antibiotics ultimately proves superior to antibiotics alone in the prevention of chronic pelvic adhesions must be resolved through multiinstitutional controlled studies using second-look laparoscopy. However, early experience with laparoscopic treatment of pelvic abscess combined with intravenous antibiotic therapy is promising and suggests that this technique may achieve better results than medical therapy alone or radical laparotomy surgery.

References

1. Simpson FF. The choice of time for operation for pelvic inflammation of tubal origin. *Surg Gynecol Obstet.* 1909;9:45–49.
2. Jansen R. Surgery pregnancy time intervals after salpingolysis, unilateral salpingostomy, and bilateral salpingostomy. *Fertil Steril.* 1980;34: 222–228.
3. Skau T, Nystrom P, Ohman L, Stendahl O. The kinetics of peritoneal clearance of *Escherichia coli* and *Bacteroides fragilis* and participating defense mechanisms. *Arch Surg.* 1986;121:1033–1040.
4. Ahrenholz DH, Simmons RL. Fibrin in peritonitis. I. Beneficial and adverse effects of fibrin in experimental *E. coli* peritonitis. *Surgery (St. Louis).* 1980;88:41–46.
5. Reich H, McGlynn F. Laparoscopic treatment of tuboovarian and pelvic abscess. *J Reprod Med.* 1987;32:747–751.
6. Reich H. Endoscopic management of tubooavarian abscess and pelvic inflammatory disease. In: Sanfilippo J, Levine R, eds. *Operative Gynecologic Endoscopy.* New York: Springer-Verlag; 1988:69–76.
7. Adducci JE. Laparoscopy in the diagnosis and treatment of pelvic inflammatory disease with abscess formation. *Int Surg.* 1981;66:359–360.
8. Henry-Suchet J, Soler A, Loffredo V. Laparoscopic treatment of tuboovarian abscesses. *J Reprod Med.* 1984;29:579–584.
9. Hudspeth AS. Radical surgical debridement in the treatment of advanced generalized bacterial peritonitis. *Arch Surg.* 1975;110:1233–1237.
10. Rivlin M, Hunt J. Surgical management of diffuse peritonitis complicating obstetric/gynecologic infections. *Obstet Gynecol.* 1986;67:652–657.
11. Raatz D, Dressler F, Zockler R, von Widekind C. [Endoscopic organ saving therapy of ascending infections: 10 years experience at the Berlin-Neukolln Gynecologic Clinic.] *Geburt Frauen.* 1990;50:982–985.
12. Mecke H, Semm K, Freys I, Gent HJ. Pelvic abscesses: pelviscopy or laparotomy. *Gynecol Obstet Invest.* 1991;31:231–234.
13. Jacobson L. Differential diagnosis of acute pelvic inflammatory disease. *Am J Obstet Gynecol.* 1980;138:1006–1012.
14. Franklin E, Hevron J, Thompson J. Management of the pelvic abscess. *Clin Obstet Gynecol.* 1973;16:66–72.
15. Sweet R, Ledger W. Cefoxitin: single-agent treatment of mixed aerobic-anaerobic pelvic infections. *Obstet Gynecol.* 1979;54:193–198.

20

Laparoscopic Suspension Procedures

Camran Nezhat, Farr Nezhat, and Ceana H. Nezhat

Uterine Suspension

Indications and Patient Selection

Uterine suspension is indicated for dyspareunia secondary to severe uterine retroversion in the absence of other cul-de-sac disease and for selected cases of severe endometriosis involving the cul-de-sac and rectum. At laparoscopy, adhesions, endometriosis, and hydrosalpinx can be corrected and the uterine suspension accomplished during the same operation.

Women with dyspareunia secondary to the uterine position will have a retroverted, retroflexed uterus, and palpation of the uterocervical junction on vaginal examination will reproduce the pain. Although some authors have advocated placing a pessary before attempting surgical correction of the retroversion,[1] others have noted that although the dyspareunia was eliminated in the patient, the male partner was disturbed by the pessary during coitus.[2] Complete or partial relief of dyspareunia from laparoscopic uterine suspension

has been reported in approximately 94% of patients,[3] although two reports showed no relief.[4,5] The three most effective techniques for performing a laparoscopic uterine suspension are the application of Falope rings, ventrosuspension of the round ligament, and the modified Olshausen uterine suspension.

Instrumentation and Techniques

Round Ligament Shortening with Falope Ring

For many years, Falope rings (Cabot Medical Corp., Langhorne, PA) have been used in laparoscopic tubal sterilization. A special instrument that fits through a 7-mm accessory trocar sleeve simultaneously grasps the tube, retracts it into the instrument, and places a small, tight silicone band around the knuckle of the tube. A similar procedure may be used to shorten the round ligaments (Fig. 20.1).[6] It may be necessary to place multiple Falope rings to achieve the proper tension on the round ligaments. Placing multiple bands on the round

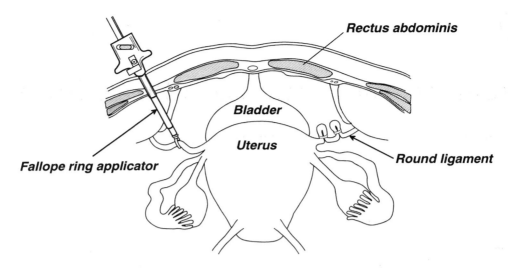

FIGURE 20.1.   Laparoscopic uterine suspension achieved by shortening the round ligaments with Falope rings.

ligaments may lacerate the broad ligament or the round ligament, and bipolar electrocoagulation should be used for hemostasis.

Ventrosuspension of the Round Ligaments

For this procedure, two 5-mm suprapubic trocars are inserted, and grasping forceps[3,7–9] or long Kelly clamps are introduced. Both round ligaments are grasped near their midpoint and the pneumoperitoneum is allowed to partially

escape. The knuckle of the round ligament is pulled gently and firmly through the incision in the fascia (Fig. 20.2). The round ligaments are sutured to the rectus fascia with 2-0 Ethibond nonabsorbable sutures. It may be necessary to extend the skin incision. The uterine position is confirmed laparoscopically, and care must be taken to avoid kinking the fallopian tubes.

Potential complications with this procedure include avulsion of the round ligament sec-

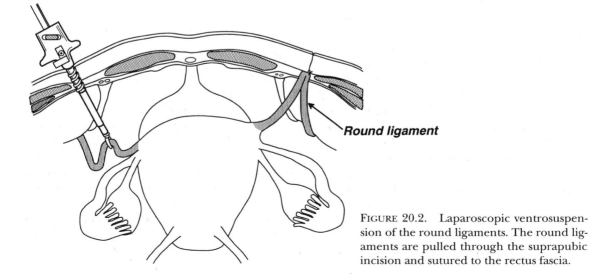

FIGURE 20.2.   Laparoscopic ventrosuspension of the round ligaments. The round ligaments are pulled through the suprapubic incision and sutured to the rectus fascia.

FIGURE 20.3. Modified Olshausen uterine suspension performed laparoscopically.

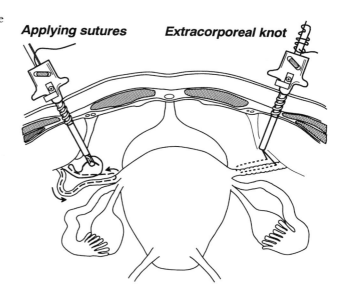

Applying sutures   **Extracorporeal knot**

ondary to an inadequate fascial incision or when attempting to position the round ligaments with a full pneumoperitoneum. The inferior epigastric vessels may be lacerated during placement of the suprapubic trocars. Intraabdominal laparoscopic evaluation of the anterior abdominal wall often helps prevent this complication but may be difficult in obese patients. The use of a nonabsorbable suture is recommended, although one of our patients presented with chronic pain at the attachment site that abated on suture removal.

For most patients, incisional pain and discomfort are managed with mild analgesics and a heating pad. Occasionally, patients who experience more significant postoperative pain secondary to spasms of the rectus abdominis muscle obtain relief with the application of local heat and the administration of muscle relaxants and analgesics. Women are advised to avoid strenuous exercise for 4 to 6 weeks postoperatively.

Lose and Lindholm[10] reported a case of intermittent urinary retention in a young woman following uterine suspension for dyspareunia and a retroverted, retroflexed uterus. At corrective surgery, the rearranged uterus appeared to cause a partial obstruction that may have been exacerbated by the patient's low voiding pressures.

Modified Olshausen Uterine Suspension

In this procedure, either a delayed absorbable or permanent suture is passed transabdominally through the suprapubic trocar site using a swaged needle. The surgeon places the round ligament on stretch, and several areas are taken where the round ligament enters the inguinal canal moving toward the uterus. Approximately 2 cm from the uterus, the direction of the needle is reversed and a similar maneuver is performed along the length of the round ligament to the inguinal canal. The needle is passed transabdominally. When both sides are completed, the pneumoperitoneum is decreased and the suture is tied above the fascia (Fig. 20.3). The result is a plication of the round ligaments.

This procedure is an alternative to the ventrosuspension of the uterus. It is associated with the same risk of complications, although the chance of round ligament avulsion is less. This procedure requires greater surgical skill than the others mentioned because intracorporeal suturing is used.

Results

Massouda et al.[6] reported three cases of successful laparoscopic uterine suspension by round ligament plication with Falope rings. Two patients presented with chronic pelvic pain and one presented with progressive pelvic pain and dyspareunia of 2 years duration. After the surgery, all three patients were relieved of pain, and one subsequently delivered a healthy infant.

In a study of 80 patients with retrodisplacement of the uterus who underwent laparoscopic uterine suspension using round ligament fixation to the rectus sheet, reduction in preoperative symptoms occurred in 74 of the patients. No ectopic pregnancies were reported after long-term follow-up, and 13 intrauterine pregnancies occurred. There was no recurrence of symptoms after either vaginal delivery or cesarean.[11]

We do not have significant experience with the modified Olshausen technique, and there are no significant data available in the literature. The original technique by laparotomy has been discouraged because of the high possibility of complications.[12]

Vaginal Vault Suspension (Sacral Colpopexy)

Indications and Patient Selection

Vaginal vault prolapse occurs when the apex of the vagina descends below the introitus. This is a rare sequela of hysterectomy that occurs in 900 to 1200 women in the United States annually because of disruption of the ligaments that maintain vaginal support.[13] Numerous surgical techniques have been proposed to prevent and correct this condition,[13–22] including abdominal sacral colpopexy with interposition of a synthetic suspensory hammock between the prolapsed vaginal vault and the anterior surface of the sacrum.[13,14,23] However, this technique usually requires a midline abdominal incision, abdominal packing, and extensive bowel manipulation with consequent morbidity, including wound separation or dehiscence and ileus or bowel obstruction.[13]

The advantages of a laparoscopic approach include a better view of the pelvis, precise hemostasis, a smaller incision, elimination of abdominal packing, and less manipulation of the viscera.[24] Sacral colpopexy involves placing a hammock of polypropylene mesh between the prolapsed vaginal vault and the anterior surface of the sacrum. Multiple permanent sutures attach one end of the mesh to the apex of the vaginal vault and the opposite end to either the hollow of the sacrum or the sacral promontory. Important patient selection factors include an ability to tolerate prolonged general anesthesia and pneumoperitoneum.

Laparoscopic sacral colpopexy is indicated when vaginal prolapse results in bothersome protrusion and symptoms of pelvic pressure and pain that worsen with ambulation and daily activity. Women may also experience coital difficulty, difficulty in walking, urinary incontinence, difficulty in voiding, fecal incontinence, or difficulty in defecating. Recurrent mucosal irritation, ulceration, cervical ulceration, and recurrent infection may be present. Physical examination should focus on the degree of prolapse and associated rectocele, cystourethrocele, and incontinence (urinary or fecal). Frequently, instructions for a preoperative mechanical and antibiotic bowel preparation are given.[24,25]

Instrumentation and Techniques

The patient is placed in the lithotomy position in Allen universal stirrups and the vagina is cleansed with an antiseptic. The laparoscope is placed through an umbilical trocar sleeve and other instruments through three suprapubic 5-mm accessory sites. The patient is placed in a steep Trendelenburg's position and tilted left to mobilize the bowel away from the operating field.

After visualization of the pelvis, the vagina is pushed up using a sponge on a ring forceps and adhesiolysis is performed as necessary.[25] Peritoneum and connective tissue are removed from the vaginal apex until the vaginal fascia and scar are identified. While holding the vaginal apex with grasping forceps, the vesical peritoneum over the vaginal apex is incised using CO_2 laser and hydrodissection or with scissors (Fig. 20.4A). The bladder is dissected from the anterior vaginal wall, and the rectum from the

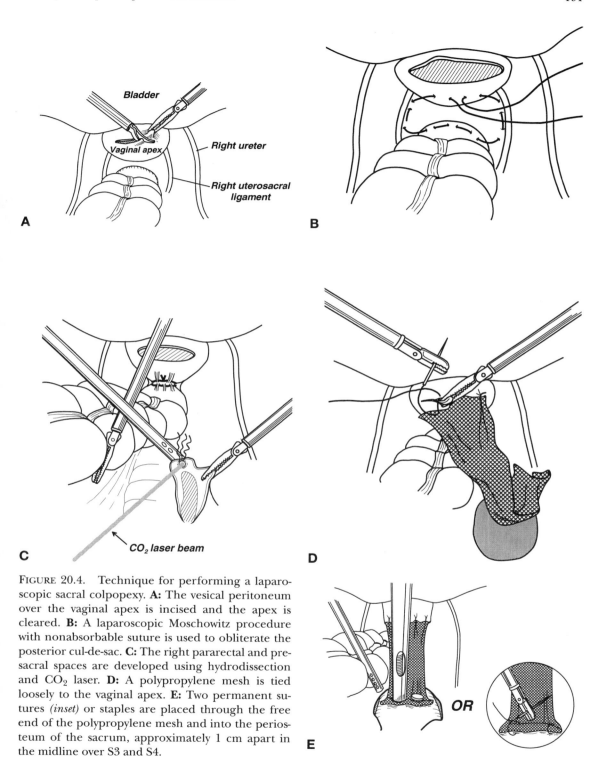

FIGURE 20.4. Technique for performing a laparoscopic sacral colpopexy. **A:** The vesical peritoneum over the vaginal apex is incised and the apex is cleared. **B:** A laparoscopic Moschowitz procedure with nonabsorbable suture is used to obliterate the posterior cul-de-sac. **C:** The right pararectal and presacral spaces are developed using hydrodissection and CO_2 laser. **D:** A polypropylene mesh is tied loosely to the vaginal apex. **E:** Two permanent sutures (inset) or staples are placed through the free end of the polypropylene mesh and into the periosteum of the sacrum, approximately 1 cm apart in the midline over S3 and S4.

posterior vaginal wall, to expose approximately 4 cm of the vaginal vault. In case of partial vaginectomy, an inflated surgical glove is placed in the vagina to help maintain pneumoperitoneum.

If a coexisting enterocele is found, the repair is performed laparoscopically by excising the sac followed by a modified Moschcowitz[26,27] posterior cul-de-sac obliteration using Ethibond (Ethicon, Somerville, NJ) (Fig. 20.4B). After the ureters are identified, the lateral peritoneum is elevated, and a continuous pursestring suture is placed through the peritoneum and passed through the cul-de-sac base, the opposite side of the peritoneum, and the anterior rectosigmoid colon serosa. For this purpose, the use of 0-polybutilate-coated polyester is preferred.

The posterior parietal peritoneum is lifted with grasping forceps and the anterior sacral fascia exposed. Care is taken to avoid injuring the presacral vessels. Bleeding is controlled with bipolar electrodesiccation, sutures, or clips. The peritoneal incision is extended downward toward the vagina through the presacral space (Fig. 20.4C). The presacral space is entered through a vertical peritoneal incision at the right pararectal area using hydrodissection combined with the CO_2 laser set at 40 to 80 W (or any other cutting modality that the surgeon chooses). The following anatomic landmarks are identified to avoid bowel, ureter, and vessel injury: the right ureter, internal iliac artery and vein, descending colon, and presacral vessels. The sigmoid colon is reflected laterally to avoid injury to vessels in the sigmoid mesentery.

The polypropylene mesh (Mersilene, Ethicon) is rolled and introduced into the abdomen through a 10-mm suprapubic port or the umbilical port after removing the laparoscope. Three to five 1-0 nonabsorbable polybutilate-coated polyester sutures are placed in a single row in the vaginal wall apex, taking care not to penetrate the vaginal mucosa, from one lateral fornix to the other (Fig. 20.4D). Each suture is then placed through one end of the polypropylene mesh and tied loosely using extracorporeal or intracorporeal knot-tying techniques.

Finally, two permanent sutures or staples (Laptak, Surgin Surgical, Tustin, CA) are placed through the remaining free end of the mesh and into the periosteum of the sacrum, approximately 1 cm apart in the midline over S3 and S4 (Fig. 20.4E). Care must be taken to avoid injury to the perforating paravertebral blood vessels in this area. Otherwise, hemostasis can be quite difficult, even by laparotomy, because of retraction of the severed vessels. The mesh is adjusted to hold the vaginal apex in the correct anatomic position without being extremely tight. The excess mesh is trimmed from the strap, and the peritoneum is closed over the strap using multiple interrupted sutures or clips.

Other supportive measures for the lower vagina often are necessary, such as retropubic urethropexy, and anterior and posterior colporrhaphy for the lower and middle third of the vagina. These procedures should be performed as indicated. Postoperatively, the patient's diet is advanced as tolerated, and a mild laxative is prescribed to prevent constipation. On discharge, patients are advised to avoid intercourse for 6 weeks.

Results

Using laparoscopic sacral colpopexy, we have treated 12 women with symptomatic posthysterectomy vaginal vault prolapse. Three had complete genital prolapse requiring hysterectomy and prophylactic vault suspension. Concomitant procedures included unilateral or bilateral adnexectomy, cholecystectomy (performed by a general surgeon at the same procedure), anterior and posterior repair, and bladder neck suspension.[28]

With the exception of one case, all procedures were completed laparoscopically. During application of the staples, one patient had significant bleeding that eventually necessitated laparotomy. After bleeding was controlled, the procedure was completed. Follow-up ranged from 6 to 36 months and was conducted by periodic examination, formal report by the referring physician, and telephone interview. All women reported complete relief of their symptoms and good vaginal vault support. One patient had mild temporary constipation that gradually resolved after a few weeks.

References

1. Donaldson JK, Sanderlin JH, Harrell WB. A method of suspending the uterus without open abdominal incision. *Am J Surg* 1942;15:537.

2. Smith DB, Kelsey JF, Sherman RL, et al. Laparoscopic uterine suspension. *J Reprod Med.* 1977;18:98.

3. Ivey JL. Laparoscopic uterine suspension as an adjunctive procedure at the time of laser laparoscopy for the treatment of endometriosis. *J Reprod Med.* 1992;37:757–765.

4. Gleeson NC, Gaffney GM. Ventrosuspension—five years of practice at the Rotunda Hospital reviewed. *J Obstet Gynecol.* 1990;10:415.

5. Yoong AFE. Laparoscopic ventrosuspension: a review of 72 cases. *Am J Obstet Gynecol.* 1990;163:1151.

6. Massouda D, Ling FW, Muram D, et al. Laparoscopic uterine suspension with Falope rings. *J Reprod Med.* 1987;32:859.

7. Steptoe PC. *Laparoscopy in Gynecology.* London: Livingstone; 1967:78.

8. Candy JW. Modified Gilliam uterine suspension using laparoscopic visualization. *Obstet Gynecol.* 1976;47:242.

9. Mann WJ, Stenger VG. Uterine suspension through the laparoscope. *Obstet Gynecol.* 1978;51:563.

10. Lose G, Lindholm P. Impaired voiding efficiency and urinary retention after laparoscopic ventrosuspension ad modum Steptoe. *Acta Obstet Gynecol Scand.* 1984;63:371.

11. Gordon SF. Laparoscopic uterine suspension. *J Reprod Med.* 1992;37:6135–6136.

12. Thompson JD. Malpositions of the uterus. In: Thompson JD, Rock JA, eds. *Te Linde's Operative Gynecology.* 7th ed. Philadelphia: JP Lippincott; 1992:823–824.

13. Timmons MC, Addison WA, Addison SB, et al. Abdominal sacral colpopexy in 163 women with post-hysterectomy vaginal vault prolapse and enterocele. *J Reprod Med.* 1992;37:323.

14. Arthure HGE, Savage D. Uterine prolapse and prolapse of vaginal vault treated by sacral hysteropexy. *J Obstet Gynaecol Br Emp.* 1957;64:335.

15. Lane FE. Repair of post-hysterectomy vaginal vault prolapse. *Obstet Gynecol.* 1962;22:72.

16. Langmade CF. Cooper ligament repair of vaginal vault prolapse. *Am J Obstet Gynecol.* 1965;92:601.

17. Richardson AC, Williams GA. Treatment of prolapse of the vagina following hysterectomy. *Am J Obstet Gynecol.* 1969;105:90–93.

18. Birnbaum SJ. Rational therapy for the prolapsed vagina. *Am J Obstet Gynecol.* 1973;115:411–419.

19. Randall CL, Nichols DH. Surgical treatment of vaginal inversion. *Obstet Gynecol.* 1971;38:327–332.

20. Beecham CT, Beecham JB. Correction of prolapsed vagina or enterocele with fascia lata. *Obstet Gynecol.* 1973;42:542–546.

21. Ridley JH. A composite vaginal vault suspension using fascia lata. *Am J Obstet Gynecol.* 1976;126:590–596.

22. Symmonds RE, Williams TJ, Lee RA, et al. Post hysterectomy enterocele and vaginal vault prolapse. *Am J Obstet Gynecol.* 1981;140:852–859.

23. Feldman GB, Birnbaum SJ. Sacral colpopexy for vaginal vault prolapse. *Obstet Gynecol.* 1979;53:399–401.

24. Nezhat CH, Nezhat F, Nezhat C. Laparoscopic sacral colpopexy for vaginal vault prolapse. *Obstet Gynecol.* 1994;84(5):885–888.

25. Nezhat C, Nezhat F, Nezhat C. Operative laparoscopy (minimally invasive surgery): state of the art. *J Gynecol Surg.* 1992;8:111–141.

26. Nezhat C, Nezhat F, Gordon S, Wilkins E, Laparoscopic versus abdominal hysterectomy. *J Reprod Med.* 1992;37:247–250.

27. Nichols DH. Enterocele and massive eversion of the vagina. In: Thompson JD, Rock JA, eds. *Te Linde's Operative Gynecology.* 7th ed. Philadelphia: JP Lippincott; 1992:855–885.

28. Nezhat CH, Nezhat F, Nezhat CR, Rottenberg H. Laparoscopic retropubic cystourethropexy. *J AGGL.* 1994;1(4):339–349.

21

Laparoscopic Hysterectomy

Harry Reich

Of the 600,000 hysterectomies performed each year, more than 60% are accomplished using an abdominal incision. Abdominal hysterectomy will probably become a rarely used procedure, however, because laparoscopy can be effectively used to accomplish a less invasive laparoscopic or vaginal hysterectomy in many cases.

Laparoscopic hysterectomy (LH), defined as the laparoscopic ligation of the uterine vessels, is an alternative to abdominal hysterectomy

with more attention to ureteral identification.[1-3] First done in January 1988,[4] laparoscopic hysterectomy stimulated a general interest in the laparoscopic approach to hysterectomy as gynecologists not trained in vaginal or laparoscopic techniques struggled to maintain their fair share of the large lucrative hysterectomy market. A watered-down version of LH called LAVH (laparoscopic-assisted vaginal hysterectomy) was taught and became known as an expensive overutilized procedure with indications for which skilled vaginal surgeons rarely found laparoscopic use necessary.

LH remains a reasonable substitute for abdominal hysterectomy. Its use, however, has presently plateaued because most managed care plans reimburse the surgeon poorly for using a laparoscopic approach. Hospitals may benefit if they are reimbursed according to diagnostic related groups (DRGs); the hospital receives more for a 1- to 2-day stay. Unfortunately, some plans reward the hospital for additional postoperative days, discouraging both hospital administrator and surgeon from encouraging short hospital stay laparoscopic surgery rather than traditional laparotomy.

Most hysterectomies currently requiring an abdominal approach may be done with laparoscopic dissection of part or all of the abdominal portion followed by vaginal removal of the specimen. There are many surgical advantages to laparoscopy, particularly magnification of anatomy and pathology, easy access to the vagina and rectum, and the ability to achieve complete hemostasis and clot evacuation during underwater examination. Patient advantages are multiple and are related to avoidance of a painful abdominal incision. They include reduced duration of hospitalization and recuperation and an extremely low rate of infection and ileus.

The goal of vaginal hysterectomy, LAVH, or LH is to safely avoid an abdominal wall incision. The surgeon must remember that if vaginal hysterectomy is possible after ligating the utero-ovarian ligaments, this should be done. Laparoscopic inspection at the end of the procedure will still permit the surgeon to control any bleeding and evacuate clots, and laparoscopic cuff suspension should limit future cuff prolapse. Unnecessary surgical procedures should not be done because of the surgeon's preoccupation with the development of new surgical skills. It should be emphasized that a laparoscopic hysterectomy is not indicated when vaginal hysterectomy is possible.

Definitions

There are a variety of operations in which the laparoscope is used as an aid to hysterectomy

TABLE 21.1. Laparoscopic hysterectomy classification

Diagnostic laparoscopy with vaginal hysterectomy
Laparoscopic-assisted vaginal hysterectomy (LAVH)
Laparoscopic hysterectomy (LH)
Total laparoscopic hysterectomy (TLH)
Laparoscopic supracervical hysterectomy (LSH), including CASH (classical abdominal Semm hysterectomy)
Vaginal hysterectomy with laparoscopic vault suspension (LVS) or laparoscopic pelvic reconstruction (LPR)
Laparoscopic hysterectomy with lymphadenectomy
Laparoscopic hysterectomy with lymphadenectomy and omentectomy
Laparoscopic radical hysterectomy with lymphadenectomy

(Table 21.1). It is important that these different procedures are clearly delineated.

Diagnostic Laparoscopy with Vaginal Hysterectomy

This term indicates that the laparoscope is used for *diagnostic* purposes to determine if *vaginal hysterectomy* is possible when indications for a vaginal approach are equivocal.[5] It also ensures that vaginal cuff and pedicle hemostasis is complete and allows clot evacuation.

Laparoscopic-Assisted Vaginal Hysterectomy

LAVH is a vaginal hysterectomy after laparoscopic adhesiolysis, endometriosis excision, or oophorectomy.[7-9] Unfortunately, this term is also used when the upper uterine ligaments (e.g., round, infundibulopelvic, or utero-ovarian) of a relatively normal uterus are ligated with staples or bipolar desiccation. It must be emphasized that in most cases the easy part of both an abdominal or vaginal hysterectomy is upper pedicle ligation.

Laparoscopic Hysterectomy

LH denotes laparoscopic ligation of the uterine arteries either by electrosurgery desiccation, suture ligature, or staples. All surgical steps after the uterine vessels have been ligated can be done either vaginally or laparoscopically, including anterior and posterior vaginal entry by transection, cardinal and uterosacral ligament division, uterine removal (intact or by morcellation), and vaginal closure (vertically or transversely). Laparoscopic ligation of the uterine vessels is the sine qua non for laparoscopic hysterectomy. Ureteral identification, often by isolation, has always been advised.

Total Laparoscopic Hysterectomy (TLH)

In TLH, laparoscopic dissection continues until the uterus lies free of all attachments in the peritoneal cavity. The uterus is then removed through the vagina, with morcellation if necessary. The vagina is closed with laparoscopically placed sutures. No vaginal surgery is done unless morcellation is necessary.[6]

Laparoscopic Supracervical Hysterectomy (LSH)

LSH has recently regained some support after suggestions that total hysterectomy results in a decrease in libido in some women.[10] The uterus is removed by morcellation from above or below.[7]

Kurt Semm's version of a supracervical hysterectomy, often referred to as the CISH procedure (classical interstitial Semm hysterectomy), leaves the cardinal ligaments intact while eliminating the columnar cells of the endocervical canal. After perforating the uterine fundus with a long sound-dilator, a calibrated uterine resection tool (CURT) that fits around this instrument is used to core out the endocervical canal. Thereafter, at laparoscopy, suture techniques are used to ligate the uteroovarian ligaments. An Endoloop is placed around the uterine fundus to the level of the internal os of the cervix and tied. The uterus is divided at its junction with the cervix and removed by laparoscopic morcellation.

Laparoscopic Pelvic Reconstruction (LPR) with Vaginal Hysterectomy

This method is useful when vaginal hysterectomy alone cannot accomplish appropriate repair for vaginal prolapse. Ureteral dissection and suture placement through the uterosacral ligaments near the sacrum, before the vaginal portion of the procedure, may be useful to achieve vaginal suspension (see following). Levator muscle plication vaginally or laparoscopically is often necessary. Retropubic Burch colposuspension can also be done laparoscopically.

Indications and Contraindications

Indications

Indications for laparoscopic hysterectomy include benign pathology such as endometriosis, fibroids, adhesions, and adnexal masses usually requiring the selection of an abdominal approach to hysterectomy. It is also appropriate when vaginal hysterectomy is not possible because of a narrow pubic arch, a constricted vagina with no prolapse, or severe arthritis that prohibits placement of the patient in sufficient lithotomy position for vaginal exposure. Laparoscopic procedures in obese women allow the surgeon to make an incision above the panniculus and operate below it. Laparoscopic hysterectomy may also be considered for stage I endometrial, ovarian, and cervical cancer.[8-10] Pelvic reconstruction procedures including cuff suspension, retropubic colposuspension, and rectocele repair may also be simultaneously accomplished through the laparoscope.

The most common indication for laparoscopic hysterectomy is a symptomatic fibroid uterus. Morcellation is often necessary and is done laparoscopically or vaginally using a scalpel. Fibroids fixed in the pelvis or abdomen without descent are easier to mobilize laparoscopically. It is important to perform current uterine size and weight measurements to confirm the appropriateness of the laparoscopic hysterectomy, as most small uteri can be removed vaginally. As an example, the normal uterus weighs 70–125 g, a 12-week (gestational age) uterus weighs 280–320 g, a 24-week uterus weighs 580–620 g, and a term uterus weighs 1000–1100 g.

Hysterectomy should not be done for stage IV endometriosis with extensive cul-de-sac involvement unless the surgeon has the skill and time to resect all deep fibrotic endometriosis from the posterior vagina, uterosacral ligaments, and anterior rectum. In these patients, excision of the uterus using an intrafascial technique leaves the deep fibrotic endometriosis behind to cause future problems. Furthermore, it becomes much more difficult to remove deep fibrotic endometriosis when there is no uterus between the anterior rectum and the bladder. After hysterectomy, the endometriosis left in the anterior rectum and vaginal cuff frequently becomes densely adherent to, or invades into, the bladder and one or both ureters.

In many patients with stage IV endometriosis and extensive cul-de-sac obliteration, it is preferable to preserve the uterus and prevent future vaginal cuff, bladder, and ureteral problems.[11] Obviously, this approach will not be effective when uterine adenomyosis is present. In these cases, after excision of cul-de-sac endometriosis, persistent pain will ultimately require a hysterectomy. Oophorectomy is not always necessary at hysterectomy for advanced endometriosis, if the endometriosis is carefully removed. Reoperation for recurrent symptoms has been necessary in fewer than 5% of my patients in whom one or both ovaries have been preserved. Bilateral oophorectomy is rarely indicated in women under age 40 undergoing hysterectomy for endometriosis.

Hysterectomy may be performed for abnormal uterine bleeding in women of reproductive age. Abnormal uterine bleeding is defined as excessive uterine bleeding, or irregular uterine bleeding, for more than 8 days during more than a single cycle or as profuse bleeding requiring additional protection (large clots, gushes, or limitations on activity). There should be no history of a bleeding diathesis or use of medication that may cause bleeding. A negative effect on quality of life should be documented. Physical examination, laboratory data, ultrasound, and hysteroscopy are frequently negative.

Hormonal or other medical treatment should be attempted before hysterectomy, and its failure, contraindication, or refusal should be documented. The presence of anemia is recorded and correction with iron supplementation attempted. If hysterectomy is chosen, a vaginal approach is usually appropriate. Laparoscopic hysterectomy is done only when vaginal hysterectomy is not feasible, including history of previous abdominal surgery and lack of prolapse (nulliparous or multiparous). TLH is considered if the surgeon has little experience with the vaginal approach; in many countries vaginal hysterectomy is not done.

Contraindications

Laparoscopic hysterectomy is not advised for the diagnosis and treatment of a pelvic mass that cannot be removed intact through a culdotomy incision or that is too large to fit intact into an impermeable sack, particularly in postmenopausal patients.[14] The largest available sack for removal of intraperitoneal masses is the LapSac (Cook Ob/Gyn, Spencer, IN), which measures 8×5 in. Although cyst aspiration is advocated by some investigators,[12,13] it is the opinion of this surgeon that postmenopausal cystic ovaries should not be subjected to aspiration before oophorectomy because the inevitable spillage may change the diagnosis from a stage Ia ovarian cancer to a stage Ic. Its effect on survival is unknown but it may be detrimental. It must be emphasized that aspiration through a small-gauge needle placed through a thickened portion of the ovary and cyst aspiration devices with surrounding suction and Endoloop placement (Cook) do not completely prevent spillage.

The medical status of the patient may prohibit surgery. Anemia, diabetes, lung disorders, cardiac disease, and bleeding diathesis should be excluded before surgery. Age alone should rarely be a deterrent.

The need for peripartum hysterectomy for placenta accreta, uterine atony, unspecified uterine bleeding, and uterine rupture are relative contraindications at present. However, laparoscopic hysterectomy may be considered for patients needing a postpartum hysterectomy. Another contraindication is stage III ovarian cancer, which requires a large abdominal incision. Finally, inexperience or inadequate training of the surgeon is a contraindication to the laparoscopic approach.

Preoperative Preparation

The preoperative use of gonadotropin-releasing hormone (GnRH) analogs for at least 2 months before hysterectomy for large myomas is encouraged. GnRH analogs may reduce the total uterine and leiomyoma volumes, making laparoscopic or vaginal hysterectomy easier.[14,15] Furthermore, the uterine circulation will also diminish. During treatment with depoleuprolide (Lupron-Depot, TAP Pharmaceutical, Deerfield, IL), at a dose of 3.75 mg IM once per month for 3 to 6 months, anemia secondary to hypermenorrhea will also resolve. Autologous blood donation can be considered before laparoscopic hysterectomy; however, it should be noted that packed red blood cells have a shelf life of 35 days if stored at $1°-6°C$. Lupron-Depot™ is often administered after ovulation in the cycle preceding surgery to avoid operating on ovaries containing a corpus luteum.

Patients are encouraged to hydrate and eat lightly for 24 hr before admission on the day of surgery. When extensive cul-de-sac involvement with endometriosis is suspected, a mechanical bowel prep is ordered, for example, with a polyethylene glycol-based isosmotic solution (GOLYTELY or Colyte). Lower abdominal, pubic, and perineal hair is not shaved. A Foley catheter is inserted during surgery and removed in the recovery room or the next morning. Antibiotics (usually cefoxitin or cefotetan) are administered preoperatively.

Instrumentation and Technique

General

All laparoscopic surgical procedures are done under general anesthesia with endotracheal intubation. The routine use of an orogastric tube is recommended to diminish the possibility of a trocar injury to a gas-filled stomach and to reduce small bowel distension during the oper-

ation. The patient remains flat (0°) on the operating table until the umbilical trocar sleeve has been inserted and then is placed in steep Trendelenburg's position (20°–30°). Lithotomy position with the hip extended (thigh parallel to abdomen) is obtained with Allan stirrups (Edgewater Medical Systems, Mayfield Heights, OH) or knee braces, which are adjusted for each individual patient before anesthesia. Examination under anesthesia is always performed before prepping the patient.

Laparoscopy was never thought to be a sterile procedure before the incorporation of video, as the surgeon operated with his head in the surgical field, attached to the laparoscopic optic. Furthermore, it is not possible to sterilize skin. Since 1983, this surgeon has maintained a policy of not scrubbing and not sterilizing or draping the camera or laser arm. Masking is optional (most surgeons in the United Kingdom do not mask for laparoscopic surgery). Infection has been rare, less than 1%.

At the completion of all my laparoscopic procedures, the umbilical incision is closed with a single 4-0 Vicryl suture opposing deep fascia and skin dermis, with the knot buried beneath the fascia. This will prevent the suture from acting as a wick, transmitting bacteria into the soft tissue or peritoneal cavity. The lower quadrant incisions are loosely approximated with a Javid vascular clamp (V. Mueller, McGaw Park, IL) and covered with Collodion (AMEND, Irvington, NJ) to allow drainage of excess Ringer's lactate solution.

Instrumentation

High-flow CO_2 insufflation, up to 15 liters/min, is beneficial to compensate for the rapid loss of CO_2 during suctioning. The ability to maintain a relatively constant intraabdominal pressure between 10 and 15 mmHg during laparoscopic hysterectomy is essential. Gasless laparoscopy with abdominal wall retractors may be used to minimize abdominal wall subcutaneous emphysema during retroperitoneal surgery, because peritoneal defects result in free communication between the peritoneal cavity and the subcutaneous space that may compromise peritoneal cavity operating space.

A useful technique is to insert a Laparolift anterior abdominal wall retractor (Origin Medsystems, Menlo Park, CA) once the vagina is opened to maintain working space.

Operating room tables capable of a 30° Trendelenburg's position are extremely valuable for laparoscopic hysterectomy. Unfortunately these tables are rare, and this author has much difficulty operating when only a limited degree of body tilt can be attained. For the past 18 years a steep Trendelenburg's position (20°–40°), with shoulder braces and the patient's arms at her sides, has been used without adverse effects.

A Valtchev uterine mobilizer (Conkin Surgical Instruments, Toronto, Canada) is the best available single instrument to antevert the uterus and delineate the posterior vagina (Fig. 21.1).[16] With this instrument, the uterus can be anteverted to about 120° and moved in an arc about 45° from the horizontal by turning the mobilizer around its longitudinal axis. An obturator that is 100 mm long and 10 mm thick, or one 80 mm long and 8 mm thick, may be used for uterine manipulation during hysterectomy.

If a Valtchev uterine mobilizer is not available, a #3 or #4 Sims curette, a Cohen acorn cannula, or a Humi is placed in the endometrial cavity to markedly antevert the uterus and stretch out the cul-de-sac. If excision of rectovaginal endometriosis is needed, a sponge on a ring forceps is inserted into the posterior vaginal fornix and a #81 French rectal probe

(Reznik Instruments, Skokie, IL) is placed in the rectum. This will also better define the posterior vagina for the performance of a culdotomy incision. Placement of the rectal probe and intraoperative rectovaginal examinations remain important techniques for defining the rectovaginal space, even when the Valtchev uterine mobilizer is available, whenever rectal location is in doubt.

Trocar sleeves are available in many sizes and shapes. For most cases, 5.5-mm-diameter cannulas are adequate. Short trapless 5-mm-trocar sleeves with a retention screw grid around the external surface (reusable, from Richard Wolf Medical Instruments, Vernon Hills, IL; or disposable, Apple Medical, Bolton, MA) are used to facilitate efficient instrument exchanges and evacuation of tissue while allowing unlimited freedom during extracorporeal suture tying.[17] With practice, a good laparoscopic surgical team will be able to make instrument exchanges fast enough so that little pneumoperitoneum is lost.

Self-retaining lateral vaginal wall retractors or Vienna retractors (Brisky–Navatril) are used for vaginal extraction of a large fibroid uterus without changing stirrups. Alternatively, after the abdominal portion of the procedure is completed, the stirrups are replaced with candy-cane stirrups to obtain better hip flexion, so that conventional vaginal side-wall retractors can be used.

Monopolar cutting current through electrosurgical electrodes that eliminate capacitance

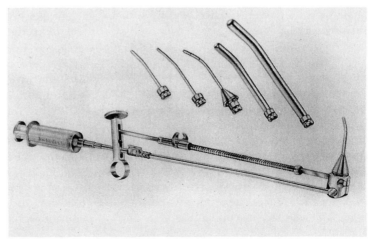

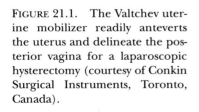

FIGURE 21.1. The Valtchev uterine mobilizer readily anteverts the uterus and delineate the posterior vagina for a laparoscopic hysterectomy (courtesy of Conkin Surgical Instruments, Toronto, Canada).

and insulation failures (Electroshield from Electroscope, Boulder, CO) is used. Bipolar forceps with high-frequency, low-voltage cutting current (20–50 W) can coagulate vessels as large as the ovarian and uterine arteries. (see Chapter 5). The Kleppinger bipolar forceps (Richard Wolf) are excellent for large vessel hemostasis. Microbipolar forceps contain a channel for irrigation and a fixed distance between the electrodes. Irrigation is used to identify bleeding sites before coagulation and to prevent sticking of the electrode to the eschar that is created. Irrigation is also used during underwater examination to dilute blood products surrounding a bleeding vessel so that it may be identified before coagulation.

Disposable stapling instruments are rarely used for laparoscopic hysterectomy because of their expense. Sutures or bipolar desiccation work better.

Procedure Specifics

The following description presents my technique for a total laparoscopic hysterectomy (TLH). Other types of laparoscopic hysterectomy (e.g., LAVH or LH) are simply modifications of this more extensive procedure.

Incisions

Three laparoscopic puncture sites including the umbilicus are used: 10-mm umbilical, 5-mm right, and 5-mm left-lower quadrant. The left-lower quadrant puncture is the major portal for operative manipulation. The right trocar sleeve is used for retraction with atraumatic grasping forceps.

Vaginal Preparation

The endocervical canal is dilated to Pratt #25, and the Valtchev uterine mobilizer (Conkin Surgical Instruments, Toronto, Canada) is inserted to antevert the uterus and delineate the posterior vagina. When the uterus is in the anteverted position, the cervix sits on a wide pedestal, making the vagina readily visible between the uterosacral ligaments when the cul-de-sac is viewed laparoscopically.

Abdominal Exploration

The upper abdomen is inspected, and the appendix is identified. If appendiceal pathology is present, such as dilatation, adhesions, or endometriosis, an appendectomy is performed (see Chapter 23).

Ureteral Dissection

Three approaches have been used for laparoscopic ureteric identification, which may be called medial, superior, and lateral. When the ureter is identified but not dissected, cystoscopy is done after vaginal closure to check for ureteral patency, 5 min after one ampule of indigo carmine dye is administered intravenously.

The Medial Approach (Reich)

If the uterus is anteflexed, the ureter can usually be easily visualized in its natural position on the medial leaf of the broad ligament provided there is no significant cul-de-sac or adnexal pathology. This allows the peritoneum immediately above the ureter to be incised to create a "window" in the peritoneum, which makes for safe division of the infundibulopelvic ligament or adnexal pedicle. Immediately after exploration of the upper abdomen and pelvis, each ureter is isolated deep in the pelvis, when possible. Ureteral dissection is performed early in the operation before the pelvic side-wall peritoneum becomes edematous or opaque from irritation by the CO_2 pneumoperitoneum or aquadissection and before ureteral peristalsis is inhibited by surgical stress, pressure, or the Trendelenburg's position.[1]

The ureter and its overlying peritoneum are grasped deep in the pelvis. An atraumatic grasping forceps is used from the opposite-side cannula to grab the ureter and its overlying peritoneum on the pelvic side wall below and caudad to the ovary, lateral to the uterosacral ligament. Scissors are used to divide the peritoneum overlying the ureter and are inserted into the defect created and spread. Thereafter one blade of the scissors is placed on top of the ureter, its blade visualized through the peritoneum, and the peritoneum divided. This is continued into the deep pelvis where the uterine vessels cross the ureter, lateral to the cardinal ligament insertion into the cervix. Connective tissue between the ureter and the vessels is separated with scissors. Bleeding is controlled with microbipolar forceps. Often the uterine artery is ligated at this time to diminish backbleeding from the upper pedicles.

The Superior Approach

The superior approach entails dissecting the colon (rectosigmoid on the left; cecum on the right) off the pelvic brim and freeing the infundibulopelvic ligament vessels from the roof of the broad ligament to allow the ureter that lies below it to be identified. The ureter is then reflected off the broad ligament and traced into the pelvis.

The Lateral Approach (Kadar)

The lateral approach makes use of the pararectal space to identify the ureter, and the ureter does not have to peeled off the broad ligament for its entire pelvic course to be visible. By displacing the uterus to the contralateral side, a pelvic side-wall triangle is identified formed by the round ligament, the lateral border by the external iliac artery, and the medial border by the infundibulopelvic ligament. The peritoneum in the middle of the triangle is incised with scissors and the broad ligament opened by bluntly separating the extraperitoneal areolar tissues. The infundibulopelvic ligament is pulled medially with grasping forceps to expose the ureter at the pelvic brim where it crosses the common or external iliac artery.[18]

The operator then searches for the ureter distal to the pelvic brim and lateral to the infundibulopelvic ligament. The dissection is carried bluntly underneath and caudad to the round ligament, until the obliterated hypogastric artery is identified extraperitoneally. If any difficulty is encountered, the artery is first identified intraperitoneally where it hangs from the anterior abdominal wall, traced proximally to where it passes behind the round ligament, and then with both its intraperitoneal portion and the dissected space under the round ligament in view, the intraperitoneal part of the ligament is moved back and forth.

Once the obliterated hypogastric artery has been identified extraperitoneally, it is an easy matter to develop the paravesical space by bluntly separating the areolar tissue on either side of the artery. The obliterated hypogastric artery is next traced proximally to where it is joined by the uterine artery, and the pararectal space is opened by blunt dissection proximal and medial to the uterine vessels, which lie on top of the cardinal ligament. Once the pararectal space has been opened, the ureter is easily identified on the medial leaf of the broad ligament, which forms the medial border of the pararectal space. The uterine artery and cardinal ligament at the distal (caudal) border of the space, and the internal iliac artery on its lateral border also become clearly visible.

Bladder Mobilization

The round ligaments are divided at their midportion using a spoon electrode (Electroscope) set at a 150-W cutting current (Fig. 21.2). Persistent bleeding is controlled with bipolar desiccation at a 30-W cutting current. Thereafter, scissors or the same electrode is

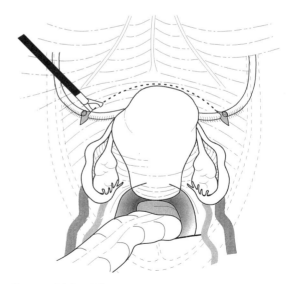

FIGURE 21.2. The round ligaments are divided at their midportion, and the vesicouterine peritoneal fold is divided starting at the left side and continuing across the midline to the right round ligament (*dotted line*).

used to divide the vesicouterine peritoneal fold starting at the left side and continuing across the midline to the right round ligament. The bladder is mobilized off the uterus and upper vagina sharply using scissors, or bluntly with the same spoon electrode, a suction-irrigator, or a endoscopic blunt tip dissector (Ethicon Endopath, Cincinnati, OH), until the anterior vagina is identified by elevating it from below with ring forceps (Fig. 21.2).

Ligation of Upper Uterine Blood Supply

When ovarian preservation is desired, the utero-ovarian ligament and fallopian tube pedicles are suture-ligated adjacent to the uterus with 0-Vicryl, using either a curved needle or a free ligature passed through a window created around the ligament (Figs. 21.3 and 21.4). When ovarian preservation is not desired, the anterior and posterior leaves of the broad ligament are opened lateral and below the infundibulopelvic ligament. A free ligature is passed through the peritoneal windows created and tied extracorporeally using the Clarke–Reich knot pusher[19] (Figs. 21.3 and 21.4). This is repeated twice until two proximal ties and one distal are placed, and the ligament is then divided. While applying traction to the cut distal pedicle, the broad ligament is divided to the round ligament just lateral to the utero-ovarian artery anastomosis using cutting current through a spoon electrode. Alternatively, the infundibulopelvic ligaments and broad ligaments may be coagulated until desiccated with bipolar forceps, at 25- to 35-W cutting current, and then divided.

Uterine Vessel Ligation

The broad ligament on each side is skeletonized down to the uterine vessels (Fig. 21.4). Each uterine vessel pedicle is suture-ligated with 0-Vicryl on a CT-1 needle (27 in.).[20] The needles are introduced into the peritoneal cavity by pulling them through a 5-mm incision.[10] The curved needle is placed around the uterine vessel pedicle at the side of the uterus or inserted on top of the unroofed ureter where it turns medially toward the previously mobilized bladder. A short rotary movement of the Cook

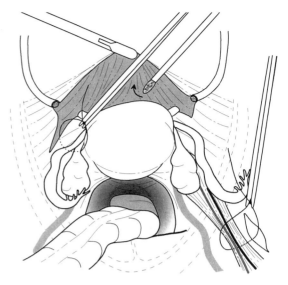

FIGURE 12.3. The bladder is mobilized off the uterus and upper vagina sharply using scissors, or bluntly with the same spoon electrode, a suction-irrigator, or a endoscopic blunt tip dissector (*depicted;* Ethicon Endopath, Cincinnatti, OH), until the anterior vagina is identified. When ovarian preservation is desired, the utero-ovarian ligament and fallopian tube pedicles are suture-ligated adjacent to the uterus with 0-Vicryl, using either a curved needle or a free ligature passed through a window created around the ligament (*left*). When ovarian preservation is not desired, the anterior and posterior leaves of the broad ligament are opened lateral and below the infundibulopelvic ligament, and a free ligature is passed through the created and tied extracorporeally (*right*).

oblique curved needle holder brings the needle around the uterine vessel pedicle. Sutures are tied extracorporeally using a Clarke–Reich knot pusher[20] (see Chapter 9). A single suture placed in this manner on each side serves as a "sentinel stitch," identifying the ureter for the remainder of the procedure.

Division of Cervicovaginal Attachments and Circumferential Culdotomy

The cardinal ligaments on each side are divided with the CO_2 laser at high power (80 W) or with the spoon electrode at 150-W cutting current. Bipolar forceps are invaluable to con-

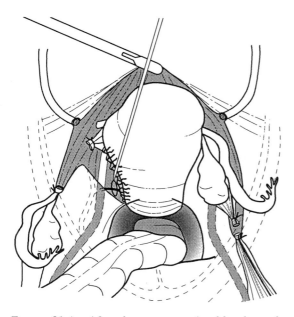

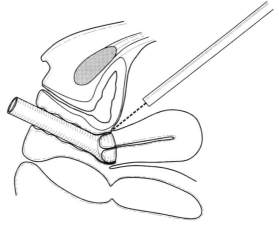

FIGURE 21.4.   After the upper uterine blood supply is secured, the broad ligament on each side is skeletonized down to the uterine vessels. Each uterine vessel pedicle is suture-ligated with 0-Vicryl.

FIGURE 21.5.   A 4-cm-diameter vaginal delineator (R. Wolf) is placed in the vagina to outline circumferentially the cervicovaginal junction, serving as a backstop for the laser and preventing loss of pneumoperitoneum. The anterior cervicovaginal junction and lateral fornices are identified and incised circumferentially with the laser. Dotted line represents laser beam.

trol bleeding from vaginal branches. The vagina is entered posteriorly over the Valtchev retractor near the cervicovaginal junction. A 4-cm-diameter vaginal delineator (R. Wolf) is placed in the vagina to outline circumferentially the cervicovaginal junction, serving as a backstop for laser work and preventing loss of pneumoperitoneum (Fig. 21.5). The vaginal delineator assists in identifying the anterior cervicovaginal junction and lateral fornices, which are incised circumferentially with the laser, to complete the culdotomy. The uterus is morcellated, if necessary, and pulled out of the vagina.

When the vaginal delineator is not available, a ring forceps is inserted into the anterior vagina above the tenaculum on the anterior cervical lip to identify the anterior cervicovaginal junction. The left-anterior vaginal fornix is entered using the laser, so that the aquapurator can be inserted into the anterior vagina above the anterior cervical lip. Following the aquapurator tip or ring forceps, and using them as a backstop, the anterior and lateral vaginal fornices are divided. The aquapurator is inserted from posterior to anterior to delineate the right

vaginal fornix, which is divided. The uterus can then be pulled out of the vagina.

Laparoscopic Vaginal Vault Closure and Suspension with McCall Culdeplasty

The vaginal delineator is placed back into the vagina for closure of the vaginal cuff, occluding it to maintain pneumoperitoneum. The left uterosacral ligament is elevated and a 0-Vicryl suture on a CT-1 needle is placed through it using an oblique Cook needle holder. The suture is then carried through the left cardinal ligament with just a few cells of the posterolateral vagina, and along the posterior vaginal epithelium, with a few bites over to the right side (Fig. 21.6).

Finally, the same suture with needle is used to fix the right posterolateral vagina and cardinal ligament to the right uterosacral ligament. This suture is tied extracorporeally and provides excellent support to the vaginal cuff apex, elevating it superiorly and posteriorly toward the hollow of the sacrum. The rest of the vagina and the overlying pubocervicovesicular fascia are closed vertically with one or two 0-

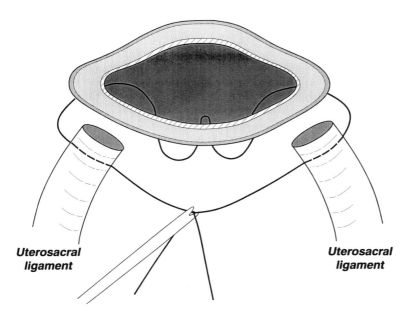

Uterosacral ligament   **Uterosacral ligament**

FIGURE 21.6. Laparoscopic vaginal vault closure and suspension with McCall culdeplasty. A 0-Vicryl suture on a CT-1 needle is placed through the left uterosacral ligament, the left cardinal ligament, the posterolateral vagina, and along the posterior vaginal epithelium. The same suture with needle is then used to fix the right posterolateral vagina and cardinal ligament to the right uterosacral ligament in a mirror fashion. This suture is tied extracorporeally.

Vicryl interrupted sutures. In most cases the peritoneum is not closed.

Underwater Examination

At the close of each operation, an underwater examination is used to detect bleeding from vessels and viscera tamponaded during the procedure by the increased intraperitoneal pressure of the CO_2 pneumoperitoneum. The CO_2 pneumoperitoneum is displaced with 2 to 5 liters of Ringer's lactate solution, and the peritoneal cavity is vigorously irrigated and suctioned until the effluent is clear of blood products. Any further bleeding is controlled underwater using microbipolar forceps to coagulate through the electrolyte solution, and at least 2 liters of lactated Ringer's solution are left in the peritoneal cavity.

Special Problems Related to Laparoscopic Hysterectomy

Very Large Fibroid Uterus

When the uterus is 16 weeks size or greater, the laparoscope is maneuvered into the deep culde-sac, and its tip may be used as a lever or rectractor to lift the uterus. The ureters are identi-

fied and isolated if possible. If endometriosis or rectal tenting is present, the peritoneum is opened and the rectum is reflected off the posterior vagina to the loose areolar tissue of the rectovaginal space. The vagina is incised between the uterosacral ligaments with a CO_2 laser beam directed through the operating laparoscope or with a spoon electrode. This incision is tamponaded with a sponge placed vaginally behind the cervix, to avoid losing pneumoperitoneum during the rest of the case.

The ovaries are examined. If oophorectomy is planned and the infundibulopelvic ligament is visible, it is ligated with 2-0 Vicryl free ties. In some cases involving a very large fibroid uterus, it is preferable to initially preserve the ovaries to avoid damaging structures at the pelvic side wall. The ovaries should be reexamined after the uterus is out and can be excised if indicated. However, when an ovary has been pulled away from its side wall by interligamentous fibroid growth, early oophorectomy may be necessary for better exposure.

The round ligament is divided with cutting current through a spoon electrode, and any bleeding is desiccated with bipolar forceps. With a large fibroid uterus, the utero-ovarian ligament and fallopian tube pedicle is generally markedly elongated. This pedicle is suture-ligated twice to prevent backbleeding. In many cases, bipolar desiccation is used and may be sufficient.

When very large fibroids are present, the bladder usually remains low in the pelvis, while the vesicouterine peritoneal fold is stretched upward. The vesicouterine peritoneal fold is divided with scissors, electrode, or CO_2 laser. This part of the procedure is generally done after ligation of the utero-ovarian ligament/round ligament/fallopian tube pedicle.

My most recent technique is to isolate and ligate the uterine artery on the side of the uterus early in the operation before upper vessel ligation to prevent backbleeding, especially if ovarian preservation is desired. The round ligament incision is extended into the ipsilateral portion of the vesicouterine peritoneal fold, and the pulsating uterine artery is identified and ligated with either a free ligature or a CT-1 needle. In these cases, the ureter is not isolated, and cystoscopy is done after cuff closure, 10 min after indigo carmine dye administration.

At this juncture, it is usually possible to incise both the anterior and posterior vagina laparoscopically and then proceed vaginally. Allan stirrups are changed to candy-cane stirrups, and the surgeon sits between the patient's legs. Vaginal clamps are applied: the uterosacral ligaments, cardinal ligaments, and uterine vessels are clamped, divided, and suture-ligated as for a vaginal hysterectomy. The uterus is then removed after extensive morcellation. The surgeon can change to the vaginal approach earlier in the procedure if vaginal access permits it.

When very large fibroids are located high above the level of the internal os of the cervix, it is often possible to manipulate the laparoscope above or beneath the large fibroid into the deep pelvis. The ureters on each side are identified using atraumatic forceps and are then separated from the uterine vessels, which are suture-ligated as previously described using curved needle techniques. The vagina is entered anteriorly and posteriorly and the cardinal ligaments are divided between these two incisions. The free uterus is removed after extensive morcellation.

Morcellation can be done laparoscopically or vaginally. For the laparoscopic technique, a #10 blade on a long handle is introduced gently through the left 5-mm trocar incision after removing the trocar. With care the uterus and its enclosed large myoma can be bivalved with the blade. The surgeon's fingers in contact with the skin prevent loss of pneumoperitoneum.

Vaginal morcellation is done after securing the ovarian arteries from above and the uterine arteries from above or below. A #10 blade on a long knife handle is used to make a circumferential incision into the fundus of the uterus while pulling outwards on the cervix and using the cervix as a fulcrum. The myometrium is incised circumferentially parallel to the axis of the uterine cavity and the serosa of the uterus. The knife is not extended through the serosa of the uterus. The incision is continued around the full circumference of the myometrium in a symmetrical fashion beneath the uterine serosa. Traction is maintained on the cervix, and the avascular myometrium is cut so that the endometrial cavity with a surrounding thick layer of myometrium is delivered with the cervix, bringing the outside of the uterus closer to the operator for further excision by wedge morcellation.[21,22]

Wedge morcellation is done by removing wedges of myometrium from the anterior and posterior uterine wall, usually in the midline, to reduce the bulk of the myometrium. After excision of a large core, the fundus is morcellated with multiple wedge resections, around either a tenaculum or an 11-mm corkscrew (WISAP, Sauerlach, Germany, or Tomball, TX). The remaining fundus, if still too large for removal, can be bivalved so that one-half can be pulled out of the peritoneal cavity, followed by the other half.

At the end of the procedure, inspection of the pelvis underwater with the laparoscope should be considered, even if a large myomatous uterus is removed using solely vaginal techniques. Bleeding from the vaginal cuff or from the stretched-out pedicles is common and can be readily coagulated laparoscopically, and blood clot seeded with vaginal organisms can be aspirated laparoscopically. Adding laparoscopy to a vaginal hysterectomy for large fibroids may reduce the morbidity of the procedure.

Stage IV and Rectal Endometriosis

In cases of severe endometriosis with cul-de-sac obliteration, the surgeon must first free the ovaries, then the ureters, and finally the rectum from the posterior vagina to the rectovaginal septum. Deep fibrotic nodular endometriosis involving the cul-de-sac requires excision of the fibrotic tissue from the uterosacral ligaments, posterior cervix, posterior vagina, and the rectum. Attention is first directed to complete dissection of the anterior rectum beneath involved peritoneum until loose areolar tissue of the rectovaginal space is reached. In all cases, a rectal probe (Reznik Instruments) is placed in the rectum.

Using the rectal probe as a guide, the rectal interface with the cul-de-sac lesion is identified and opened at this junction with CO_2 laser or scissors. Careful blunt dissection is then done using the aquadissector for aquadissection and suction-traction. Laser or scissors are used for sharp dissection until the rectum, with or without some fibrotic endometriosis, is separated from the posterior uterus and upper vagina and is identifiable below the lesion in the loose areolar tissue of the rectovaginal space. Only after the rectum is fully mobilized should excision of the fibrotic endometriosis be attempted from the posterior vagina, uterosacral ligaments, and rectum. Full-thickness excision of the vaginal nodular areas usually results in relief of the patient's pain and bleeding.[9]

Nodules in the muscularis of the anterior rectum can usually be excised laparoscopically. Full-thickness penetration of the rectum can occur during hysterectomy surgery, especially when excising rectal endometriosis nodules. Following identification of the nodule or rent in the rectum, a closed circular stapler [Proximate ILS curved intraluminal stapler (Ethicon, Stealth)] is inserted into the lumen just past the lesion or hole, opened 1 to 2 cm, and held high to avoid the posterior rectal wall. The proximal anvil is positioned just beyond the lesion or hole that is invaginated into the open-

ing and the device closed. Circumferential inspection is made to ensure the absence of encroachment of nearby organs and posterior rectum in the staple line and the lack of tension in the anastomosis. The instrument is fired, then removed through the anus.

The surgeon must inspect and ensure that the fibrotic lesion or a doughnut of tissue representing the excised hole is contained in the circular stapler. Once verified, anastomotic inspection is done laparoscopically underwater after filling the rectum with indigo carmine solution.

Laparoscopic Uterosacral-Vaginal Suspension

It is possible to suspend the vagina after hysterectomy using laparoscopic surgical techniques. In cases in which hysterectomy is done for vaginal and uterine prolapse, the ureters are dissected laparoscopically before vaginal hysterectomy to better identify the ventral aspect of the uterosacral ligaments, close to the sacrum. Sutures are applied to these firm ligaments adjacent to the sacrum and upper rectum. The suture material is left long in the peritoneal cavity for later fixation.

After vaginal removal of the uterus, the previously applied sutures are grasped transvaginally with the surgeon's index finger and brought into the vagina. These sutures are then inserted into the vaginal cuff using free curved needles. They are then tied after completion of the vaginal closure repair, elevating the vaginal cuff to a higher position than would be obtainable with conventional vaginal surgery only.

Laparoscopic Rectocele Repair

Enterocele and rectocele are amenable to a laparoscopic repair. Laparoscopic plication of the levator ani muscles above the anal sphincter results in excellent vaginal and rectal support. To carry out this procedure, the rectovaginal space is opened with aquadissection or retroperitoneal space expanders (Preperitoneal Distention Balloon, Origin Medsystems, Menlo Park, CA). Separation of the rectum bilaterally results in identification of the levator ani muscles. These are brought together across the midline with the placement of 0-Vicryl or Ethibond in an interrupted fashion. Thereafter, the vaginal vault is suspended to the uterosacral ligaments overlying the levator plate and sacrum, as described earlier, using a combined laparoscopic and vaginal approach.[23]

Postoperative Considerations

The vaginal cuff is checked for granulation tissue between 6 and 12 weeks postoperatively, as sutures are usually absorbed by then. Patients usually experience some fatigue and discomfort for approximately 2 to 4 weeks after the operation, but may perform gentle exercise such as walking and may return to routine activities between 2 and 6 weeks postoperatively. Sexual activity may be resumed when the vaginal incision has healed, usually after 6 weeks.

Risks and Complications

Complications of laparoscopic hysterectomy are those of hysterectomy and laparoscopy in general: anesthetic accidents, respiratory compromise, thromboembolic phenomenon, urinary retention, injury to vessels, ureters, bladder, and bowel, and infections, especially of the vaginal cuff.[24] Complications unique to laparoscopy include large vessel injury and subcutaneous emphysema. Since the introduction of prophylactic antibiotics, vaginal cuff abscess, pelvic thrombophlebitis, septicemia, pelvic cellulitis, and adnexal abscesses are rare. Abdominal wound infection is rare, but the incidence of incisional hernias after operative laparoscopy is greatly increased if 10-mm or larger trocars are placed at extraumbilical sites. These sites should be closed. If the incision is lateral to the rectus muscle, the deep fascia is elevated with skin hooks and suture repaired. If the incision is through the rectus muscle, the peritoneal defect is closed with a laparoscopically placed suture. For a further discussion of laparoscopic complications, please see Chapter 25.

Febrile morbidity associated with a vaginal hysterectomy is about half that of the abdominal procedure. Laparoscopic evacuation of all blood clots and the sealing of all blood vessels after the uterus has been removed should further reduce the infection rate. Morcellation during laparoscopic or vaginal hysterectomy results in a slightly increased risk of fever, especially if prophylactic antibiotics are not used.

Conclusions

It is difficult to extrapolate indications for the role of laparoscopy in hysterectomy from present publications because the surgeons most skilled in the laparoscopic approach are referred the difficult cases and rarely see those that could be easily performed vaginally. The future role of laparoscopic hysterectomy will be determined by the increased familiarity and skill of surgeons with vaginal procedures, stimulated by doing the difficult part of a "laparoscopic-assisted vaginal hysterectomy" vaginally.

It is possible that more than 50% of indicated hysterectomies can be performed using the vaginal route only without laparoscopy; the laparoscope may convert more than one-half of the remaining cases to a vaginal procedure. It is probable that vaginal hysterectomy, after an initial diagnostic laparoscopy, will be possible in one-half of those patients who present with some relative contraindication to the vaginal approach. One-half of the remaining indicated hysterectomies will require laparoscopic oophorectomy or adhesiolysis of the upper portion to be removed, i.e., an LAVH. Of the remaining 12.5% of the total, the skilled laparoscopic surgeon will consider laparoscopic hysterectomy in fewer than 1% of cases.

References

1. Reich H. Laparoscopic hysterectomy. *Surgical Laparoscopy and Endoscopy*. Vol. 2. New York: Raven Press; 1992:85–88.
2. Liu CY. Laparoscopic hysterectomy: a review of 72 cases. *J Reprod Med.* 1992;37:351–354.

3. Liu CY. Laparoscopic hysterectomy. Report of 215 cases. *Gynaecol Endosc.* 1992;1:73–77.

4. Reich H, DeCaprio J, McGlynn F. Laparoscopic hysterectomy. *J Gynecol Surg.* 1989;5:213–216.

5. Kovac SR, Cruikshank SH, Retto HF. Laparoscopy-assisted vaginal hysterectomy. *J Gynecol Surg.* 1990;6:185–189.

6. Reich H, McGlynn F, Sekel L. Total laparoscopic hysterectomy. *Gynaecol Endosc.* 1993;2: 59–63.

7. Lyons TL. Laparoscopic supracervical hysterectomy. In: Hunt RB, Martin DC, eds. *Endoscopy in Gynecology.* Proceedings of the World Congress of Gynecologic Endoscopy, AAGL 20th Annual Meeting, Las Vegas, NV. Baltimore: Port City Press; 1993:129–131.

8. Reich H. Laparoscopic extrafascial hysterectomy with bilateral salpingo-oophorectomy using stapling techniques for endometrial adenocarcinoma. AAGL 19th Annual Meeting, Orlando, FL. 1990.

9. Reich H, McGlynn F, Wilkie W. Laparoscopic management of Stage I ovarian cancer. *J Reprod Med.* 1990;35:601–605.

10. Canis M, Mage G, Wattiez A, Pouly JL, et al. Does endoscopic surgery have a role in radical surgery of cancer of the cervix uteri? *J Gynecol Obstet Biol Reprod.* 1990;19:921.

11. Reich H, McGlynn F, Salvat J. Laparoscopic treatment of cul-de-sac obliteration secondary to retrocervical deep fibrotic endometriosis. *J Reprod Med.* 1991;36:516–522.

12. Reich H, McGlynn F, Sekel L, Taylor P. Laparoscopic management of ovarian dermoid cysts. *J Reprod Med.* 1992;37:640–644.

13. Parker WH, Berek JS. Management of selected cystic adnexal masses in postmenopausal women by operative laparoscopy: a pilot study. *Am J Obstet Gynecol.* 1990;163:1574–1577.

14. Stovall TG, Ling FW, Henry LC, Woodruff MR. A randomized trial evaluating leuprolide acetate before hysterectomy as treatment for leiomyomas. *Am J Obstet Gynecol.* 1991;164: 1420–1425.

15. Schlaff WD, Zerhouni EA, Huth JA, Chen J, Damewood MD, Rock, JA. A placebo-controlled trial of a depot gonadotropin-releasing hormone analogue (leuprolide) in the treatment of uterine leiomyomata. *Obstet Gynecol.* 1989; 74:856–862.

16. Valtchev KL, Papsin FR. A new uterine mobilizer for laparoscopy: Its use in 518 patients. *Am J Obstet Gynecol.* 1977;127:738–740.

17. Reich H, McGlynn F. Short self-retaining trocar sleeves. *Am J Obstet Gynecol.* 1990;162:453–454.

18. Kadar N. A laparoscopic technique for dissecting the pelvic retroperitoneum and identifying the ureters. *J Reprod Med.* 1995;40:116–122.

19. Clarke HC. Laparoscopy—New instruments for suturing and ligation. *Fertil Steril.* 1972;23: 274–277.

20. Reich H, Clarke HC, Sekel L. A simple method for ligating in operative laparoscopy with straight and curved needles. *Obstet Gynecol.* 1992;79:143–147.

21. Lash AF. A method for reducing the size of the uterus in vaginal hysterectomy. *Am J Obstet Gynecol.* 1941;42:452–459.

22. Kovac SR. Intramyometrial coring as an adjunct to vaginal hysterectomy. *Obstet Gynecol.* 1986; 67:131–136.

23. Zacharin RF. Pulsion enterocele: Review of functional anatomy of the pelvic floor. *Obstet Gynecol.* 1980;55:135–140.

24. Woodland MB. Ureter injury during laparoscopy-assisted vaginal hysterectomy with the endoscopic linear stapler. *Am J Obstet Gynecol.* 1992;167:756–757.

22

Laparoscopic Retropubic Colposuspension Procedures

Andrew I. Brill

Despite the fact that the majority of women suffering from urinary incontinence will not seek professional help for reasons of embarrassment or ignorance of available therapeutic options, the treatment of this clinical disorder continues to be one of the most frequent facets of contemporary gynecologic care. Conservative estimates indicate that nearly 20% of women aged from 40 to 60 years old and 35% of noninstitutionalized women older than 60 years suffer from urinary incontinence.[1]

As the health care paradigm of the 1990s establishes its footing, each physician will be progressively held accountable for adhering to standards that will decrease cost and improve the quality of care. Reward and penalty will be linked to how effectively care is delivered in an ambulatory setting. Nonsurgical alternatives and outpatient strategies will be hailed while inpatient services are strictly scrutinized. In this spirit, as the role of endoscopic surgery for the treatment of genuine stress incontinence continues to be demonstrated, gynecologic surgeons with advanced laparoscopic skills are behooved to apply minimally invasive surgical techniques to perform indicated antiincontinence surgeries traditionally performed by laparotomy.

The laparoscopic approach is ideally suited to performing surgery in the retropubic space. It promises to produce results equivalent to those attained by laparotomy, reduce operating room time and postoperative pain, accelerate recovery of the voiding mechanism, and minimize social and economic disability by shifting therapy to an outpatient setting. Global costs should be substantially reduced without compromising clinical outcome.

Since it was first reported by Vancaillie and Schuessler in 1991,[2] a number of publications have confirmed the ability to laparoscopically perform a retropubic urethropexy without added morbidity and with similar results in the short term.[3-9] Laparoscopic retropubic colposuspension simply accomplishes the traditional laparotomic procedure by a different means of surgical access. As with other advanced laparoscopic surgical procedures, technical requirements are more demanding than its laparotomic counterpart. Advanced laparoscopic skills are a necessity.

Advantages of the laparoscopic approach include elimination of the abdominal incision, unhindered visual access, and exposure of the anatomic structures of the space of Retzius. The visual clarity and magnification of tissues permits more precise dissection, refined hemostasis by means of identification of blood vessels before transection, less trauma to the periurethral tissues, more accurate placement of sutures, avoidance of injury to the urinary tract and neurovascular structures, and identification of associated herniations of the anterior endopelvic fascia. Postoperative complications including wound infection, retropubic hematoma, and detrusor instability may be reduced.

The laparoscopic approach has yet to be widely embraced secondary to the absence of prospective and long-term comparative studies that utilize urodynamic assessments and the laparotomic approach as the gold standard and because of the technical demands of the procedure. Endoscopic suturing in the space of Retzius can be laborious and frustrating. The loss of depth of field and peripheral vision from monocular vision must be overcome. Suture placement is hampered by unstable needle holders, the tenacity of Cooper's ligament, and restrictions in instrument mobility and angle of freedom. Extracorporeal knot tying has to be mastered. Overcoming these challenges requires practice, patience, and skilled assistance in the operating theater.

As more innovative surgeons continue to tackle the laparoscopic approach, modifications in technique will evolve to simplify this procedure. For example, the traditional Burch technique is modified by eliminating suturing into Cooper's ligament, using staples instead to secure the lateral suture strand to this structure.[9] Suturing can be completely eliminated by anchoring a piece of Prolene mesh between the pubocervical fascia and Cooper's ligament with endoscopic staples.[5]

Patient Selection and Preoperative Evaluation

Preoperative Evaluation

A carefully orchestrated diagnostic plan maximizes accuracy, directs the choice of proper therapy, helps ensure long-term therapeutic efficacy, and should minimize the performance of unwarranted surgery. The severity and magnitude of urinary incontinence is best objectified by having the patient complete a voiding diary for 1 to 3 days to ascertain voiding habits, frequency and volume of fluid intake, episodes of incontinence including precipitants, and bladder capacity.

The patient interview should strive to elucidate the past obstetric history (e.g., macrosomia, operative deliveries, prolonged second stage), gynecologic history (e.g., surgery, symptomatic anatomic defects, pelvic irradiation), the presence of significant medical problems (e.g., cardiac, pulmonary, neurological disease), and the use of medications (especially substances that affect detrusor function such as anticholinergics and alpha or beta sympathomimetics). Because urinary tract infection can masquerade as incontinence, a clean urine should be sent for culture and sensitivity. After voiding, the bladder is catheterized to measure the residual volume.

The pelvic examination should be performed at rest and while standing and should be site specific, examining the uterus or vault for prolapse, the anterior vaginal wall for midline and lateral defects, the posterior wall for rectocele, and the perineal body for length and mobility. The presence of a urethral diverticulum or lower urinary tract fistula should be ruled out. Overall estrogen effect should be noted. The Q-tip test can be used to measure the anatomic support of the proximal urethra; it is valuable for establishing hypermobility at the urethrovesical junction (greater than 30° rotation from the horizontal plane). The lower genital exam is completed by looking for deficiencies of the sacral reflexes and dermatomes (S2–S4) and assessing the ability to isolate and contract the levator ani muscles.

The diagnosis of genuine stress incontinence is definitively established by demonstrating the involuntary loss of urine when the intravesical pressure exceeds urethral pressure in the absence of a bladder contraction. Cystometry is the test of choice to evaluate the pressure–volume relationships of the detrusor muscle and to elicit uninhibitable bladder contractions. Although the presence of detrusor instability does not preclude the need for surgery, failure to diagnose vesical instability preoperatively has been identified as one reason for unsuccessful incontinence surgery. On completion of the cystogram, the patient is asked to cough with a symptomatically full bladder. A positive cough stress test with a negative preceding cystometrogram is close to being 100% specific and sensitive for the diagnosis of genuine stress incontinence.

Further testing with multichannel urodynamics should be performed for patients who have undergone prior antiincontinence surgery or pelvic irradiation, for those who had a positive cystometrogram, for elderly patients, and when incontinence coexists with urinary retention to rule out intrinsic sphincteric deficiency (low-pressure urethra). Cystourethroscopy should be performed in women who suffer from persistent irritative symptoms of the lower urinary tract, are suspected to have a urethral diverticulum, or have undergone prior antiincontinence surgery that utilized permanent suture materials.

Preoperative Preparation

Before surgery, a diligently completed informed consent should review the usual risks of retropubic surgery and include the risks of transperitoneal entry, the possibility of conversion to laparotomy, injury to the urinary tract, and postoperative voiding dysfunction. The patient should be taught to perform self-catheterization in case of postoperative bladder instability and supplied with straight catheters.

Indications and Patient Selection

Although genuine stress incontinence has been traditionally treated by surgery, current data and accepted recommendations suggest that all patients should first be given the opportunity to undergo a trial of nonsurgical therapy. Available options include the use of behavioral therapy, mechanical devices, and pharmacologic therapy. Although a minority of these patients will be entirely cured of their symptoms, many women attain enough improvement that surgical therapy is no longer desirable as a treatment option.

A number of surgical strategies have been proverbially used to treat genuine stress incontinence. To varying degrees of success, all these techniques attempt to reestablish anatomic support for the urethra from a vaginal hammock to recreate the efficient transmission of intraabdominal pressure to the proximal urethra. In the most comprehensive review to date, Jarvis[10] reported the collective results of antiincontinence surgeries performed on 1439 patients that excluded cases with detrusor instability, were limited to the treatment of objectively established genuine stress incontinence, included pre- and postoperative urodynamic assessments, and had at least 1 year of follow-up. These data demonstrated that the retropubic colposuspension as described by Burch and the Marshall–Marchetti–Krantz procedure produced the highest objective cure rates as measured by total continence of urine (89.8% and 89.5%, respectively).

Regardless of these findings, no surgical procedure is ideal for all patients. In each case the physician must take into account the patient's age, degree of physical frailty, hormonal status, weight, preoperative urodynamic findings, relative vaginal mobility and capacity, and the existence of concomitant pelvic floor defects, prolapse, or urethral scarring.

The suburethral sling is the most effective technique for restoring continence in women undergoing subsequent procedures for recurrent stress incontinence. Women with low urethral closure pressures (<20 cmH$_2$O) are at significant risk for treatment failure after colposuspension and are better served undergoing either a suburethral sling procedure or periurethral collagen injections. By itself, the Marshall–Marchetti–Krantz procedure may be insufficient to completely correct severe anterior vaginal wall herniation.

Consideration must be given to potential alterations in the continence mechanism created by procidentia, severe cystocele, and vault prolapse. Simple repair of these anatomic defects can decrease urethral resistance caused by kinking from the prolapse and may unmask predisposing factors for stress incontinence. These women are best managed with a combined approach using a transvaginal repair with a needle suspension procedure. Surgical implantation of an artificial urinary sphincter is reserved for women who have failed multiple antiincontinence surgeries or suffer from neuropathic incontinence and who face the potential for long-term indwelling catheter drainage or undergoing a urinary diversion procedure.

Instrumentation and Techniques

A single dose of an appropriate prophylactic antibiotic should be administered no more than 1 hr before surgery. After induction of general anesthesia or regional block, the legs are positioned to facilitate a retropubic urethropexy with the aid of vaginal manipulation. This is accomplished by adjusting the patient's torso and extremities to a low dorsal lithotomy position with the legs and feet supported by Allen Universal Stirrups (Allen Medical, Mayfield, OH), or by keeping the legs in a flat position and flexing the knees and abducting the thighs to oppose the plantar surfaces of the feet in a "frog-leg" position.

After appropriate antiseptic preparation of the vagina and operative field, the patient is draped with a combined laparotomy and lithotomy drape for access to both the abdomen and perineum during surgery. A three-way 24-Fr. Foley catheter is placed in the bladder and the bulb is inflated to 20 cc to help identify the urethrovesical junction during surgery.

Trocar Considerations

The umbilical trocar site is used for a conventional or operating laparoscope and the placement of mechanical balloon dissectors. Accessory trocar sheath diameters are dictated by the endoscopic instrumentation specific to each method for colposuspension. All ports can be used for the interchange of ancillary instruments such as the suction irrigator, grasping forceps, needle holder, curved monopolar scissors, bipolar forceps, and Kittner sponge dissector. A 10–11 trocar is used for the unhindered passage of typically used suture needles and the endoscopic stapling gun.

Depending on the surgeon's comfort level, two to three accessory trocars are placed in the usual fashion: during the transperitoneal approach, one trocar is placed in the midline, midway between the umbilicus and pubic symphysis. One to two additional trocars are placed lateral to the inferior epigastric vessels, halfway between the anterior iliac spine and the umbilicus (Fig. 22.1). Trocar placements during the extraperitoneal technique are logically similar but limited to the outer visual limits of the insufflated retroperitoneal space.

Pertinent Anatomy

With an intact urinary tract and normal intrinsic urethral function, the involuntary loss of urine during sudden rises in abdominal pressure is normally prevented by the passive transmission of abdominal pressure to the proximal urethra; urinary continence is maintained by the creation of a positive pressure gradient between the urethra and bladder. This dynamic transfer of intraabdominal pressure is dependent on the native anatomic position and mobility of the proximal urethra.

The middle and proximal urethra is supported by a suspensory hammock composed of suburethral endopelvic fascia (pubocervical) and the anterior vaginal wall (Fig. 22.2). At this level of the pelvis, the vagina is suspended to the lateral pelvic side walls by a mesentery-like

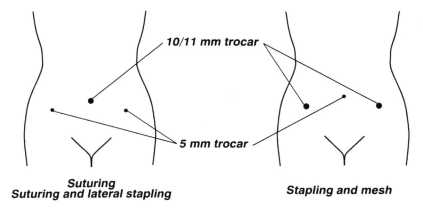

FIGURE 22.1. Trocar placement sites for performing laparoscopic retropubic colposuspension procedures: *left,* for either suturing or suturing and lateral stapling; or *right,* for stapling and mesh placement.

sling of endopelvic fascia that attaches posteriorly to the medial border of the levator ani muscles and anteriorly to the arcus tendineus fasciae pelvis (the "white line"). Connective tissue damage at the level of the pubocervical fascia releases the proximal urethra from the sphere of intraabdominal pressure transmission, resulting in stress-induced incontinence. This is clinically manifested as a cystocele and proximal urethral hypermobility.

A complete understanding of the anatomic boundaries and interior components of the retropubic space will minimize surgical morbidity and ensure the best operative results. The space of Retzius is a large potential area bounded inferiorly by the pubic symphysis and ischial spine, medially by the rich perivesical venous plexus and fat, and laterally by the obturator internus muscle and obturator neurovascular bundle (Fig. 22.3). Laparoscopic

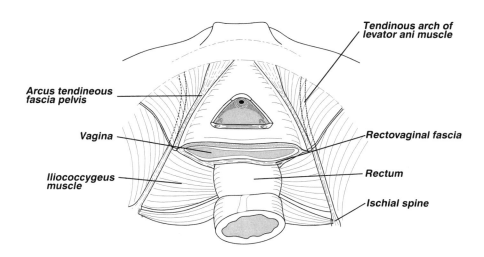

FIGURE 22.2. Anatomy of urethral support. The middle and proximal urethra is supported by a suspensory hammock composed of suburethral endopelvic fascia (pubocervical) and the anterior vaginal wall.

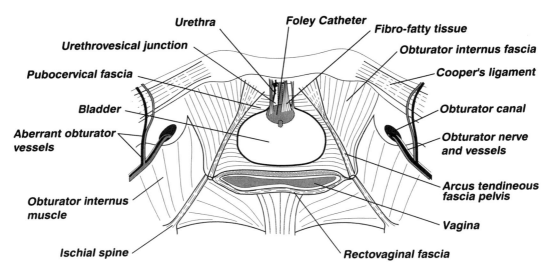

Urethra — Foley Catheter — Fibro-fatty tissue
Urethrovesical junction — Obturator internus fascia
Pubocervical fascia — Cooper's ligament
Bladder — Obturator canal
Aberrant obturator vessels — Obturator nerve and vessels
Obturator internus muscle — Arcus tendineous fascia pelvis
Vagina
Ischial spine — Rectovaginal fascia

FIGURE 22.3. Anatomy of retropubic space. The space of Retzius is a large potential area bounded inferiorly by the pubic symphysis and ischial spine, medially by the rich perivesical venous plexus and fat, and laterally by the obturator internus muscle and obturator neurovascular bundle.

dissection of this space anteriorly exposes the urethra, urethrovesical junction, anterior wall of the bladder, and underlying glistening pubocervical fascia. More laterally, the arcus tendineus fasciae pelvis, or white line, is exposed as it travels from the undersurface of the pubic bone to the ischial spine.

Dissection of the loose areolar and connective tissue on the inner superior surface of the pubic symphysis uncovers Cooper's ligament. Further dissection laterally exposes the obturator neurovascular bundle as it descends along the inner surface of the symphysis to exit through the obturator canal. Accessory obturator vessels arising from the inferior epigastric vessels run along the lateral surface of Cooper's ligament to laterally anastomose with the obturator vessels. There are two approaches to the space of Retzius: transperitoneal and extraperitoneal, as discussed next.

Transperitoneal Approach

Advantages and Disadvantages

Advantages of the transperitoneal approach to the space of Retzius include the ability to concomitantly correct other pelvic pathology by laparoscopy, to visualize and correct other defects in pelvic support, and to perform a prophylactic culdoplasty. Relative disadvantages include the need for general anesthesia, Trendelenburg positioning, the inherent risk of injury to visceral and vascular structures, the potential for needing to abort the procedure secondary to dense intraabdominal adhesions, the risk of bladder injury secondary to the need for incision in the supravesical peritoneum, and the physiologic sequelae and postoperative pain related to pneumoperitoneal carbon dioxide.

Technique

After placing the trocars in the usual fashion, the patient is placed in a 20° Trendelenburg's position. The laparoscope is inserted, and the pelvic viscera and trocar sites are inspected for injury. Surgery is performed to correct other pelvic pathology.

Before incising the anterior peritoneum to enter the retropubic space, the superior extent of the bladder dome can be ascertained by temporarily inflating the bladder with 200cc of saline or sterile milk. Using the urachus to identify the midline, the anterior abdominal wall peritoneum is grasped approximately 1 in. above the pubic symphysis, incised transversely using monopolar endoscopic scissors or laser energy, and extended laterally to both the obliterated umbilical ligaments. Care must be taken to avoid transecting the inferior epigastric vessels as they course parallel to these structures.

Once entered, the retropubic space can be opened down to the pubic symphysis by a combination of gentle blunt and sharp dissection using curved monopolar electrosurgical scissors, the irrigator probe, the laparoscope, aquadissection, an endoscopic Kittner sponge, or laser energy. To prevent troublesome pooling of blood and staining of tissues, hemostasis should be meticulous by discrete identification of blood vessels and prophylactic coagulation with monopolar or bipolar electrosurgery. Staying close to the back of the pubic bone, the space is progressively dissected to sequentially separate the anterior bladder, vaginal wall, and urethra in a downward fashion.

Digital pressure within the vaginal vault is used to facilitate further dissection. Two fingers are placed in the vagina, one on each side of the catheterized urethra, to elevate the fornices so as to identify the bladder neck and underlying pubocervical fascia.

Starting laterally, the bladder is dissected medially and upward from the underlying fascia by using blunt dissection over the surgeon's fingers as the vagina is displaced anteriorly and laterally. This can be accomplished either by static digital traction and active endoscopic blunt dissection, or by static endoscopic traction and active traction with the surgeon's fingers. It is imperative to protect the delicate neurovascular plexus and musculature at the urethrovesical junction by keeping all dissection at least 1 to 2 cm lateral and away from the urethra and to avoid injuring the rich, thin-walled vascular plexus around the urethra.

To promote scarification, fibrofatty tissue can be cleared from the vaginal wall as it is dissected to expose the underlying pubocervical fascia and removed through an accessory trocar. As it is highly vascular, prevesical fat is best dissected with the help of electrosurgery or laser energy. Using the aberrant and primary obturator vessels as the outer limits of dissection, preparation of the retropubic space is completed by identifying Cooper's ligament bilaterally and clarifying excessive fat and areolar tissue. The space is actively lavaged, and hemostasis is accomplished with directed bipolar desiccation.

Extraperitoneal Approaches

Advantages and Disadvantages

The comparative advantages of the extraperitoneal approach include the ability to use regional anesthesia and supine patient positioning, unhindered entry into the retropubic space in the presence of significant intraabdominal adhesions, entering the retropubic space by blunt rather than sharp dissection, the reduced risk for herniation at trocar sites, the virtual elimination of the risks from peritoneal entry, decreased operating time, and reduced postoperative pain. Relative disadvantages of this approach include the cost of disposable mechanical devices, lower accessory trocar positions, potentially difficult deep rectus dissection in obese patients, failure to enter the retropubic space secondary to scarring of the abdominal wall after prior laparotomy, and the inability to perform a prophylactic culdoplasty. Furthermore, the space of Retzius may become physically obstructed by a protuberant pneumoperitoneum accidentally created by peritoneal entry during the dissection of the preperitoneal space. Once recognized, the obstruction can be reduced by placing a small trocar into the peritoneal cavity to continuously vent the intraperitoneal carbon dioxide. In some cases, conversion to a transperitoneal approach will be necessary.

Techniques

Extraperitoneal entry into the space of Retzius can be accomplished using either blunt operative dissection or disposable balloon distension systems. Once the retropubic space is surgically or mechanically developed, further mobilization of the bladder, urethra, and paravaginal tissues is accomplished using the same surgical techniques as described for the transperitoneal approach. While the factors affecting trocar size and anatomic positions are similar to the transperitoneal technique, trocar placements are limited by the lateral and superior extent of the insufflated retropubic space.

Blunt surgical dissection into the retropubic space is initiated at the umbilicus. A subumbilical skin incision of several centimeters is made transversely and carried into the subcutaneous tissues. The rectus fascia is cleared, incised transversely, and suture-tagged at both edges for countertraction and to affix a Hasson trocar. Using the index finger, the subrectus preperitoneal space is bluntly dissected toward the symphysis pubis in the midline. A Hasson trocar is then inserted and secured in the usual fashion.

A conventional or operating laparoscope is directed into the preperitoneal space, which is insufflated and initially dissected with carbon dioxide at a setting of 8 to 10 mmHg. Under direct vision the laparoscope is advanced over the anterior surface of the posterior rectus sheath to the midline of the pubic symphysis. The retropubic space is bluntly cleared of areolar tissues using the laparoscope or instruments inserted through the operating channel. Alternatively, after externally identifying the

midline of the symphysis pubis as an anatomic target, the laparoscope is aimed and blindly advanced horizontally along the preperitoneal space into the space of Retzius. The space is then dissected by sweeping the laparoscope bilaterally in a slightly curvilinear fashion.

The space of Retzius can also be approached in an extraperitoneal fashion after completion of an intrapelvic laparoscopic procedure. The laparoscope is withdrawn into the subumbilical preperitoneal space and under direct vision redirected caudally to progressively dissect the areolar tissue above the posterior sheath into the retropubic space. Using the laparoscope to alternatively visualize intraperitoneal and extraperitoneal sites, each accessory trocar is withdrawn from the peritoneal cavity and tunneled into the space of Retzius.

Mechanical balloon distension systems are an efficient method to bluntly and atraumatically dissect the retropubic space (Fig. 22.4). After creating a 10-mm vertical or elliptical infraumbilical incision, the preperitoneal space is sharply entered and digitally developed as performed in blunt surgical dissection. The balloon–trocar system is lubricated at its distal

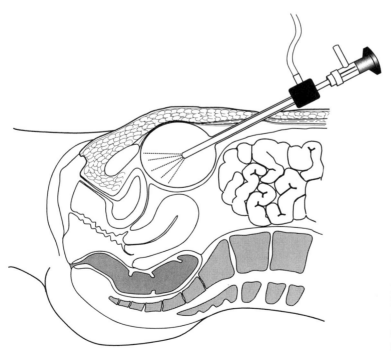

FIGURE 22.4. Mechanical balloon distension systems are an efficient method to bluntly and atraumatically dissect the retropubic space.

end and inserted beneath the underbelly of the rectus muscle. While staying in a horizontal plane slightly lateral to the linea alba, the preperitoneal space is gently dissected downward aiming toward the posterior symphysis pubis. The balloon is then inflated either under direct vision with air (Preperitoneal Distention System, Origin Medsystems, Menlo Park, CA) or blindly with saline (Spacemaker Balloon Dissector, General Surgical Innovations, Portola Valley, CA) to mechanically dissect the retropubic space. After 1 to 2 min of resting time, the balloon (and laparoscope) is removed after deflation. A blunt-tipped trocar is then inserted into the developed preperitoneal space and secured with a skin seal. The laparoscope is inserted down the cannula, and the retropubic space is insufflated with carbon dioxide at a setting of 8 to 10 mmHg.

Methods for Colposuspension

Suturing Techniques

After adequate mobilization of the urethra and fascial attachments of the bladder from the underlying pubocervical fascia, laparoscopic retropubic colposuspension is performed using the same time-honored principles practiced during the laparotomic technique. Both O-Vicryl and O-Ethibond on a CT-2 needle (Ethicon/Summerville, NJ) or #2 Gore-Tex on a THX-26 needle (W. L. Gore/Flagstaff, AZ) can be used as suture materials. Proponents of using permanent suture argue that retropubic fibrosis and scarring are maximized by using materials with greater longevity. Both types of needles can be passed down the sheath of a 10–11 trocar by grasping the suture strand with a needle holder 2 cm from the swedge point and passing it through the cannula into the surgical field.

Larger curved needles or smaller trocar sheaths can be accommodated by passing the needle directly into the surgical field. After removing the trocar sleeve from the abdominal wall, a needle holder is inserted into the sleeve and the terminal end of the suture is pulled up and out of the sheath. The needle holder is reinserted and the suture is grasped 2 to 3 cm from the swedge point. Any suture slack is reduced by gentle traction on the terminal end. The needle holder is then inserted directly through the abdominal incision with the curved needle following in step. The trocar sleeve is then pushed back into the abdominal wall over the needle holder. The needle is then properly positioned into the needle holder with the help of the assistant.

Before suturing the vagina, it should be digitally lifted upward and forward to confirm that the mobility of the urethrovesical junction is adequate for repositioning to its normal location. Laparoscopic suturing is least encumbered when the available area of the anterior vaginal wall is maximized. This is best accomplished by elevating the fornix anterolaterally, with a finger placed vaginally, while the bladder and proximal urethra are simultaneously displaced medially using a blunt probe from the midline or contralateral port (Fig. 22.5).

The suture needle is placed into the surgical field using a midline 10–11 or contralateral 5-mm port. Two sets of full-thickness figure-of-eight stitches are sequentially placed into the vagina just short of the mucosa, driven into Cooper's ligament, and tied extracorporeally.

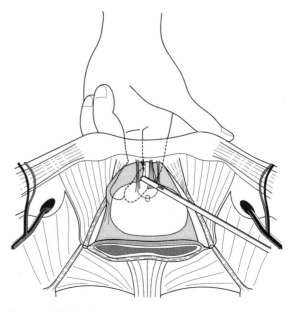

FIGURE 22.5. Laparoscopic mobilization of periurethral tissues before laparoscopic suturing.

Although suturing into the pubocervical fascia can be adequately performed through the midline or contralateral trocar ports, using the needle holder through a port ipsilateral to Cooper's ligament provides the best leverage for driving, turning, and bringing the needle out of this fibrous structure by permitting a perpendicular angle of attack.

Guided by the surgeon's or assistant's first and second fingers in the elevated vaginal fornix, the first stitch is placed distally, 1 to 2 cm opposite the bladder neck, and driven through the tissue mediolaterally to minimize the chance for urethral injury (Fig. 22.6). A sterile sewing thimble can be used to protect against accidental needle injury. Bleeding from perforation of the large veins that run along the vaginal wall is usually controlled when the sutures are tied. If the suture penetrates the vaginal canal, the mucosa will grow over it and tension will inevitably pull it inward and away from the vaginal canal.

After securing the vagina, the suture is driven through Cooper's ligament in an antero-posterior direction, immediately above the location of the vaginal wall stitch (Fig. 22.7). The suture is then tied extracorporeally with an endoscopic knot pusher by passing four to six alternating hitches to secure vaginal elevation as the assistant pushes his or her fingers upward toward Cooper's ligament (Fig. 22.7, inset). Alternatively, a double-clinch slip knot as described by Weston,[11] which can be locked at any point, is tied outside the trocar and pulled into the retropubic space to be cinched into position as the vagina is digitally elevated. After cutting both suture strands, the ligature is reinforced by intracorporeally tying a square knot. Excessive tension must be avoided to reduce the risk of necrosis at the suture site, suture release, and compressing or kinking the urethra; the vaginal wall should not come in contact with Cooper's ligament, and the urethra should be drawn no closer than 1 cm to the symphysis pubis.

A second proximal stitch is similarly placed into the vagina 1 to 2 cm cephalad and lateral to the first, driven through Cooper's ligament (carefully noting the well-perfused aberrant obturator vessels), and tied. The colposuspension is completed by repeating all steps with another set of sutures on the contralateral side.

The techniques used for removing needles from the retropubic space are dictated by the needle size and the diameter of the largest trocar sheath. Before tying to Cooper's ligament, a CV-2 or THX-26 needle is removed by reversing the order of events used for their insertion through a 10–11 trocar. When using larger curved needles or smaller trocars, each needle is cut off, leaving 4 cm of attached suture, and temporarily set in the retropubic space. The freed strand is grasped and pulled out of the trocar sheath. After tying, each needle is re-

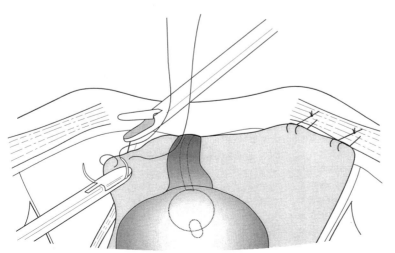

FIGURE 22.6. Placement of periurethral stitch. Elevating the vaginal fornix transvaginally, the first stitch is placed distally, 1–2 cm opposite the bladder neck, and driven through the tissue mediolaterally to minimize the chance for urethral injury.

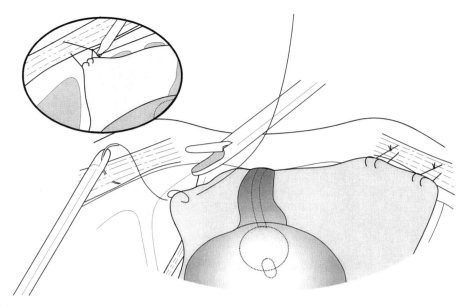

FIGURE 22.7. Suturing and approximation of the bladder to Cooper's ligament. After securing the vagina, the suture is driven through Cooper's ligament in an anteroposterior direction, immediately above the location of the vaginal wall stitch. The suture is then tied extracorporeally with an endoscopic knot pusher by passing four to six alternating hitches to secure vaginal elevation as the assistant pushes his or her fingers upward toward Cooper's ligament (*inset*).

moved by grasping the end of the suture tail and removing the trocar sheath, grasper, and needle together with one continuous motion out of the abdominal wall.

Suturing and Lateral Stapling

Suturing into Cooper's ligament, for many physicians the most difficult technical task during laparoscopic colposuspension, is eliminated by using endostaples to affix the lateral suture strand to this ligamentous structure.[9] After placing the suture into the vaginal fascia, the lateral suture arm is grasped by the assistant and laid flat along Cooper's ligament directly above the vaginal suture site. The suture is secured to the ligament with two or three staples by using the EMS Endostapler (Ethicon/Endosurgery, Cincinnati, OH) through the midline 10–11 trocar (Fig. 22.8). The staples function as a pulley to elevate the vaginal wall as the suture is removed. Each suture is tied extracorporeally with an endoscopic knot pusher

or using a double-clinch slip knot that is then backed up with a square knot.

Colposuspension Using Prolene Mesh

The use of suturing to perform a laparoscopic colposuspension is entirely eliminated by using a laparoscopic stapling gun to secure a piece of Prolene mesh as a permanent suspensory hammock between the vagina and Cooper's ligament.[5] Despite appearing to significantly deviate from traditional teaching, this technique preserves the fundamental surgical principles of retropubic colposuspension.

Prolene mesh has been successfully used by general surgeons for more than 20 years to perform open, and more recently laparoscopic, herniorrhaphy without significant morbidity. Used in the retroperitoneal space, this material is highly inert, essentially nonallergenic, and withstands infection. The fine double-knitted construction beneficially promotes fibroepithelial invasion and fixation among its interstices, stimulating retropubic scarring and

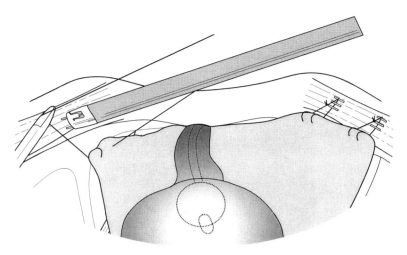

FIGURE 22.8. Stapling suture to Cooper's ligament. After placing the suture into the vaginal fascia, the lateral suture arm is grasped by the assistant and laid flat along Cooper's ligament directly above the vaginal suture site. The suture is then secured to the ligament with two or three staples by using the EMS Endostapler (Ethicon/Endosurgery, Cincinnati, OH) placed through the midline 10- or 11-mm trocar.

fibrosis that should be sustained. This obviates the need to tediously remove the well-vascularized retropubic fat to promote scarification.

Two strips of Prolene mesh, 1.5 × 5 to 6 cm, are prepared with scissors and bathed in a cephalosporin solution to minimize the chance of introducing infection. Each strip is then grasped and introduced into the prepared retropubic space through a contralateral trocar port. While the assistant holds the distal end of the strip with a grasper, it is flattened and held parallel to the urethra. The surgeon displaces the vaginal fornix anterolaterally to identify the areas for attachment while the mesh is stabilized. The EMS Endostapler is placed through the ipsilateral 10–11 trocar, and the stapler head is positioned over the distal mesh 1 to 2 cm lateral to the midurethra.

Two staples are fired into the pubocervical fascia.

The proximal end of the strip is then stabilized by the assistant and two more staples are fired into the vagina 1 to 2 cm lateral to the urethrovaginal junction (Fig. 22.9A). This procedure is repeated on the contralateral side using the same trocar port logic. Before affixing the segments of mesh to Cooper's ligament, cystoscopy can be performed to inspect for staples in the bladder wall. If encountered, staples can be laparoscopically removed with a staple remover (Endopath Endoscopic Staple Remover, Ethicon Endosurgery, Cincinnati, OH).

While digitally tenting the vaginal fornix toward Cooper's ligament, the proximal end of the mesh is grasped and placed on tension over the ligament above the site of attachment

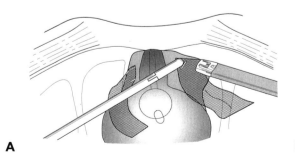

A

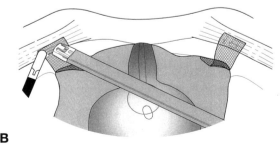

B

FIGURE 22.9.   Colposuspension using prolene mesh. **A:** The prolene mesh is stapled to the pericervical fascia. **B:** The mesh is then stapled to Cooper's ligament.

lateral to the bladder neck. A lubricated Q-tip can be placed in the urethra to help guide the degree of vaginal elevation. Traction is terminated on attaining a horizontal angle. The surgeon should strive to leave at least a 1-cm gap between the urethra and pubic symphysis, which is fortuitously the approximate diameter of the endostapler nose. The stapling gun is placed through the contralateral 10–11 port, and with the head over the mesh three more staples are fired into Cooper's ligament (Fig. 22.9B). This is repeated on the contralateral side in a similar fashion. Excess mesh is trimmed away with scissors and removed through the trocar sheath.

Concerns about potentially adverse effects of metal staples in the vaginal wall are logically unfounded. The firing mechanism of the endoscopic stapling gun is duplex, initially extending the arms of the staple followed by rapid enfolding. This essentially prevents entry into the vaginal canal. In the rare instance of transmural application, they will become well epithelialized just like suture materials. The widespread use of titanium staples in general surgery has consistently demonstrated their inertness and lack of migratory sequelae. Furthermore, the forces of tension tending to pull the staples out will always be directed cephalad. Downward forces exerted on the mesh by increases in abdominal pressure will be opposed by the tenacious hold of the staples to Cooper's ligament. Therefore, any movement of the paravaginal staples should be upward and away from the vaginal vault.

Closure

On completion of the colposuspension, the retropubic space is thoroughly lavaged to remove clots and tissue debris and assessed for hemostasis under varying degrees of insufflation pressure or by underwater examination. Bleeding points are coagulated with bipolar desiccation. A suprapubic catheter can be placed under direct vision. The transperitoneal approach is completed by closing the peritoneal defect with 2-0 or 3-0 absorbable suture in a pursestring fashion or with the remaining endostaples.

Cystoscopy may be performed to evaluate the integrity of the ureters (preceded by intravenous injection of 5cc of indigo carmine) and to rule out the presence of sutures or staples in the bladder wall. On withdrawal of all instruments from the surgical field and peritoneal cavity, fascial and subcutaneous stitches are placed at all trocar sites larger than 10 mm and adhesive strips across all 5-mm trocar sites.

Adjunctive Reparative Surgeries

A prophylactic culdoplasty can be performed in conjunction with a retropubic colposuspension. The incidence of postoperative enterocele formation after retropubic colposuspension has been reported to range from 3% to 17%.[12] This results from a number of factors that include the effects of altering the axis of the posterior vaginal wall in relation to abdominal pressure, intrinsic collagen deficiencies, and the presence of unrecognized early vault prolapse.

Laparoscopic culdoplasty requires transperitoneal entry of the laparoscope and ancillary instruments, and for maximal surgical access should be performed before the colposuspension. The cul-de-sac is obliterated by using permanent suture materials that are tied extracorporeally. Culdoplasty can be accomplished using either a modified McCall procedure by placing several stitches to plicate the uterosacral ligaments side to side while incorporating the peritoneum of the cul-de-sac, or a Moschowitz procedure to concentrically occlude the cul-de-sac by successively taking bites of the lateral pelvic peritoneum, anterior serosa of the rectum, and peritoneum of the cul-de-sac. Both procedures require careful identification of the ureters to prevent entrapment or kinking. See Chapter 20 for a more detailed discussion of these procedures.

Laparoscopic entry into the space of Retzius provides an invaluable opportunity to evaluate the endopelvic fascia for lateral avulsion of the anterolateral vaginal sulcus from the arcus tendineus fasciae pelvis. Pneumoperitoneal pressure in the retropubic space serendipitously accentuates these defects. Failure to concomitantly repair associated lateral weaknesses of the endopelvic fascia condemns the patient to incompletely corrected anterior vaginal wall prolapse and may decrease the longevity of the urethropexy by colposuspension. If a lateral herniation is noted, the paravaginal defect can be repaired in a fashion similar to the traditional laparotomic approach. The vaginal wall is digitally placed on medial traction to accentuate the defect and maximize surgical access. Beginning 1 cm above the ischial spine, four or five figure-of-eight stitches are successively placed to restore the attachment of the paravaginal tissue to the fascia overlying the obturator internus muscle and tied extracorporeally.

Anterior herniations of the endopelvic fascia are commonly found in association with other defects in pelvic support. Any clinically significant rectocele or enterocele should be repaired by the usual surgical approach. The longevity of a retropubic colposuspension is inherently related to the surgical correction of these associated pelvic floor herniations.

Postoperative Care

Because periurethral and perivesical dissection is minimized during laparoscopic development of the retropubic space, in most cases postoperative urinary drainage is unnecessary. If a suprapubic catheter is placed intraoperatively, it can be removed within 24 to 48 hr after the patient can comfortably void and the residual volume is less than 100 cc.

Otherwise, the patient is asked to void in the recovery room and a postvoid residual volume

is measured. If less than 100 cc, she is discharged home with a set of straight catheters for potential voiding difficulties. If she is unable to void or found to have a significant residual volume, either a 12-Fr. pediatric catheter is inserted or self-catheterization directions are reviewed with instruction to stop when the postvoid residual volume is less than 100 ml. In either case, the patient is scheduled to be reevaluated in the office in 48 hr. She is asked to refrain from sexual intercourse and significant physical activity for the next 4 weeks.

Results

Complications specific to laparoscopic colposuspension are related to peritoneal entry, dissection of the retropubic space, and surgical manipulation of the urinary tract. Potential intraoperative complications include hemorrhage, enterotomy, cystotomy, urethral injury, accidental stapling or suturing into the bladder or urethra, and ureteral kinking or urethral compression from overcorrecting the urethrovesical angle. Postoperatively, voiding may be disrupted by dysuria, infection, detrusor instability, and urinary retention. Although less apt to occur after the laparoscopic approach, both retropubic hematoma and abscess may result from inadequate hemostasis. If left unclosed, larger fascial defects at trocar sites may cause entrapment and obstruction of the underlying bowel.

More than 400 cases of laparoscopic retropubic urethropexy have been reported. Direct

TABLE 22.1. Results of laparoscopic retropubic colposuspension procedures.

Study[a]	Number of patients	Clinical continence	Longest follow-up (months)
Albala et al. (1992)[3]: A	32	32 (100%)	12
Liu and Paek (1993)[4]: A	107	104 (97.2%)	27
Ou et al. (1993)[5]: C	40	40 (100%)	16
Underwood and Smith (1993)[6]: A	69	62 (90%)	18
Nezhat et al. (1994)[7]: A	62	56 (90%)	30
McKinney et al. (1994)[8]: C	83	81 (97.5%)	27
Lyons and Winer (1995)[9]: A,B	20	18 (90%)	12
Totals:	413	393 (95%)	

[a]Letters after each reference refer to the method of colposuspension: A, suturing; B, suturing and lateral stapling; C, Prolene mesh.

comparisons between these studies are difficult owing to the wide range of physician experience, sample size, follow-up interval, variations in techniques, and in many instances the absence of pre- and postoperative urodynamic assessments. Taking these variables into account, laparoscopic colposuspension resulted in 95% patient satisfaction for as long as 30 months after the procedure (Table 22.1). Although patient satisfaction does not necessarily equate with objective continence, these preliminary results compare favorably with the results of the laparotomic alternatives.

References

1. Thomas TM, Plymatt KR, Blanin J, Mead TW. Prevalence of urinary incontinence. *Br Med J.* 1980;281:1243–245.
2. Vancaillie TG, Schuessler W. Laparoscopic bladderneck suspension. *J Laparoendosc Surg.* 1991; 1:169–173.
3. Albala DM, Schuessler WW, Vancaillie TG. Laparoscopic bladder neck suspension. *J Endourol.* 1992;6:137–141.
4. Liu CY, Paek W. Laparoscopic retropubic colposuspension (Burch procedure). *J Am Assoc Gynecol Laparosc.* 1993;1(1):31–5.
5. Ou CS, Presthus J, Beadle E. Clinical correspondence: laparoscopic bladder neck suspension using hernia mesh and surgical staples. *J Laparoendosc Surg.* 1993;3(6):563–564.
6. Underwood L, Smith M. Minimally invasive management of stress urinary incontinence. World Congress of Gynecological Endoscopy, AAGL 22nd Annual Meeting, San Francisco, CA, November 1993.
7. Nezhat CH, Nezhat F, Nezhat CR, Rottenberg H. Laparoscopic retropubic cystourethropexy. *J Am Assoc Gynecol Laparosc.* 1994;1(4):339–349.
8. McKinney T, Burns J, Kessler B, Woodland M. Laparoscopic retropubic urethropexy. World Congress of Gynecological Endoscopy, AAGL 23rd Annual Meeting, New York, NY, November 1994.
9. Lyons TL, Winer WK. Clinical outcomes with laparoscopic approaches and open Burch procedures for urinary stress incontinence. *J Am Assoc Gynecol Laparosc.* 1995;2(2):193–198.
10. Jarvis GJ. Surgery for genuine stress incontinence. *Br J Obstet Gynaecol.* 1994;101:371–374.
11. Weston PV. A new clinch knot. *Obstet Gynecol.* 1991;77:6–9.
12. Wiskind AK, Creighton SM, Stanton SL. The incidence of genital prolapse after the Burch colposuspension. *Am J Obstet Gynecol.* 1992;187(2):399–405.

23

Laparoscopic Intestinal Procedures

Daniel S. Seidman, Farr Nezhat, Ceana H. Nezhat, and Camran Nezhat

The application of laparoscopy to bowel surgery began with appendectomy, which was developed by gynecologists more than a decade ago[1] and adopted to routine care.[2] More complex laparoscopic bowel operations include colostomy, ileostomy, partial and total rectosigmoid colon resection with reanastomosis, hemicolectomy, abdominoperineal resection, and the repair of planned and unplanned bowel entry.[3–11]

Advantages of Laparoscopic Bowel Surgery

The benefits of laparoscopic intestinal surgery include less postoperative pain, lower risk of wound dehiscence, early ambulation, and generally more rapid convalescence. This approach may allow a quicker return of bowel function and decreased use of analgesics. The risk of adhesion formation is reduced with laparoscopic surgery.[12]

Basic surgical principles must always be observed, and include appropriate patient selection and preoperative evaluation, excellent exposure of the operative field, avoiding spillage of enteric contents in the peritoneal cavity, and retrieving the specimen intact for complete pathological analysis.[8] The anastomosis must be well vascularized, free of tension, and circumferentially intact.[8]

Disadvantages of Laparoscopic Bowel Surgery

One of the major restrictions of laparoscopic bowel surgery is poor tactile feedback because direct palpation is not possible. The use of a colonoscope during surgery can reduce this shortcoming by improving the operator's ability to locate and assess bowel lesions. Laparoscopic sonography using specially designed probes may help identify structures beneath the visualized surface, and it is an important intraoperative diagnostic tool. Additional limitations of the laparoscopic approach include difficulty in achieving optimal retraction of the adjacent organs and possible challenge of the surgeon's depth perception by the two-dimensional vision of video.[13]

Indications

The most frequent indications for bowel surgery observed by gynecologists are intestinal involvement with endometriosis, adhesions, or gynecologic malignancy that can be managed laparoscopically by an experienced surgeon. Traumatic bowel injury can be repaired with laparoscopic primary repair or segmental resection. Closure of ileostomy or colostomy can be performed laparoscopically.

The carbon dioxide (CO_2) laser has long been used to ablate endometriotic implants on the peritoneum and other intraabdominal organs.[14] Observation and accessibility to the upper abdomen, including the diaphragm, and deep pelvis are better at videolaparoscopy. This improved access and observation combined with magnification may facilitate identification and treatment of lesions.

Contraindications to laparoscopic colon surgery include diffuse fecal peritonitis, unprepared bowel, massive obesity, extensive multiple adhesions, and large bulky tumors. Relative contraindications include large phlegmon, acute inflammatory bowel disease, liver cirrhosis, and large abdominal aortic aneurysm.

Patient Selection and Preoperative Evaluation

Severe endometriosis may include widespread implants that penetrate deep into the retroperitoneal surface and affect every organ in the abdominal cavity, from the urinary bladder to the diaphragm. This chapter is primarily based on our experience with laparoscopic intestinal procedures performed for endometriosis. Recent achievements by general surgeons in intestinal laparoscopic operations are also discussed.

Careful patient selection for laparoscopic bowel surgery is important,[8,15] although absolute contraindications have not been formally defined.[10] By respecting the contraindications noted here and their own skill and experience, surgeons can decrease complications associated with the procedure. The more experienced laparoscopist may regard some of the previously described contraindications as support for performing, rather than avoiding, laparoscopic surgery. Additionally, improved instrumentation and operative techniques may increase the margin of safety for operative laparoscopy.

All patients should undergo outpatient mechanical and antibiotic bowel preparation. Two days before the operation, the patient consumes only clear liquids. The day before surgery, the patient drinks a gallon of GoLytely (Braintree Laboratories, Inc., Braintree, MA) over a 3- to 4-hr period. GoLytely and NuLytely are oral solutions containing polyethylene glycol 3350, sodium chloride, bicarbonate, and potassium chloride. The night before surgery, the patient should undergo a Fleet enema and take 1 g of metronidazole orally. Two grams of cefoxitin sodium (Mefoxin, Merck Sharp & Dohme, West Point, PA) are administered intravenously 30 min before the scheduled procedure.

Instrumentation and Techniques

Laparoscopic Operative Setup

Laparoscopy is performed under general endotracheal anesthesia. A uterine manipulator is inserted to allow adequate mobilization and stabilization of the uterus. This is especially important when access to the rectovaginal area is required, demanding sharp anteflexion of the uterus. We commonly use either the HUMI (Unimar, Wilton, CT) or the Cohen cannula in combination with a single-toothed tenaculum applied to the anterior cervical lip.

A 10-mm trocar is directly inserted infraumbilically. An operating videolaparoscope is inserted and a camera is attached to the laparoscope (Circon ACMI, Stamford, CT). After visual verification that the trocar has been properly placed in the peritoneal cavity, pneumoperitoneum is induced. Under direct guidance, three 5-mm suprapubic trocars are placed, one each in the lower-left and -right quadrants lateral to the inferior epigastric vessels, and one in the midline, 5 to 6 cm above the pubic symphysis. The number, size, and location of the trocars may be modified depending on the procedure. The grasping forceps are inserted through the lower-right sleeve, the bipolar electrocoagulator through the midline, and the suction-irrigator probe through the lower-left port. Then, using the video laparoscope through the umbilical channel, the pelvic and abdominal organs are examined. If the CO_2 laser is to be used, a direct lens–laser coupler is attached to the laparoscope. The laser (Coherent, Palo Alto, CA) is placed through the operating channel of the laparoscope and is used for cutting and for coagulating small blood vessels. Electrosurgery, sharp scissors, or any other cutting modality can replace the CO_2 laser. The power of the CO_2 laser is set between 40 and 80 W. Hemostasis is accomplished with the laser or bipolar electrocoagulation.

Laparoscopic Appendectomy

Procedure Specifics

The appendix is examined and mobilized after lysis of periappendiceal or pericecal adhesions. This is done carefully because there may be attachment to the lateral pelvic wall or a retrocecal appendix. Next, the bipolar electrocoagulator and sharp scissors or CO_2 laser are used sequentially to desiccate and cut the mesoappendix 1.5 cm from the ileocecal area (Fig. 23.1). The bipolar forceps is withdrawn and the Endoloop applicator is inserted through the suprapubic midline puncture. Two chromic or polydioxanone Endoloop sutures (PDS, Ethicon, Somerville, NJ) are passed to

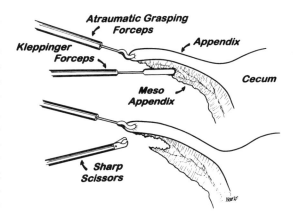

FIGURE 23.1. With an atraumatic grasping forceps (Storz No. 26177AG) placed through the right-lower quadrant suprapubic incision, the appendical tip is grasped and placed on traction. Using a bipolar forceps placed through the midline suprapubic incision, the mesoappendix is desiccated to a point 0.5 cm below the junction of the appendix and cecum (*top*). Care should be used to keep the bipolar forceps 0.5 cm away from the cecum proper. Using sharp scissors, the mesoappendix is progressively incised as it is cauterized (*bottom*).

the base of the appendix, 3 to 5 mm from the cecum, and tied one on top of the other (Fig. 23.2). Both suture ends are cut. A third Endoloop suture is applied 1 cm distal to the other sutures, and cut, leaving a 15-cm tail to facilitate retrieval should the appendix inadvertently fall into the pelvic well (Fig. 23.3). The appendix is then cut between the second and third sutures. Luminal portions of the appendiceal stump and the removed appendix are seared with the bipolar or the CO_2 laser. The abdomen is irrigated copiously with lactated Ringer's. We recently have begun omitting the third Endoloop, thoroughly coagulating the distal part of the appendix using bipolar forceps.

The appendix is removed from the abdomen with a long grasping forceps passed through the operating channel of the laparoscope or a suprapubic port and submitted for pathology. If available, an appendix extractor is placed through the central port, after replacing the central 5-mm trocar with a 10-mm one, and used to withdraw the cut appendix. Instru-

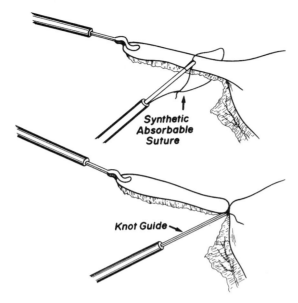

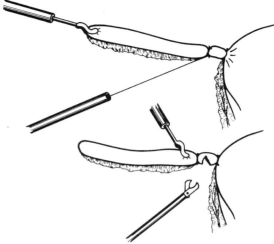

FIGURE 23.3. Using the atraumatic grasper, the appendiceal base is grasped and milked to push fecal matter into the cecum. A loop ligature (0-Vicryl, Dexon, or chromic) is placed through the midline puncture. The appendiceal tip is regrasped and pulled through the loop, using a micrograsping forceps (WISAP No. 7678) to direct the ligature toward the base of the appendix. Three loop ligatures are placed.

FIGURE 23.2. Using the atraumatic grasping forceps, the appendix is milked toward the tip, and a third loop is applied approximately 1 cm distal from the tied appendiceal base. The appendix is then cut with sharp scissors. The severed appendiceal end is passed to a claw forceps (WISAP No. 7655KG or WOLF No. 8385) placed through a 10-mm suprapubic incision and the appendix removed. The scissors, grasper, and claw forceps are then removed from the operating field. The exposed mucosa of the appendiceal stump are lightly bipolared or painted with iodine.

ments, possibly contaminated, are removed from the surgical field. No adjunctive therapy is used. Last, the appendiceal and other operative sites are inspected for hemostasis by completely emptying the abdominal cavity of CO_2 gas. This will decrease the intraabdominal pressure and allow any noncontained bleeding to become apparent. The abdomen is then reinflated and the cavity thoroughly irrigated with lactated Ringer's.

Results

In our first 100 cases, appendectomies were accomplished in 4 to 21 min.[2] No major intraoperative complications occurred. All patients were discharged from the hospital within 24 hr of surgery. Seven remained overnight because of patient preference or because the surgery was

performed late in the day; the average hospital stay was 14 hr. All patients resumed oral intake the day after surgery. Except for mild periumbilical ecchymosis and one febrile morbidity, no apparent postoperative complications were noted in the study group. In a series of 254 cases, 1 woman postoperatively developed a pelvic abscess that required surgical intervention.

A number of techniques are employed for laparoscopic appendectomy, and the procedure is common.[13,16-17] Although this operation has a favorable cost–benefit ratio, complications including stump blowout, wound infection, hemorrhage, and postoperative ileus have been described.[18]

Laparoscopic Repair of Enterotomies of the Small Bowel, Colon, and Rectum

Intentional or inadvertent enterotomies created during diagnostic or therapeutic laparoscopy can be corrected successfully using the laparoscopic approach.

Procedure Specifics

Direct Repair with Sutures

The pelvic and abdominal cavity is thoroughly irrigated and any bowel contents are removed. The location of the enterotomy is evaluated and necrotic tissue is removed. We usually perform repairs with a single-layer closure incorporating mucosa, submucosa, and serosa using 0-Dexon or Vicryl (Ethicon) on a curved or straight needle, with intracorporeal or extracorporeal knot tying. The repair can be vertical or transverse, depending on the size of the enterotomy. Care should be taken to avoid bowel stricture. If the laceration is extensive, it is safer to resect the injured portion of the bowel. The bowel is mobilized laparoscopically, and resection and reanastomosis are completed with a stapler or through a minilaparotomy incision. The same principles of laparotomy are observed, except that they are performed laparoscopically.

Direct Endoloop Closure of Bowel Enterotomies

In patients with prepared bowel, if the opening is less than 0.5 cm, one Endoloop suture (0-polydioxanone, Ethicon) is used for enterorrhaphy in either the small or large bowel. The single loop is applied tightly around the perforation and the closure verified using the methods described. This technique is less complicated and therefore faster than a running suture.

Bowel Repair with a Stapling Device

Some large and possibly small bowel injuries can be repaired using a laparoscopic stapling device (EZ35W, Ethicon, Inc.). The device is inserted into the abdominal cavity through a 12-mm abdominal port or transvaginally if the rectum is injured. After the defect is evaluated, the edges of the bowel are brought together using atraumatic grasping forceps. The stapling device is introduced to the abdominal cavity and passed across the bowel defect. The edges are confirmed to be even and completely within the stapler's jaws, and the device is fired. The integrity of the repair is evaluated underwater as described. It is imperative that bowel stricture be avoided. Our limited experience with this technique to repair the rectosigmoid colon has been positive.

After repair, the bowel is evaluated using one of the following methods. To assess the integrity of small bowel and colonic closures, the abdominal and pelvic cavities are filled with lactated Ringer's. The bowel is observed under fluid for the presence of air bubbles, indicating that the closure is not airtight. To evaluate rectal and rectosigmoidal repairs, the posterior cul-de-sac is filled with lactated Ringer's, sigmoidoscopy is performed, and the rectum is inflated with air via sigimoidoscope, again observing for air bubbles.

Postoperatively patients receive 1 g cefoxitin for two to three doses every 8 hr. They are given clear liquids orally after bowel function resumes, and the postoperative course is closely monitored.

Results

In 26 women who had laparoscopy for endometriosis (18 women), pelvic adhesions (7 patients), and adhesions with Crohn's disease (1 woman), enterotomies were repaired laparoscopically. All women had preoperative antibiotic and mechanical bowel preparation as described. In 23 patients, enterotomies had occurred secondary to CO_2 laser vaporization or excision of endometriosis or lysis of adhesions adjacent to or involving the bowel wall, and in 3 patients, following trocar insertion. The enterotomies related to trocar insertion occurred in women who had prior abdominal surgery. The injuries included 9 small bowel, 4 colonic, and 13 rectal enterotomies.

All patients tolerated solid low-residual diets within 72 hr of surgery. Twenty-three patients were discharged from the hospital within 24 hr of surgery. There were no clinical complications related to the laparoscopic bowel repair, and no patients developed infection or obstruction. No fistulas occurred, and all repairs healed without clinical evidence of infection.

Twelve enterotomies (5 small bowel and 7 large bowel) that resulted from CO_2 laser, cold scissors, or trocars were repaired using direct Endoloop closure of the bowel perforation, without complication. Care should be taken to avoid strangulation of the bowel tissue, which may lead to local necrosis. We believe enterotomies of the small bowel, colon, and rectum that occur during laparoscopic procedures in patients who have had preoperative bowel preparation may be repaired laparoscopically. The results of repair in unprepared bowel, as might occur with penetrating trauma, have not yet been determined.

Laparoscopic Treatment of Infiltrative Endometriosis Involving the Rectosigmoid Colon and the Rectovaginal Septum

The posterior cul-de-sac is the site most often involved with infiltrating endometriosis. This area includes the posterior aspect of the cervix; the posterior vagina and the anterior rectum in the midline; and the pararectal area, uterosacral ligaments, and lower portion of the posterior aspect of the broad ligaments laterally. Superficial endometrial implants on the peritoneum or retroperitoneally can be easily treated by vaporization or excision. However, infiltrative lesions are usually proximal to or involving structures such as ureters, uterine and lower pelvic vessels, and rectum. The recognition and thorough treatment of these implants are challenging and requires familiarity with anatomy and surgical skill, so as to not only remove the lesions completely but also to appropriately manage injuries that may occur during treatment.

Severe and infiltrative lesions result in anatomic distortion of the posterior cul-de-sac. Affected uterosacral ligaments are often retracted and attached to the cervix. The ureters can be retracted medially. When the posterior broad ligament is involved, it may result in periureteral fibrosis and stricture, and, rarely, partial or complete ureteral obstruction. Partial or complete posterior cul-de-sac obliteration occurs when endometriosis of the back of the vagina, pararectal area, and lower rectum is present, and there is retraction and attachment of the rectum to the uterosacral ligaments, posterior aspect of the vagina, cervix, and uterus, either laterally or centrally.

This attachment usually is associated with different degrees of infiltrative endometrial implants and nodules that are found after the rectum is separated from the cervix and vagina.

The lesions may involve the different layers of the rectal wall, penetrate to the pararectal area below the uterosacral ligaments toward the levator ani muscles or toward the rectovaginal septum, and occasionally penetrate the entire vaginal wall.

Procedure Specifics

The assistant should stand between the patient's legs and perform rectovaginal examination with one hand. With the other hand, the assistant holds the uterus up with a rigid uterine elevator while both assistant and surgeon observe the monitor. For rectovaginal septum and uterosacral ligament endometriosis, 5 to 8 ml of dilute vasopressin (10 U in 100–200 ml of lactated Ringer's) are injected into an uninvolved area with a 16-gauge laparoscopic needle. The peritoneum is opened and a plane is created in the rectovaginal septum using hydrodissection.

It is imperative that the ureters be located before continuing with this procedure. Any alteration in the direction of the ureters should be identified. Because the ureters are lateral to the uterosacral ligaments, the surgeon should attempt to operate between the ligaments as much as possible. With the aid of hydrodissection, a relaxing incision is made lateral to the uterosacral ligament, allowing the ureters to retract laterally. Ureterolysis often is necessary to free the ureters from the surrounding fibrotic diseased tissue and from endometriosis. Hydrodissection with the CO_2 laser and blunt dissection can be used for ureterolysis, enterolysis, and ovarian resection.

While the assistant examines the rectum, the involved area is completely excised or vaporized until the loose areolar tissue of the rectovaginal space and the normal muscularis layers of the rectum are reached (Fig. 23.4). In women whose rectum is pulled up and attached to the back of the cervix between the uterosacral ligaments, the uterus is anteflexed sharply and an incision is made at the right or left pararectal area, then extended to the junction of the cervix and the rectum. If the rectal involvement is more extensive and the assistant's finger is not long enough, a sigmoidoscope, a sponge on forceps, or a rectal probe is

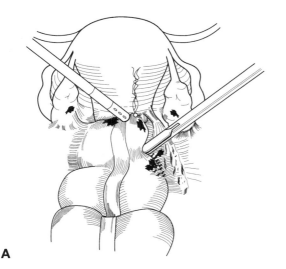

A

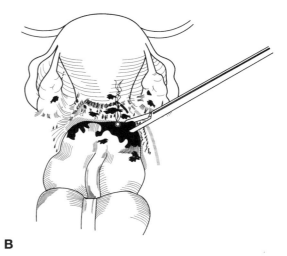

B

FIGURE 23.4. Laparoscopic treatment of infiltrative endometriosis (black areas) involving the rectosigmoid colon and the rectovaginal septum. **A:** The peritoneum overlying the rectovaginal septum is opened, and a plane is created using hydrodissection. A relaxing incision is made lateral to the uterosacral ligament allowing the ureters to retract laterally. It is imperative that the ureters be first located. **B:** While the assistant examines the rectum, the involved area is completely excised or vaporized until the loose areolar tissue of the rectovaginal space and normal muscularis layers of the rectum are reached.

used. The use of the sigmoidoscope also aids in identifying bowel perforation, because air bubbles can be seen passing from the air-inflated rectum into the posterior cul-de-sac when the latter is filled with irrigation fluid. The insertion of these devices should be done gently and cautiously to prevent rectal perforation.

While the assistant guides the surgeon by rectovaginal exam, the rectum is completely freed from the back of the cervix. Generalized oozing and bleeding can be controlled with the injection of 3 to 5 ml dilute vasopressin (1 ampule in 100 ml), laser, or bipolar electrocoagulator. Occasional bleeding from stalk vessels coming from the hypogastrics, caused by dissection or vaporization of the fibrotic uterosacral ligaments and pararectal areas, is controlled with the bipolar electrocoagulator.

Endometriosis rarely penetrates the mucosa of the colon, but commonly involves the serosa, subserosa, fatty tissue, and the two muscularis layers. This involvement begins with an implant on the outermost surface and progresses toward the mucosa layer by layer. We use the UltraPulse CO_2 laser set at 40 to 80 W and between 25 and 200 millijoules (mJ) to excise or vaporize the lesion. When significant portions of both serosal and muscularis layers have been excised or vaporized and the mucosa is reached, the bowel wall may be reinforced by one to three 0-polydioxanone or polyglactin sutures. The rectum is thoroughly evaluated by a digital examination and sigmoidoscopy and, if a perforation is detected, it is repaired laparoscopically as described. Consultation with a colorectal surgeon is usually recommended.

Postoperatively, the patient gradually advances her diet from clear liquids to solid food. Oral laxatives are prescribed to avoid constipation, and rectal manipulation is avoided for 6 weeks.

Results

The management of 185 patients, ages 25 to 41, who had endometriosis of the lower colon, rectum, uterosacral ligaments, or rectovaginal septum were reviewed retrospectively with a follow-up of 1 to 5 years.[7] All were referred for treatment because previous surgical or hormonal management failed to relieve their discomfort. Excluding 9 patients with bowel perforation and 1 with a partial bowel resection, all were discharged within 24 hr. The procedures lasted from 55 to 245 min. All patients had benign disease, and a large number underwent additional surgical procedures including ureterolysis, presacral neurectomy, hysterectomy with unilateral or bilateral oophorectomy, myomectomy, and appendectomy. The patients were instructed to have nothing by mouth for 24 hr postoperatively except for sips of water, and if no complications were noted the diet was gradually increased. Patients with bowel perforation or resection had nothing by mouth until they passed flatus and were instructed to avoid constipation by eating a high-fiber diet.

Minor complications were shoulder pain, abdominal wall ecchymosis, urine retention, and dyschezia for 1 to 2 weeks. Eleven patients were lost to follow-up. Of the remaining 174, 162 reported moderate to complete pain relief, 12 reported persistent or worse pain, 7 eventually underwent total hysterectomy, 4 had bowel resections, and 1 had salpingo-oophorectomy. Of 61 infertility patients, 25 achieved pregnancy; 14 women (73%) had AFS scores of 10 to 40, 10 (33%) scored from 40 to 110, and 1 (8%) had a score of more than 116.

Laparoscopic Bowel Resection

When the endometriotic lesion involves the full thickness or a major portion of the rectum, sigmoid colon, or any other portion of the small or large intestine, or if the lesion has caused significant stricture, segmental or complete resection of the affected bowel may be necessary in symptomatic patients. One of four techniques is used depending on the location and the extent of the disease.

Procedure Specifics

Disk Excision of Full-Thickness Anterior Rectal or Sigmoidal Wall Lesions and Primary Repair with Suture

The following technique for total laparoscopic resection of part of the colon wall and repair of the defect eliminates the need for stapling devices. It is used to treat selected cases of infiltrative symptomatic intestinal endometriosis. The extent of bowel involvement is evaluated and the need for full-thickness disk excision is determined. We use a sigmoidoscope to completely clean the rectum, to further delineate the lesion, and to guide the surgeon. If the lesion is low enough, an assistant can identify it by performing a rectal examination. After the ureters are identified in each side, the lower colon is mobilized. Depending on the location of the lesion, the right and/or left pararectal area(s) are separated from adjacent organs. Any bleeding that is not controlled with the CO_2 laser is managed with bipolar electrocoagulation.

Full-thickness excision begins above the area of visible disease. After identifying normal tissue, the lesion is held at its proximal end with grasping forceps inserted through the right-lower quadrant trocar. An incision is made through the bowel serosa and muscularis, and the lumen is entered (Fig. 23.5A). The lesion is completely excised from the anterior rectal wall (Fig. 23.5B). Following complete excision of the lesion, the pelvic cavity is thoroughly irrigated and suctioned. The lesion is removed from the abdomen through the operative channel of the laparoscope or sigmoidoscope using a long grasping forceps and submitted for pathological examination.

The bowel is repaired transversely in one layer. Two traction sutures are applied to each side of the bowel defect, transforming it into a transverse opening (Fig. 23.6A). The stay sutures are brought out via the right- and left-lower quadrant trocar sleeves. The sleeves are removed then replaced in the peritoneal cavity next to the stay sutures, and the sutures are secured outside the abdomen. The bowel is then repaired by placing several interrupted through-and-through sutures spaced 0.3 to 0.6 cm apart (Fig. 23.6B,C). We use 0-polyglactin laparoscopic sutures and a straight or curved needle with extracorporeal knot tying. For patients in whom the bowel defect is less than 4 cm long and 1 cm wide, we repair the rectum vertically, without having had problems with bowel stricture.

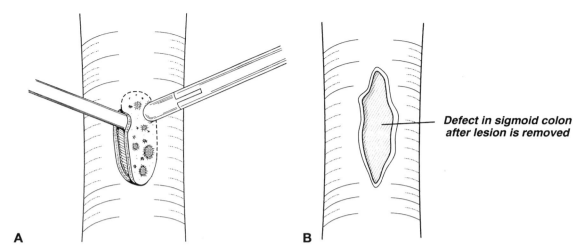

A   **B**

Defect in sigmoid colon
after lesion is removed

FIGURE 23.5.   Disk excision of anterior rectal or sigmoidal wall endometriosis implants and primary repair with suture. **A:** An incision is made through the bowel serosa and muscularis and the lumen is entered. **B:** The lesion is completely excised from the anterior rectal wall.

At the end of the procedure, we carefully examine the rectosigmoid colon, using the sigmoidoscope as described earlier, to confirm that the closure is airtight and to ensure that there is no bowel stricture. Neither a Jackson–Pratt drain nor a nasogastric tube is used routinely. The Foley catheter is removed the day of surgery. Oral feeding is resumed after the spontaneous release of flatus, usually on the first or second postoperative day. All patients are released from the hospital between postoperative days 2 and 4, when they are able to tolerate clear liquids well. Low residual diet is begun after the patient has a bowel movement.

Partial Transanal or Transvaginal Resection

For small, isolated lesions in the lower rectum near the anus, the following technique can be used. The rectovaginal septum is delineated by the assistant who performs simultaneous vaginal and rectal examination. The rectum is mobilized along the rectovaginal septum anteriorly to within 2 cm of the anus, using scissors and blunt dissection, or the CO_2 laser and hydrodissection. Mobilization is continued along the left and right pararectal spaces by coagulating and dividing branches of the hemorrhoidal artery, if necessary.

When the rectum is sufficiently mobilized, the lesion is prolapsed transvaginally to the level of the introitus (Fig. 23.7A) or transanally (Fig. 23.7B). The perineal body is retracted and an RL 30 (Ethicon) multifire stapler is applied across the segment of the anterior rectal wall containing the nodule. Two staple applications usually are required to traverse the width of the involved mucosa. The affected area is excised, and two additional interrupted 2-0 polyglactin sutures are applied along the staple line. Resection can be performed without the multifire stapler, instead using primary resection and suturing for repair.

The rectum is returned to the pelvis under direct observation. Integrity of the anastomosis is verified by insufflation of air into the rectum while the cul-de-sac is filled with lactated Ringer's.

Complete Segmental Resection with
Transanal or Transvaginal Prolapse

When there are multiple lesions or a larger portion of the bowel is involved, an entire segment of bowel is resected. The technique used depends on the location of the lesion. If the lesion is in the rectum or lower rectosigmoid colon, the bowel is mobilized by entering the pararectal area, rectovaginal septum, and posterior rec-

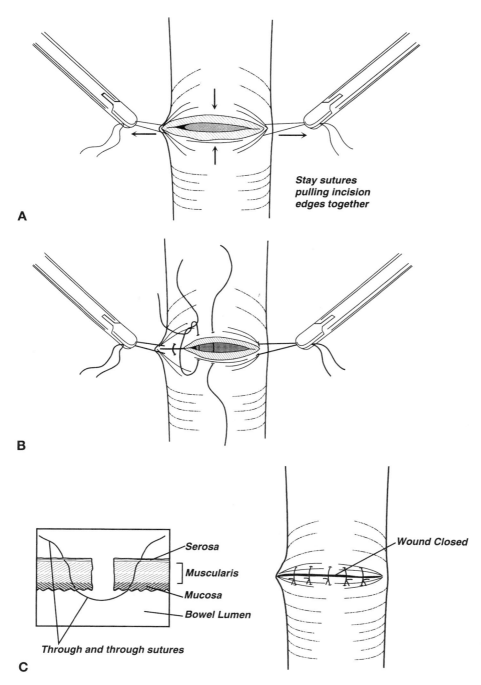

FIGURE 23.6. **A:** Two traction sutures are applied to each side of the bowel defect, transforming it into a transverse opening. **B:** The bowel is repaired by placing several interrupted through-and-through sutures in 0.3- to 0.6-cm increments. **C:** The bowel is completely repaired.

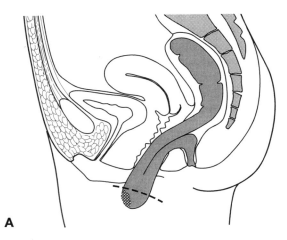
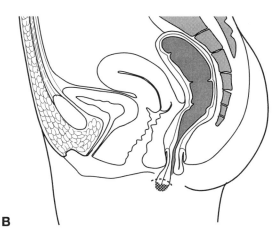

A   **B**

FIGURE 23.7. Partial transanal or transvaginal re-section. After the rectum is mobilized, the lesion (*hatched area*) is prolapsed transvaginally to the level of the introitus (**A**) or transanally (**B**). The affected area is then excised.

tosigmoid colon from the presacral space to the levator muscles, as is done via laparotomy. The branches of the inferior mesenteric vessels are electrodesiccated and cut if necessary. The involved segment is prolapsed either transvaginally (Fig. 23.8A) or transrectally.

The rectum is transected distal to the lesion (Fig. 23.8B) and again transected proximal to the lesion (Fig. 23.8C). The anal (distal) portion of the transected rectum is replaced into the pelvic cavity. The resected segment is sent for pathologic diagnosis, and a 2-0 polypropylene pursestring suture is placed around the circumference of the proximal limb of the bowel. The anvil of an ILS 29 or -33 stapler (Ethicon) is placed through the pursestring into the proximal bowel, and the proximal limb of bowel is replaced into the pelvis (Fig. 23.8D). Using Babcock clamps, the distal rectal segment is prolapsed through the anal canal, closed with an RL60, and replaced through the anal canal into the pelvis.

The ILS circular stapler is then placed into the rectum (Fig. 23.8D), and the anvil trocar within the proximal bowel is inserted into the stapling device using the laparoscope and a laparoscopic anvil holder (Fig. 23.8E). The device is fired, creating an end-to-end anastomosis (Fig. 23.9A,B). A proctoscope is used to examine the anastomosis for structural integrity and bleeding. The pelvis is filled with lactated Ringer's and observed with the laparoscope as the rectum is insufflated with air to check for leakage. Air leaks may be corrected using 2-0 polyglactin sutures placed transanally or laparoscopically. This technique is identical to resection at laparotomy, with the bipolar electrocoagulator and laser replacing suture and scissors.

Intraabdominal Segmental Resection

After the bowel is completely mobilized, a 60-mm Endostapler (Ethicon) is placed and fired distal to the lesion (Fig. 23.10A). The proximal limb of the colon is delivered from the abdomen and exteriorized through a small incision (Fig. 23.10B). The lesion is amputated, and the anvil of the stapler is inserted into the lumen following placement of a pursestring suture. At this stage, anastomosis is completed with the ILS stapler gun (see Fig. 23.8E).

Segmental Resection Through a Minilaparotomy

When the lesion is high on the sigmoid or other part of the colon, or if a large portion of bowel must be removed (e.g., diverticulitis or cancer), this technique is utilized. The portion of bowel to be resected is mobilized using the CO_2 laser or scissors for cutting and bipolar,

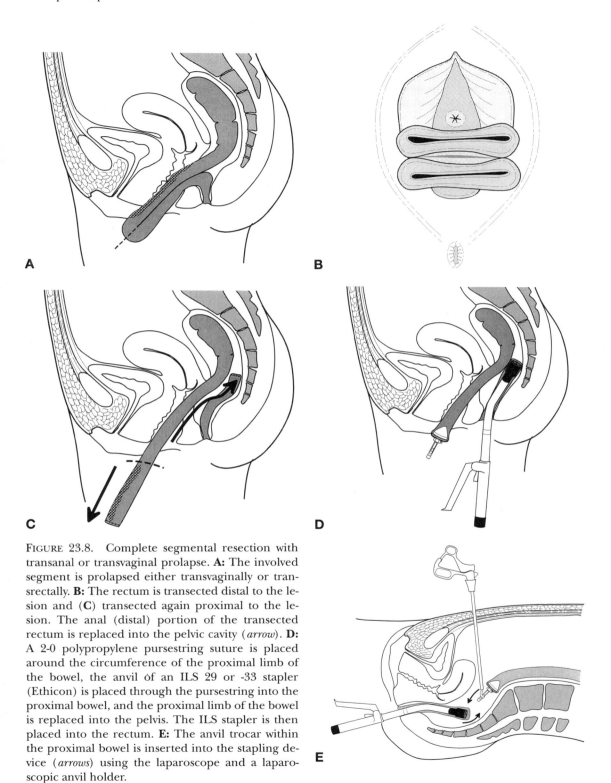

FIGURE 23.8. Complete segmental resection with transanal or transvaginal prolapse. **A:** The involved segment is prolapsed either transvaginally or transrectally. **B:** The rectum is transected distal to the lesion and (**C**) transected again proximal to the lesion. The anal (distal) portion of the transected rectum is replaced into the pelvic cavity (*arrow*). **D:** A 2-0 polypropylene pursestring suture is placed around the circumference of the proximal limb of the bowel, the anvil of an ILS 29 or -33 stapler (Ethicon) is placed through the pursestring into the proximal bowel, and the proximal limb of the bowel is replaced into the pelvis. The ILS stapler is then placed into the rectum. **E:** The anvil trocar within the proximal bowel is inserted into the stapling device (*arrows*) using the laparoscope and a laparoscopic anvil holder.

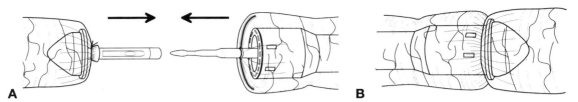

A **B**

FIGURE 23.9. The circular stapler is used for end-to-end bowel anastomosis. **A:** The anvil trocar is in-serted into the stapling device. **B:** The device is fired, creating an end-to-end anastomosis.

surgical clips, or laparoscopic stapler (EZ35W, Ethicon, Inc.) to desiccate or clip the meso-colon attachment and vasculature. The loca-tion and size of the ancillary incision are modi-fied on the basis of the area of the involved colon. A minilaparotomy is performed in the midsuprapubic, left-, or right-lower quadrant by extending the corresponding ancillary inci-sion. The bowel is guided to the minilaparo-tomy with grasping forceps. After resection and reanastomosis are completed, the bowel is returned to the abdominal cavity. The integrity of the repair is evaluated underwater by inject-ing air through a proctoscope as described.

We have used this technique for resection and reanastomosis for small bowel injuries with a trocar, during lysis of small bowel adhesions, or to correct small bowel strangulation through a Richter herniation. At times, in these situations, resection and reanastomosis can be done through an umbilical incision that is enlarged vertically or transversely.

Results

In a series of 356 women who underwent lap-aroscopic treatment of superficial or deep bowel endometriosis using the different tech-niques just presented, two cases were converted to laparotomy early in our experience. The first was for repair of an enterotomy after treatment of infiltrative rectal endometriosis. The second

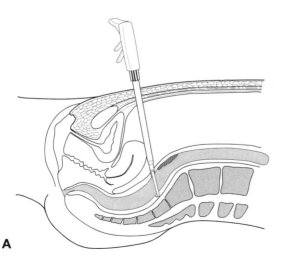

A

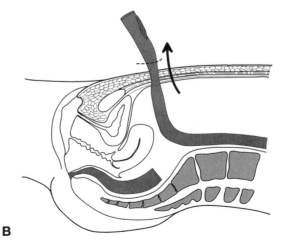

B

FIGURE 23.10. Intraabdominal laparoscopic bowel resection. **A:** After the bowel is completely mobi-lized, a 60-mm Endostapler (Ethicon) is fired distal to the lesion. **B:** The proximal limb of the colon is delivered from the abdomen and exteriorized (*arrows*) through a small incision.

required laparotomy for anastomosis following an unsuccessful attempt to place a pursestring suture around a patulous rectal ampulla.

Significant postoperative complications occurred in 1.7% of patients. Two women developed leaks and pelvic infections. One required temporary colostomy (performed laparoscopically) with subsequent takedown and repair by laparotomy, and the other was managed by prolonged drainage. One patient had bowel stricture requiring resection and reanastomosis by laparotomy. Another developed a pelvic abscess that did not respond to drainage; she underwent laparoscopic right salpingo-oophorectomy. Finally, a fifth patient had an immediate rectal prolapse that was reduced without surgical management. Her bowel symptoms persisted, and she eventually underwent a total colectomy. Minor complications included skin ecchymosis, temporary urinary retention, temporary diarrhea or constipation, and dyschezia.

For multiple and extensive lesions, and those that affect a large portion of the rectum or rectosigmoid colon, the bowel is mobilized laparoscopically. Resection and reanastomosis are performed through a minilaparotomy incision, vaginally or transanally, depending on the location of the disease. For the small bowel and ileocecum, after the bowel is mobilized laparoscopically, the resection and reanastomosis are performed laparoscopically or through a minilaparotomy. Appendiceal endometriosis is managed by appendectomy.

The laparoscopic approach can be used for most intestinal surgery performed by the gynecologic surgeon. Numerous techniques have been proposed for laparoscopic colon surgery, and modifications are constantly devised.[12,14] Generally, the technique of laparoscopic bowel resection is identical to that used in the past, except that access is by laparoscopy, rather than laparotomy.

Conclusions

Endometriosis is a chronic disease, and unfortunately, despite medical and surgical advances in its treatment, recurrence of the disease or symptoms is not uncommon. The symptoms caused by endometriosis sometimes are not specific to the involved organ. Careful patient selection for a specific treatment, and patient consultation and follow-up, are recommended.

At present, we treat bowel endometriosis by vaporizing and excising the lesions using the CO_2 laser, providing they are isolated and involve only serosa, subserosa, or muscularis without mucosal penetration. The bowel is repaired and reinforced whenever there is a deep defect. For deeply infiltrative lesions, wedge resection of the anterior colon or rectum is performed. Depending on the size of the defect, the bowel is repaired transversely or vertically. If the lesion is low in the rectum, close to the anus, the rectovaginal septum is entered and completely dissected. The lower portion of the rectum is mobilized, and the nodule is brought out through the vagina or anus and resected.

References

1. Semm K. Kie endoskopische appendektomie. *Gynäkol Prax.* 1983;7:26–30.
2. Nezhat C, Nezhat F. Incidental appendectomy during videolaseroscopy. *Am J Obstet Gynecol.* 1991;165:559–564.
3. Nezhat C, Pennington E, Nezhat F, et al. Laparoscopically assisted anterior rectal wall resection and reanastomosis for deeply infiltrating endometriosis. *Surg Laparosc Endosc.* 1991; 1(2):106–108.
4. Redwine DB, Koning M, Sharpe DR. Laparoscopically assisted transvaginal segmental resection of the rectosigmoid colon for endometriosis. *Fertil Steril.* 1996;65(1):193–197.
5. Nezhat F, Nezhat C, Pennington E. Laparoscopic proctectomy for infiltrating endometriosis of the rectum. *Fertil Steril.* 1992;57: 1129–1132.
6. Nezhat F, Nezhat C, Pennington E, et al. Laparoscopic segmental resection for infiltrating endometriosis of the rectosigmoid colon: a preliminary report. *Surg Laparosc Endosc.* 1992; 2:212–216.
7. Nezhat C, Nezhat F, Pennington E. Laparoscopic treatment of lower colorectal and infiltrative rectovaginal septum endometriosis by the technique of videolaseroscopy. *Br J Obstet Gynaecol.* 1992;99:664–667.

8. Wexner SD, Johansen OB. Laparoscopic bowel resection: advantages and limitations. *Ann Med.* 1992;4:105–110.

9. Nezhat C, Nezhat F, Ambroze W, et al. Laparoscopic repair of small bowel, colon, and rectal endometriosis: a report of twenty-six cases. *Surg Endosc.* 1993;7:88–89.

10. Ambroze WL, Orangio GR, Armstrong D, et al. Laparoscopic surgery for colorectal neoplasms. *Semin Surg Oncol.* 1994;10:398–403.

11. Nezhat C, Nezhat F, Pennington E, et al. Laparoscopic disk excision and primary repair of the anterior rectal wall for the treatment of full-thickness bowel endometriosis. *Surg Endosc.* 1994;8:682–685.

12. Nezhat C, Nezhat F, Metzger DA, et al. Adhesion reformation after reproductive surgery by videolaseroscopy. *Fertil Steril.* 1990;53: 1008–1011.

13. Nezhat C, Nezhat F, Luciano AA, et al. *Operative Gynecologic Laparoscopy: Principles and Techniques.* New York: McGraw-Hill; 1995.

14. Nezhat C, Crowgey S, Nezhat F. Videolaseroscopy for the treatment of endometriosis associated with infertility. *Fertil Steril.* 1989;51: 237–240.

15. Franklin ME Jr, Ramos R, Rosenthal D, Schuessler W. Laparoscopic colonic procedures. *World J Surg.* 1993;17:51–56.

16. Semm K. *Operationslehre für endoskopische Abdominalchirurgie.* Stuttgart: Schattauer, 1984.

17. Götz F. Die endoskopische Appendektomie nach Semm bei der akuten und chronischen Appendizitis. *Endosk Heute.* 1988;2:5–7.

18. Nezhat C, Nezhat F, Nezhat C. Operative laparoscopy (minimally invasive surgery): state of the art. *J Gynecol Surg.* 1992;8:111–141.

24

Office Laparoscopy Under Local Anesthesia

Steven F. Palter

The practice of modern operative gynecology was revolutionized by the advent of laparoscopy, which has undergone progressive advancement from simple diagnostic work to present-day advanced operative procedures. Office microlaparoscopy under local anesthesia is one of the most recent advances in minimally invasive surgery, representing the merging of two technologies. The first, microlaparoscopy, is the use of small-caliber (often 2-mm) laparoscopes and accessory instrumentation. The second is a technique to perform laparoscopy under local anesthesia, often in nontraditional (i.e., non-operating room) settings such as the hospital procedure room or a physician's office.

Each of these innovations can be performed alone and provide benefits for practitioners and patients. For example, microlaparoscopy can be performed in the operating room under general anesthesia. Similarly, traditional laparoscopic instrumentation can be used for office-based operative procedures under local anesthesia. Together, however, these two techniques create a synergism that allows radical new ideas and modifications of laparoscopic technique and procedures. The technique of office laparoscopy under local anesthesia is especially suited to meet the current pressures of quality versus cost in an era of managed care. It is likely that this technique will soon become a major part of the practicing gynecologist's diagnostic and operative armamentarium.

Advantages of office microlaparoscopy under local anesthesia can be separated into those realized by the practitioner, the patient, and the managed care provider (Table 24.1). Nonetheless, office microlaparoscopy under local anesthesia has several inherent disadvan-

TABLE 24.1.   Advantages of office microlaparoscopy under local anesthesia.

Patient	Practitioner	Managed care providers
Decreased scheduling delays	Decreased scheduling delays	Decreased procedure costs
Decreased preoperative delays	Decreased preoperative delays	Increased rate of recovery
Elimination of preoperative blood tests, interviews, delays	Elimination of operative paperwork	
Reduction in operative costs	Elimination of travel time and delays	
Decreased postoperative morbidity		
Increased rate of recovery		
High rates of patient acceptance		

TABLE 24.2.   Disadvantages of office microlaparoscopy under local anesthesia.

Limited therapeutic options
Limited backup
Limited field of view
Limited operative time
Patient not paralyzed
Patient not asleep
Fragile equipment
Additional training requirements
Startup costs

tages (Table 24.2) related to the use of smaller and more fragile equipment, the elimination of general anesthesia, and the therapeutic limitations of the alternative operative location.

History of Microlaparoscopy Under Local Anesthesia

Laparoscopy under local anesthesia traces its conception closely with the development of laparoscopy itself. Contrary to common belief, laparoscopy was initially developed as a procedure under local, and not general, anesthesia.[1] A remarkable publication by Short in the *British Medical Journal* in 1925 was the first description of laparoscopy in England as well as of its performance under local anesthesia outside a traditional hospital setting.[2]

Microlaparoscopy refers to the inspection of internal organs via small-caliber telescopes. In general, the term "microlaparoscope" refers to those scopes (and accessory instruments) less than 5 mm in diameter and most recently has been reserved for instrumentation of 2 mm or less in diameter. The first generation of micro-

laparoscopes created almost 20 years ago suffered from poor-quality optics, and visualization was both significantly compromised and inadequate for full inspection of the pelvis. These "optical catheters" however were the precursors of today's miniaturized fiberoptic laparoscopes.

One of the only reported studies using this first generation of microlaparoscope was by Steege, who performed office laparoscopic (multiple early-interval, second-look) procedures under local anesthesia. In doing so, lysis of developing adhesions was performed with the laparoscope itself in a single puncture technique.[3] He reported a high success rate of symptom relief in patients with chronic pelvic pain as well as reduced adhesion scores after multiple repeat-look laparoscopies. The protocol employed has limited generalizability, however, in that it required an indwelling Tenckoff catheter to be left in place. This is not the case with current protocols.

Indications and Patient Selection

In general, office laparoscopy under local anesthesia is primarily indicated for diagnostic and simple operative procedures. The scope of office laparoscopy procedures currently being performed or under development are listed in Table 24.3. In gynecology, diagnostic laparoscopy for the evaluation of chronic pelvic pain, diagnostic laparoscopy for the evaluation of infertility, and tubal ligation are the only procedures for which tolerance and efficacy data exist. Other procedures must be considered investigational at this time. Operative indications have purposely been limited to

TABLE 24.3. Potential uses for office microlaporoscopy under local anesthesia.

Gynecologic	General surgical
Diagnostic laparoscopy	Evaluation of acute abdomen
Infertility evaluation: chromopertubation	Evaluation of abdominal trauma
Evaluation of pelvic pain: conscious pain mapping	Herniorrhaphy
Lysis of adhesions	Catheter placement
Assisted Reproductive Technologies: GIFT/ZIFT/TET	Directed biopsy
Second-look laparoscopy	Evaluation of chronic abdominal pain
Emergency room evaluation	Diagnosis of acute appendicitis
Tubal ligation	

decrease the risk of operation-related complications. There exist few published criteria regarding patient selection for office laparoscopy. In general, the exclusion criteria are similar to those of laparoscopy in general. Patient selection is therefore based on anesthesia-related factors, operation-specific factors, and patient tolerance factors.

The American Society of Anesthesiologists (ASA) grading system was established to stratify patient anesthetic risk on the basis of underlying systemic illness. Patients of grade I or II have at most mild systemic illnesses, and we have limited office-based laparoscopy to these patients only. This greatly decreases the risk of anesthesia and stress-related complications (mainly cardiac and respiratory) and simplifies the monitoring requirements of the procedure.

Patient obesity makes laparoscopy under local anesthesia more difficult. Morbid obesity makes trocar insertions more difficult and increases the possibility of preperitoneal insertion and insufflation. For most operators, a Veress needle with a specialized covering sheath is used as a trocar. Therefore, in cases of morbid obesity, an extralong Veress may be necessary. More so than when using traditional-sized equipment, reinsertion after preperitoneal insertion is especially difficult when using miniaturized equipment. The use of low-level insufflation (often 0.5–1 liter total) also may be inadequate in obese patients. Without muscle relaxation and higher insufflation volumes, the weight of the abdominal wall becomes a limiting factor for visualization. In this regard, the use of microlaparoscopy under local anesthesia is effectively limited to patients under 200 pounds.

Similarly, previous abdominal surgery, especially midline abdominal incisions, as well as a history of peritonitis increase the risk of the procedure and are relative contraindications for some surgeons. Such a history will increase the risk of inadvertent injury to vital structures, most notably the bowel and the bladder. Specialized insertion techniques (i.e., left-upper quadrant) are effective and may be required for safe access in these situations.

Perhaps the most important requirement for successful laparoscopy under local anesthesia is proper patient counseling. We discuss with our patients all aspects of the procedure to avoid surprise and alleviate anxiety. Anecdotal reports exist of patients who were improperly prepared or medicated and who had dissociative reactions during the procedure. Because patient cooperation is vital to perform a safe, controlled procedure under local anesthesia, psychiatric illness in general, and anxiety disorders in specific, may be considered relative contraindications. In our experience however these patients do not have more difficulty or tolerate the procedure less well provided they are extensively counseled and prepared preoperatively.

Techniques

Instrumentation

Traditional laparoscopes are constructed from a series of rigid glass lenses or rod–lens assemblies. These are surrounded by a thick metal sheath and incorporate an assembly of fiberoptic light bundles. Laparoscopes of this type range from 5 mm to 12 mm in diameter and may include an operative channel. Recent refinements in fiberoptic technology have allowed the creation of laparoscopes in which the optical element is composed of fused bundles of fiberoptic cables (Fig. 24.1). These modern fiberoptic scopes may have 10,000 to 30,000 optical image fibers as well as additional light-carrying bundles. Fiberoptic scopes of this type range from 25 to 27 cm working length and have a field of view of 60° to 75°. All currently available microlaparoscopes have a 0° direct forward direction of view, and their outer diameters range from less than 1 mm to 4 mm. Certain manufacturers have employed designs that require the laparoscope to be affixed to a rigid insertion sheath which increases the effective outer diameter. Laparoscopes of this type are currently available from manufacturers including Imagyn Medical, Inc., U.S. Surgical Corporation, Olympus, Origin Medsystems, MIST, Storz, and Optimed. Image quality, laparoscope durability, and system flexibility vary considerably among the different designs. We have observed a dramatic decline in image quality and sturdiness with current scopes less than 2 mm in diameter. Depending on design, these fiberoptic laparoscopes may be as durable and sturdy as rigid lens scopes.

Accessory 2 mm diameter instruments are now available for microlaparoscopy (see Fig. 24.1). In our experience, the most commonly used accessory instruments are the rigid blunt probe and a grasper. With the micrograspers, however, care must be taken because the small jaw size results in a large force transmission to the tissue and may produce a laceration if incorrectly applied. Various configurations of biopsy devices are available that will provide a 1-mm sample of superficial tissue which is adequate to diagnose endometriosis. Scissors are also available; however, to date all are of the reusable type and become dull with minimal use. As such, they are not economical or reliable. Various manufacturers are currently addressing this issue with the development of fully, or partially, disposable devices.

The greatest limitation in microlaparoscopy instrumentation is an energy source for hemostasis. Various prototype unipolar and bipolar devices are available; however, their small size limits their usefulness. Power settings, durability, and insulation strength are currently being investigated. Similarly, while other energy sources theoretically can be developed in a 2-mm size (laser, argon beam coagulator, etc.), their safety and cost-effectiveness in the office setting are questionable.

In addition to a laparoscope (miniaturized or standard-sized), the following equipment is required for office laparoscopy (Fig. 24.2): (1) videocamera and monitor, (2) light source, (3) accessory instrumentation and access devices, (4) a table capable of achieving Trendelenburg position, (5) a crash cart and resuscitation equipment, (6) intravenous setup and medications, (7) sterile drapes and gown, and (8) a trained operative assistant as well as one

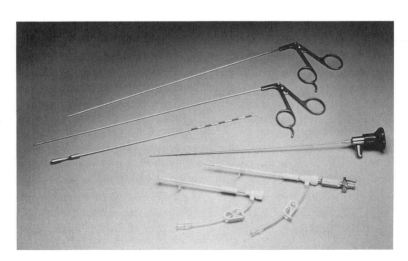

FIGURE 24.1. Two-millimeter (2-mm) office laparoscopy equipment (Imagyn Medical, Inc., Laguna Miguel, CA).

FIGURE 24.2.   Room setup for office laparoscopy under local anesthesia.

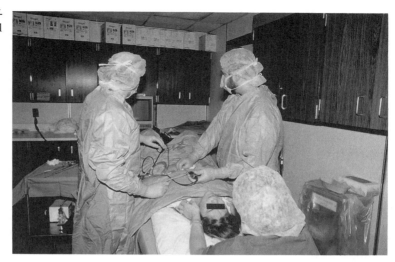

individual dedicated to monitoring the patient's vital signs and administering the intravenous sedation.

Anesthesia

Traditional thought in the United States has dictated that laparoscopy is a procedure which requires general anesthesia. Many arguments are given in support of this, including: (1) General anesthesia is required for adequate intraoperative pain control. (2) Creation of a pneumoperitoneum compromises diaphragmatic excursion and dictates intubation and mechanical ventilation to ensure adequate oxygenation. (3) There is a need for paralysis of the patient to prevent intraoperative movement and inadvertent injury. (4) There is a need for mechanical ventilation to clear CO_2 absorbed from the pneumoperitoneum. Each of these arguments is based on anecdote and speculation rather than actual data. In fact, there is a long history to support the safety, feasibility, and advantages of laparoscopy under local anesthesia refuting these arguments.[4-6]

Most of the laparoscopic procedures under local anesthesia that have been reported were performed with some degree of supplemental intravenous (IV) sedation in addition to local anesthesia.[3,5-10] In these reports, the term local anesthesia is used liberally to differentiate the procedures from those performed under general anesthesia, even if supplemental IV agents were used. The prime consideration in the use of IV (or "conscious") sedation is the preservation of patient alertness and responsiveness. In doing so, the patient will independently preserve the integrity of her own airway and maintain adequate ventilation. In contrast, under general anesthesia, there is partial or complete loss of protective reflexes. Should the patient not remain responsive to verbal instructions, the line into deep sedation or general anesthesia has been crossed and the risk of the procedure increases dramatically.

Procedures can be performed under strict local anesthesia; however, this results in diminished operative time tolerance and prohibits all but the most simple procedures. Historically, laparoscopy under strict local anesthesia (using traditional-sized instrumentation) was limited to 10 to 15 min of operative time before patient discomfort became limiting. We have found that by using the microlaparoscopes and adding supplemental IV sedation we can usually extend operative times to 30 to 45 min. We routinely administer intravenous fentanyl and midazolam for conscious sedation. These agents are titrated to the patient's weight, comfort level, level of consciousness, and vital signs.

We have found that for patients with chronic pelvic pain the average dosage of medication administered was 91 mcg of fentanyl and 4 mg of midazolam, while patients being evaluated for infertility required significantly less medication (75 mcg of fentanyl and 2.7 mg midazolam; $p < .05$).[9] To date, no studies have directly addressed pain tolerance of traditional-sized versus microlaparoscopes, or strict local anesthesia compared to local plus supplemental IV sedation.

Procedure Specifics

Both laparoscopy under local anesthesia and microlaparoscopy require unique skills. A history of successful advanced laparoscopy is not sufficient to ensure success with these new techniques, and practitioners are recommended to pursue a formal educational program. We perform office laparoscopy under local anesthesia in an office-based procedure room. All video and insufflation equipment is placed on a traditional operating room-type equipment cart. We keep two tables adjacent to the patient, one for vaginal equipment and one for abdominal. We begin by placing the patient in dorsal lithotomy position and preparing the vagina and perineum with an antiseptic solution. Next, a paracervical block is administered and a uterine manipulator inserted. We use a standard Cohen uterine manipulating cannula and have found that it is better tolerated than uterine manipulators that have a distal balloon.

The abdomen is prepared with an antiseptic solution, and the patient sterilely draped. Next, a field block is administered to the umbilicus. This allows insertion of the specialized insufflation trocar over a Veress needle. This Veress needle passes through the center of the sheath, which includes an insufflation port (Fig. 24.1). The entire assembly is inserted as one and the Veress removed leaving the sheath in place. The Veress needle/sheath assembly is inserted in the same fashion as a standard Veress needle; however, extreme care must be taken to monitor the insertion angle and force. Furthermore, elevation of the abdominal wall (with the operator's hand) is required when working under low anesthesia with low insufflation volumes.

The abdomen is next insufflated with CO_2 gas until an adequate "visual window" is cre-

ated. While pressure can be regulated, it is an inaccurate measure of insufflation adequacy in a patient without muscle paralysis. Instead, a maximum pressure of 15 mm is set, and "active insufflation" used to maintain the visual window. In this process, the gas flow is continually adjusted, started, and stopped, to keep adequate visualization and to maintain patient comfort. In total, 0.5 to 2 liters are usually used for insufflation although in selected cases we have had to use volumes as great as 6 liters. Secondary 2-mm trocars are inserted in a similar manner, again requiring elevation of the anterior abdominal wall. Absolute care must be taken to insert these slowly under direct visualization because the tip of the trocars will pass close to the viscera and pelvic vessels.

During the course of the operation the patient is placed in Trendelenburg's position to aid displacement of the bowel from the cul-de-sac. In general, 10° to 25° is sufficient. Should excessive local internal discomfort be experienced, local anesthetics can be directly applied; however, care must be taken to avoid administering large volumes that might cause systemic toxicity. We follow the same dose per body weight recommendations as would be used for the injection of any of these agents.

Traditional-sized laparoscopic instrumentation can also be used for office laparoscopy under local anesthesia. Its use, however, is potentially more dangerous because of the larger degree of trauma that would result from a trocar injury. Similarly, we have found significantly increased patient comfort (and increased tolerance of the length of operative procedures) using the miniaturized instrumentation. We use 2-mm secondary ports and instrumentation for all office procedures with the exception of tubal ligation.

Results

Laparoscopic Sterilization Under Local Anesthesia

Perhaps the greatest wealth of literature related to laparoscopy under local anesthesia was published in the 1970s in conjunction with the development of laparoscopic methods of female sterilization. Numerous publications described methods of laparoscopic tubal occlusion with cautery, bands, or clips. In fact, many techniques for laparoscopic tubal ligation were initially developed under local anesthesia using traditional 10- or 12-mm laparoscopes with operative channels.[7,8]

A remarkable series of 250,000 consecutive laparoscopic tubal ligations were performed P.V. Methaly over a 9-year period using silastic rings.[4] The procedures were carried out in improvised rural Indian sterilization camps in an assembly-line fashion. Simple wooden benches placed on blocks to achieve Trendelenburg's position were used as the operative tables. Despite this setting and the use of boiling water for sterilization of equipment, success and complication rates were similar to those in the west! The authors reported 74 cases of abdominal wall bleeding (0.03%), 4 cases of bowel trauma requiring subsequent laparotomy (0.002%), and 12 deaths within the first 30 days after the procedure (0.005%). There were no major vessel injuries reported. More importantly, none of the deaths was an immediate consequence of the operative procedure. The failure rate in this series was 0.1%, and the overall incidence of major complications (requiring admission to a hospital) was 0.003%.

Today, laparoscopic sterilization under local anesthesia is generally performed via this traditional one-puncture technique or via a two-puncture method. In two-puncture office laparoscopic sterilization, a 5-mm secondary trocar is inserted and a standard clip applied or bipolar cauterization performed. Comfort is maintained through the application of clips or bipolar coagulation by dripping 2 to 5 ml of local anesthetic directly onto the tubal surface approximately 5 min before the ligation is performed. Newer techniques for dual 2-mm procedures using rings, clips, cautery, or loops are currently under development. Currently, most operators are performing this procedure with standard 10- and 12-mm laparoscopes. Anecdotally, the use of 2-mm endoscopes results in increased patient comfort and lower operative risk, although these results are not yet confirmed.

Use of Office Microlaparoscopy in the Evaluation of Chronic Pelvic Pain and the Technique of Conscious Pain Mapping

We have conducted a prospective cohort study on patients presenting with chronic pelvic pain (CPP; $n = 17$) who underwent diagnostic office microlaparoscopy performed under local anesthesia as compared with patients undergoing diagnostic evaluations for infertility ($n = 11$; Table 24.4).[9] Patients were queried preoperatively and at 30 min and 1 week postoperatively with a specially designed questionnaire and a modification of the McGill Pain Inventory scale. A specific subset of questions evaluated the recovery period and time until return to usual activities, including diet, work, and sexual activity.

TABLE 24.4. Results of office microlaparoscopy under local anesthesia for chronic pelvic pain (CPP) and infertility (INF).

Factor	ALL	CPP	INF	p value
Age (years)	35.33	36.45	34.56	NS
Gravidity	0.96	1.55	0.56	<.05
Operative time (min)	20.85	23.91	18.75	NS
Recovery Time (min)	51.65	51.64	51.67	NS
Fentanyl (mcg)	81.48	90.91	75.00	.05
Versed (mg)	3.20	4.00	2.66	<.05
Pain scale score	5.87	7.00	5.04	<.05
30-min postoperative pain score	1.48	3.17	0.53	<.005
Time to normal activity (days)	1.88	1.73	2.01	NS
Time to return to work (days)	1.70	2.23	1.29	<.05
Time to resume intercourse (days)	4.61	5.42	4.21	NS
Postoperative medication usage (tablets ibuprofen)	4.88	9.45	1.53	<.005

ALL

The technique of "conscious pain mapping" was developed for use during office laparoscopy under local anesthesia in patients with CPP.[9] The pelvis is systematically inspected and the major structures (i.e. large and small bowel, round ligaments, ovaries, uterine fundus, anterior and posterior cul de sac, pelvic sidewalls, and uterosacral ligaments) grasped or probed in a standardized fashion. Any visible areas of pathology (e.g., endometriosis, adhesions, or scarring) are also probed. Patients are asked to rate the pain of this grasping with a weighted 0–10 point scale. It is noted if the pain experienced can be localized to a specific point or if it is generalized throughout the pelvis and abdominal cavity. If the patient experiences local pain with the manipulation of viscera, lidocaine is directly applied topically to that area and the pain is rerated.

Conscious pain mapping demonstrated a distinct pattern of pain in the majority of patients with severe CPP: a generalized visceral hypersensitivity in all areas of the pelvis and abdominal cavity. In this case, all areas probed elicit pain regardless of the presence of visualized pathology. Local application of anesthetic to areas of evoked pain (1% lidocaine dripped onto the peritoneal surface) was able to reduce the level of pain and allow the procedure to continue but it did not completely eliminate the pain. This pattern was not seen in any of the patients undergoing office laparoscopy for infertility. Perhaps the most important use of conscious pain mapping is to identify foci of pain that may not be clearly visible on routine examination, such as in areas of previous surgical excision or questionable endometriosis. This focal distribution of pain sensitivity is the second pattern observed in some patients with chronic pelvic pain.

Office Microlaparoscopy for the Evaluation of Infertility

We performed a cohort study on all patients requiring diagnostic laparoscopy as part of their general infertility evaluation ($n = 27$) to determine whether a complete laparoscopic infertility evaluation (including chromopertu-

bation) could be performed under local anesthesia in an office setting.[10] Here, office microlaparoscopy under local anesthesia is performed with one or two secondary 2-mm punctures. The pelvis and abdomen are inspected in the same fashion as in traditional laparoscopy. A dilute solution of indigo carmine dye is then injected via the uterine manipulator. Care must be taken to inject the dye slowly to avoid the risk of tubal spasm and false-positive findings. All these patients reported that they were highly satisfied with the procedure; 96% would repeat the procedure in the office under local anesthesia, and 93% preferred the office laparoscopy to a previous traditional operating room-based laparoscopy.

There were no procedures that could not be performed as the result of patient or equipment failures, and no procedures required general anesthesia. All aspects of the infertility investigation, including chromopertubation, biopsy of endometriosis, and inspection of all areas of the pelvis and abdomen, could be successfully performed. The average procedure length was 18 min, ranging from 8 to 50 min. Furthermore, patients were stable for discharge in fewer than 50 min. The average patient required minimal to no postoperative medication and returned fully to usual activities within 24 hr. Analysis of costs demonstrated an approximate 75% reduction in costs as compared with traditional laparoscopy. These results would suggest that the use of office microlaparoscopy may allow diagnostic laparoscopy to be considered earlier in the infertility investigation. In this setting, appropriate patient selection is vital to reduce the possibility that operative interventions will be required.

Possibilities for the Future

Careful assessments must be made of this new technology as it is introduced. It is imperative that we not only report on what "can" be done but rather critically assess new technologies in terms of efficacy, cost-effectiveness, tolerance, and acceptance. There will undoubtedly be procedures that do not translate well into surgery under local anesthesia. For example, diagnostic office laparoscopies must be performed with a technique that allows full visualization of all areas of the pelvis which would be visualized with traditional laparoscopy. Similarly, office or procedure room appendectomies must be shown to be advantageous when compared to a traditional laparoscopic approach to be a viable option. The danger with any rapidly proliferating new technology (especially when there are financial incentives to choose it) is to accept the procedure on the basis of anecdote without objective documentation of efficacy and safety. It is the goal of those who are currently developing these techniques to ensure the progression of office laparoscopy under local anesthesia from a novelty to a gynecologic standard.

References

1. Gunning JE. The history of laparoscopy. *J Reprod Med.* 1974;12:222–226.
2. Short AR. The use of celioscopy. *Br Med J.* 1925;2:254.
3. Steege JF. Repeated clinic laparoscopy for the treatment of pelvic adhesions: a pilot study. *Obstet Gynecol.* 1994;83:276–279.
4. Metha PV. A total of 250,136 laparoscopic sterilizations by single operator. *Br J Obstet Gynaecol.* 1989;96:1024–1034.
5. Peterson HB, Hulka JF, Spielman FJ, Lee S, Marchbanks PA. Local vs. general anesthesia for laparoscopic sterilization: randomized study. *Obstet Gynecol.* 1987;70:903–908.
6. Brown DR, Fishburne JI, Roberson VO, Hulka JV. Ventilatory and blood gas changes during laparoscopy with local anesthesia. *Am J Obstet Gynecol.* 1976;124:741–745.
7. Wheeless CR Jr. Outpatient laparoscopic sterilization under local anesthesia. *Obstet Gynecol.* 1972;39:767–770.
8. Alexander GD, Goldrath M, Brown EM, Smiler BG. Outpatient laparoscopic sterilization under local anesthesia. *Am J Obstet Gynecol.* 1973;116:1065–1068.
9. Palter S, Olive D. Office laparoscopy under local anesthesia for chronic pelvic pain: utility, acceptance, and cost-benefit analysis. *J Am Assoc Gynecol Laparosc.* 1996;3:359–364.
10. Palter SF, Olive DL. Office laparoscopy under local anesthesia for infertility: utility, acceptance, and cost-benefit/outcome analyses. *Fertil Steril.* 1995;64:S8–S9.

25

Minimizing, Recognizing, and Managing Laparoscopic Complications

Samuel Smith

This chapter describes the most common complications associated with laparoscopic surgery, with an emphasis on prevention and management. Reference texts published by Borten[1] and by Corfman et al.[2] provide comprehensive reviews of laparoscopic complications, and every gynecologic endoscopic surgeon should review these or a similar text.

Complications of Operative Laparoscopy

The First Annual Report of the Complications Committee of the American Association of Gynecologic Laparoscopists (AAGL) reviewed 12,182 laparoscopies performed in 1972 (Table 25.1).[3] Eighty-two major complications were reported for a rate of 6.8 per 1,000 procedures. In addition, 3 deaths occurred (25.0 per 100,000 cases). The AAGL had a 24% response rate to its 1988 membership survey on operative laparoscopy (Table 25.2),[4] with a total of 36,928 operative laparoscopies reported; 568 major complications (15.4 per 1,000 procedures) and 2 deaths (5.4 per 100,000 cases) were noted. This complication rate may actually be an underestimation of the true complication rate because 76% of AAGL members failed to respond to the survey, which may be a source of ascertainment bias.

The 1991 AAGL survey had a 17% response rate with a total of 56,536 procedures, a 1.5-fold increase over 1988. Complications appeared to be increased over the 1988 rates. Unintended laparotomies to manage hemorrhage, bowel, or urinary tract injuries were increased 1.5 fold. Particularly worrisome is a 5.3-fold increase in the rate of spillage of unsuspected ovarian cancer. The death rate continued to be very low (Table 25.2).[5]

From these reports it appears that major laparoscopic complications are more common today, probably related to the greater diversity of

TABLE 25.1. 1973 Report of the American Association of Gynecologic Laparoscopists (AAGL) on 12,182 laparoscopies.

Complication	Rate/1000 cases
Major	6.8
Anesthetic	0.7
Laparotomy for surgical trauma	3.2
Mesosalpingeal bleeding	1.9
Gastrointestinal	0.5
Electrocoagulation injury	2.3
Gastrointestinal	2.2

Adapted from Hulka JF, Soderstrom RM, Corson SL, et al. Complications Committee of the American Association of Gynecological Laparoscopists: first annual report. *J Reprod Med.* 1975;10:301–306.

operative endoscopic procedures being performed. It is incumbent upon our readers to take this trend very seriously. Surgeons need to recognize how quickly and unexpectedly complications may occur even with good technique. We must do our best to avoid complications and be ever ready to recognize and manage them. The principles minimizing complications during operative laparoscopy are summarized in Table 25.3.

Anesthetic Complications

Complications of anesthesia are rare during laparoscopy. Although the 1975 AAGL survey noted 9 anesthetic incidents and 9 insufflation difficulties (1.4 per 1000),[3] anesthesia complications now occur with about one-tenth the frequency. More than 50% of anesthesia-related deaths are related to hypoventilation. In the past, failed intubation and esophageal intubation were major causes of anesthesia-related death during laparoscopy.[6] Inadvertent endobronchial intubation resulting in ventilation of a single lung may also occur, as the hilum of the lung is displaced upward in the deep Trendelenburg position.[1] The use of short endotracheal tubes minimizes this risk.

The Trendelenburg position and the increased intraabdominal pressure used with laparoscopy are associated with an increased risk of regurgitation of gastric contents.[1] However, Trendelenburg's position also reduces the risk of aspiration of regurgitated material into the airway because of the beneficial effect of gravity. Cuffed endotracheal tubes should be used in all laparoscopies to prevent aspiration pneumonitis.[1]

Excessive intraabdominal CO_2 insufflation producing intraperitoneal pressures exceeding 20 mmHg may lead to adverse cardiorespiratory effects.[1] During tension pneumoperitoneum, the anesthesiologist may observe an increased resistance to ventilation. The insufflation of CO_2 and Trendelenburg's position should be reduced. Many new insufflators will automatically cut off gas flow when intraabdominal pressure exceeds a designated pressure, generally 12 to 16 mmHg. When using insufflators that do not have automatic cutoffs, intraperitoneal pressure should be frequently checked and abdominal tension monitored.

TABLE 25.2. Comparison of complication rates between two AAGL surveys.

Complication	Rate/1000 cases		Change since 1988
	1988 survey	1991 survey	
Major	15.4	NA	—
Laparotomy for surgical trauma	4.2	8.9	1.5-fold
Hemorrhage	2.1	6.8	2.6-fold
Bowel or urinary tract	1.6	2.8	1.7-fold
Nerve injury	0.5	0.5	NC
Spill of unsuspected ovarian cancer	0.5	3.2	5.3-fold
Death rate	5.4/100,000	1.8/100,000	−3.0-fold

NA, Not available; NC, no change.
Adapted from Peterson HB, Hulka JF, Phillips JM. American Association of Gynecologic Laparoscopists 1991 membership survey. *J Reprod Med.* 1990;35:590–591; and Hulka JF, Peterson HB, Phillips JM, Surrey MW. Operative laparoscopy—American Association of Gynecologic Laparoscopists 1991 membership survey. *J Reprod Med.* 1993;38:569–571.

TABLE 25.3. Guidelines for minimizing complications during operative laparoscopy.

During anesthesia:
    Use cuffed endotracheal tube
    Use nasogastric drainage
    Avoid overforceful mask ventillation
    Use complete muscle paralysis
In positioning patient:
    Place in frog-leg lithotomy position
    Avoid excessive hip or knee flexion or extension
    Avoid excessive pressure on inner thighs
    Use soft shoulder padding, if any
    Use knee- and foot-supporting stirrups
    Empty and continuously drain bladder
    Maintain arm on surgeon's side (usually the left) parallel alongside the body
    Avoid excessive Trendelenburg's position
    Lower operating table to level of the surgeon's elbows or hips to maximize control during insertion of umbilical or auxiliary trocars
In establishing pneumoperitoneum:
    Percuss left-upper quadrant to detect gastric distension
    Elevate umbilical skin before making skin incision
    During Veress needle insertion:
        Test spring mechanism before placement
        Leave valve open
        Direct to hollow of the sacrum
        Advance only 2–3 mm after piercing the parietal peritoneum
        Perform saline aspiration test
    Do not insufflate CO_2 at more than 1 liter/min initially
    If no loss of dullness to percussion over the liver edge is observed after insufflation of 1 liter of CO_2, suspect preperitoneal or omental insufflation
    Avoid overinsufflation of the abdominal cavity; generally maintain intraabdominal pressure at less than 16 mmHg
During laparoscope insertion and withdrawal:
    During trocar insertion:
        Maintain patient horizontal
        Extend index finger to within 3 cm of trocar tip to protect against sudden deep penetration
        Use controlled twisting motion
        Direct trocar tip toward sacral hollow
        Advance no more than 2 cm beyond parietal peritoneum
    When withdrawing trocar sheath, replace laparoscope (not trocar) first, after emptying the abdominal cavity of excess CO_2
During auxiliary trocar insertion:
    Transilluminate for visualization of epigastric vessels
    Identify at laparoscopy the inferior epigastrics on the anterior lateral to the umbilical artery remnants; they usually arise just medial to where the round ligaments enter the internal inguinal ring
    Place trocars as high above the symphysis as cosmetically possible, but never less than 3 cm
    Insert under direct laparoscopic visualization
    Direct downward, toward uterine fundus, not laterally
    If peritoneum tents around trocar tip, direct cranially along the anterior abdominal wall into the umbilical sleeve
    Consider radially expanding sleeves when large-diameter trocars and sleeves must be placed, especially laterally
During endoscopic surgery:
    Minimize use of unipolar electrocautery
    Disconnect or turn off all electrosurgical or laser units when not in use, even temporarily
    Identify ureters before any surgery on the pelvic side wall
    Mobilize the ovaries completely before performing a cystectomy
    Minimize forceful blunt dissection, especially when adhesions involve bowel serosa
    Use traction/countertraction to identify tissue planes
    Spread jaws of scissors to develop tissue planes, in lieu of cutting across the tissues
    Avoid cautery of bowel serosa
    Cauterize/coagulate vessels before transection
    Avoid scissor action ("crossed swords") between different instruments to minimize the risk of pinching or traumatizing bowel or omentum
    Do not cut any tissue before fully identifying the anatomy

Improper anesthetic techniques may contribute to the development of endoscopic complications. Complete muscle relaxation must be maintained at all times during operative laparoscopy procedures. Movement, retching, or coughing increases the risk of laceration or thermal injury when it occurs during the procedure, and if it occurs before closure of the umbilical incision may lead to herniation of small bowel. Excessive and forceful mask ventilation during a difficult intubation may lead to gastric distension and subsequent perforation by the umbilical trocar. The left-upper quadrant should always be percussed before Veress needle insertion; if it is found to be tympanic, a nasogastric tube is placed. Nasogastric tubes should be considered for any patient in whom there is a question of gastric enlargement by air or liquid.

Diagnostic and therapeutic procedures utilizing 2-mm laparoscopes are currently undergoing evaluation. Local and in some instances regional anesthesia is being utilized for these procedures. Vagal reactions have been observed during the periods of induced pneumoperitoneum and during manipulations of the peritoneum. Arrhythmias may also occur when gas is being insufflated under local anesthesia.

Laparoscopy is rarely associated with mortality. Potentially life-threatening emergencies do occur, however, and it is the responsibility of the surgeon and the anesthesia personnel to be aware of the major complications that can lead to sudden falling blood pressure or oxygen concentration, or to cardiac arrest, such as gas embolism (discussed later), or to pneumothorax or pneumopericardium caused by extremes of subcutaneous insufflation of CO_2 gas (discussed later).

Complications of Pneumoperitoneum and Insufflation

Complications associated with Insertion of the Veress Needle

The majority of laparoscopic complications (whether operative or diagnostic) occur during placement of the Veress needle or the tro-

cars.[6] Leaving the valve of the needle open during insertion allows room air to enter the abdominal cavity, encouraging the peritoneal contents to fall away from the needle tip. Moreover, once the needle is felt to penetrate the fascia and parietal peritoneum, it should be advanced only 2 to 3 mm more. In this manner the Veress needle tip has minimal opportunity to lacerate an omental or mesointestinal vessel, become buried within the omentum or loops of bowel, enter the retroperitoneal space, or completely transect an adherent loop of bowel. A variety of techniques are described to minimize the potential for incorrect needle placement, including listening for the "hissing" sound, the aspiration test, the "hanging drop" method, and the readings of intraabdominal pressure.[7,8] The hissing sound refers to the sound made by a Veress needle, when properly positioned within the abdominal cavity, on elevation of the abdominal wall. A drop of saline may also be placed in the needle hilt and the abdomen elevated, the so-called hanging drop test. The intraabdominal pressure is usually less than 1 mmHg. Generally, fluctuations in intraabdominal pressure can be detected on the insufflator manometer accompanying the patient's respirations.[7,8]

The most important safety maneuver to determine adequate placement of the Veress needle is the aspiration test.[1,7] The hilt of the Veress needle is attached to a syringe and, as soon as the needle is felt to be within the peritoneal cavity, gently aspirated. Normally no fluid should be recovered. Second, a small amount of saline is injected and reaspirated. Recovery of fluid suggests that the saline has been injected into a closed space, usually within the abdominal wall, or subperitoneally. Initial recovery of blood indicates that there either is free blood in the peritoneal cavity or that the tip of the needle has entered a blood vessel. Carbon dioxide should not be insufflated before these two entities are differentiated. In the case of obvious vascular injury, laparotomy to manage hemorrhage is the standard of care.[9]

Aspiration of intestinal fluid through the Veress needle suggests puncture of the intestinal tract, generally the small bowel (whose contents are more liquid, green, and usually sterile, compared to the large intestine). If accidental puncture of the small or large bowel has occurred with the Veress needle, the needle can be removed and a new one inserted, with laparoscopy then performed in the usual manner.[1] The site of gastrointestinal injuries should then be identified and inspected as soon as possible. In most cases, an intestinal puncture with the Veress needle will heal spontaneously without complication. Close observation for 24 to 48 hr, however, is indicated to rule out peritonitis.[1,8] Traditionally the patient is observed as an inpatient. Observation as an outpatient is not supported by any medical literature, although some physicians under managed care directives or incentives may be tempted to do so.

If urine is aspirated through the Veress needle, the needle can be withdrawn, a new needle inserted, and laparoscopy performed. Bladder punctures generally heal spontaneously. An indwelling catheter is usually left in place for 1 to 3 days.[1] Some surgeons suggest leaving the Veress needle in place in the event of intestinal contents or urine being reaspirated, so that the site is easily identifiable when laparoscopy is performed through a second site. However, this may result in the extension of a simple puncture into a laceration.[1] Others recommend omitting the Veress needle altogether and inserting the laparoscopic trocar directly into the abdominal cavity without the aid of prior pneumoperitoneum. Several large series describe this technique as safe, even in obese patients or women who have had prior laparotomy.[10–13] For example, the risk of bowel injury in women with previous laparotomy in one series was 1 per 416 procedures.[11]

Extraperitoneal Insufflation

Extraperitoneal insufflation of CO_2 usually occurs preperitoneally, in the abdominal wall, but may also occur retroperitoneally (i.e., beneath the posterior parietal peritoneum) if the needle has been inserted too deeply. Accumulation of gas extraperitoneally can technically complicate continuation of the laparoscopic procedure and results in greater patient morbidity. Once the Veress needle is felt to be in place, CO_2 should be insufflated at no more than 1 liter/min initially. This allows time to determine insufflation is occurring in a normal manner. Intraabdominal pressure is close to 1 mmHg before the influx of gas; it slowly rises as more gas is insufflated. After about 0.5 liter is insufflated you can accurately detect lower abdominal tympany by raising the abdominal wall several inches with one hand and percussing with the opposite hand. Hepatic dullness to percussion generally disappears once 1 liter of CO_2 is insufflated. Intraabdominal pressures are generally below 10 mmHg during insufflation, and most surgeons set the insufflation cutoff pressure between 12 and 14 mmHg. Rapid flow insufflation (>2.5 liters/min) should not be started until the aforementioned changes in tympany can be appreciated. Extraperitoneal or omental insufflation should be suspected when these signs are missing.

Subcutaneous emphysema results when the Veress needle fails to penetrate the rectus fascia (Fig. 25.1). Crepitation can be felt in the abdominal wall as CO_2 extends upward toward the loose areolar tissue of the neck or downward to the inguinal region. If the error is recognized early, the Veress needle is removed and reinserted. If the error is only recognized after a large volume of gas has been insufflated, disconnecting the gas tubing from the Veress needle, without removing the needle, will allow much of the gas to escape. If the error is first identified by laparoscopic visualization, the gas tubing should be disconnected from the trocar sheath; withdrawing the laparoscope then allows the gas to escape. Postoperative patient discomfort will be reduced if the amount of subcutaneous emphysema is decreased by these techniques.[1]

Insufflation of gas below the rectus fascia but outside the peritoneal cavity creates preperitoneal emphysema (see Fig. 25.1). This is less likely than subcutaneous emphysema to be identified before insertion of the laparoscopic trocar. The aspiration test is critical to detect preperitoneal location of the Veress needle tip. Saline may run in under pressure as the preperitoneal tissue is a loose connective type, but you will usually be able to reaspirate 1 ml or more of saline back. If you inadvertently insufflate, high insufflating pressures may not be

FIGURE 25.1. Sites where abnormal insufflation of CO_2 gas may occur: *a*, subcutaneous; *b*, preperitoneal; *c*, omental; *d*, retroperitoneal.

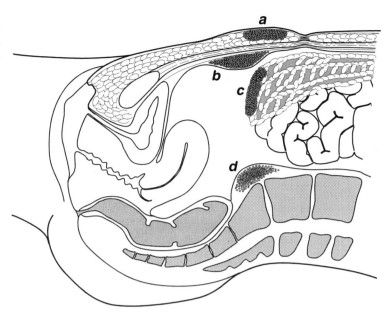

seen because the preperitoneal tissues offer little resistance to the gas. In addition, the expected loss of liver dullness to percussion can occasionally be seen.[1] Large volumes of preperitoneal gas will make it very difficult to insert the laparoscopic trocar.

Preperitoneal insufflation is usually identified when the laparoscope is placed and the peritoneum is merely displaced by the insufflated gas. Once diagnosed, an 18-gauge spinal needle, or similar aspirating needle, can be inserted into the preperitoneal space and the emphysema reduced under direct vision. Pressing on the abdominal wall seldom facilitates escape of the gas and usually results in lateral extension of the gas. Many times the preperitoneal insufflation is first recognized when trying to insert the laparoscopic trocar. The laparoscope is placed, and the preperitoneal insufflation is observed instead of the normal intraabdominal contents. Attempts at penetration of the peritoneum through the emphysema are discouraged because of the risk of damage to intraabdominal structures. The sleeve can be left in place and the gas escape valve opened to allow escape of the CO_2. Large quantities of gas can be evacuated in this manner. Some surgeons will try a direct insertion technique at this point. When this technique

fails it is usually because the peritoneum has been stripped from the posterior rectus fascia and the trocar's safety shield snaps in place after fascia has been penetrated but before the peritoneum is penetrated. Further attempts at direct insertion are probably ill advised at this point.

Pneumoperitoneum following preperitoneal insufflation can be established through the intraumbilical insertion of needle and trocar, a site where all tissue layers are fused.[14] Insertion of the Veress needle through the cul-de-sac may also be helpful.[8] Occasionally, with the use of an operating laparoscope the ballooned-out peritoneum can be incised under direct visualization; however, extreme caution is advised because of the potential to cause injuries intrabdominally. As intraperitoneal insufflation of gas occurs, the increasing intraabdominal pressure will slowly push the preperitoneal gas through the spinal needle or previously placed trocar.[1] Preperitoneal insufflation is one of the more common problems encountered in obese patients because of the greater thickness of their abdominal wall. Elevating the abdominal wall, inserting the Veress needle in a more vertical direction through the base of the umbilicus, and use of longer needles reduces the likelihood of preperitoneal insufflation.[14]

Recently marketed optical trocars that allow direct visualization of tissue layers are now available (Visiport, US Surgical, Norwalk, CT) to further increase safety. These trocars allow the surgeon to visualize, on the video monitor, a layer-by-layer entry into the peritoneal cavity. They are extremely useful in cases of preperitoneal insufflations that would otherwise be difficult to manage. In the past, as many as 3% of laparoscopies failed because an adequate pneumoperitoneum could not be established.[8] Occasionally we have to abandon a procedure because of "failed pneumoperitoneum" just to be safe.

Retroperitoneal insufflation or emphysema is uncommon (see Fig. 25.1). Small accumulations of retroperitoneal gas can be left in situ to reabsorb. Larger volumes should be aspirated under direct vision with an aspiration needle. Always consider that vascular damage may have also occurred.[1] Omental insufflation is not uncommon (Fig. 25.1), although it is seldom extensive and rarely interferes with the planned laparoscopic procedure. It is associated with greater postoperative patient discomfort.

Gas Embolism

Gas embolism is a clinically rare and potentially fatal event. Minor amounts of CO_2 gas or air entering the circulatory system may be absorbed and excreted without clinical recognition. Gas emboli are usually filtered by the pulmonary capillaries so that there is little risk of arterialization of venous gas embolism. Accidental puncture of a blood vessel and direct insufflation into the vessel is the most likely explanation for fatal embolization, although a variety of theories have been described.[6] If the patient is supine, gas is most likely to embolize to the coronary arteries and cause cardiac arrhythmias. In the Trendelenburg position, gas bubbles may be trapped in the splanchnic vascular bed or left ventricle only to later embolize with a change of position. Embolization to the brain occurs if the patient is upright. If gas embolization is suspected because of the sudden development of cardiac symptoms, gas flow should be stopped, and a central venous line should be advanced into the right atrium

or superior vena cava to try to aspirate gas from the cardiovascular system.[1] Additional supportive measures include 100% oxygen and fluids. Gas embolization is a rare and largely preventable problem. Air should not be injected during a saline aspiration test, and CO_2 insufflation rates should be kept low until the surgeon is certain of the proper intraabdominal location of the Veress needle.

Complications of Trocar Insertion

Insertion of sharp trocars rarely causes injury to intraabdominal structures. Placement of the laparoscopic trocar is more likely than auxiliary trocars to produce intraabdominal injury because it is so difficult to predict the presence of bowel or omental adhesions to the anterior abdominal wall. The Veress needle can be moved laterally during insufflation; observing a sudden rise in insufflation pressure suggests the needle tip is touching omentum, bowel, or adhesions.[7] Semm's probing test may also be used as a safety check before inserting the laparoscopic trocar.[7] For this test a 20-gauge spinal needle is attached to a 10-ml syringe filled with 3 to 4 ml of saline. The needle is inserted through the umbilical incision into the abdominal cavity. As the plunger is withdrawn, gas bubbles up into the saline. If no gas is recovered, the needle tip is probably in omentum or bowel. This test helps the surgeon map out a path of trocar entry when adhesions to the anterior abdominal wall are suspected. Insertion of the umbilical trocar should be directed toward the hollow of the sacrum. The patient should be completely flat, so as to maximize the distance between the umbilicus and the aorta (see following). The auxiliary trocars should be inserted under direct visualization.

The laparoscopic and auxiliary trocars should be inserted with controlled, twisting motions that minimize the risk of uncontrolled deep intraabdominal penetration and injury. Conical-tipped trocars were specifically designed for a twisting insertion, while pyramidal tips were designed for direct insertion, producing a self-closing X-shaped (flapped) opening in the fascia. However, both trocars can be inserted in a twisting fashion. An index finger extended over the trocar stem will limit the depth of penetration.[1] Trocars that are slightly dulled pose an important risk for injury. Dulled trocars require greater force to penetrate the abdominal wall than sharp trocars, and there is a greater likelihood of an uncontrolled thrust by the laparoscopist.[15] This principle applies to both the primary and auxiliary trocars. Disposable safety-shield trocars, marketed in a variety of sizes, require less force to penetrate the abdominal wall than reusable trocars.[16] They appear to offer an added measure of safety to trocar insertion. The "direct view" optical trocars (Visiport, US Surgical) also appear to add safety once their use is learned.

Vascular Injuries

Vascular injuries account for 30% to 50% of surgical trauma at laparoscopy.[15] Mintz' 1977 survey of 100,000 laparoscopic procedures reported only 34 injuries to major internal blood vessels (0.34 per 1,000 cases).[17] Unfortunately, major vascular complications are much more common today, according to the AAGL data (see Table 24.2). The pneumoperitoneum needle accounts for about 36% of vascular injuries, and the primary and auxiliary trocars account for about 32% each.[15] Additional bleeding can occur during the course of operative laparoscopic procedures. However, this type of bleeding is usually amenable to laparoscopic management.[1]

Superficial Epigastric Artery

The superficial epigastric artery, a branch of the femoral artery, pierces the femoral sheath and fascia lata to course in the subcutaneous tissues toward the umbilicus.[1] It is at greatest risk of injury during insertion of auxiliary trocars. Transillumination of the abdominal wall with the intraperitoneal laparoscopic light may identify the superficial epigastric artery and other large subcutaneous vessels and guide the placement of auxiliary trocars.[1]

Injury to deep subcutaneous vessels may be managed by occlusive pressure or by clamping and ligating the vessel through a small skin incision. Overnight hospitalization is recommended if the injury is treated by pressure be-cause recognition of subcutaneous bleeding is frequently delayed.[1]

Inferior Epigastric Vessels

The midline linea alba of the abdominal wall is relatively avascular. Lateral to the linea alba lie the rectus muscles, whose blood supply derives from the inferior and superior epigastric arteries, branches of the external iliac artery and internal mammary artery, respectively.[1] The inferior epigastric artery, which lies between the rectus muscle and its posterior fascia (see Fig. 10.2), is particularly prone to injury during placement of auxiliary trocars. With the exception of thin patients, this vessel generally cannot be identified by transillumination of the abdominal wall.[1] Thus, the paramedian insertion of the auxiliary trocar may be blind with regard to the inferior epigastric vessels unless they can be seen by direct laparoscopic visualization just lateral to the ligaments of the obliterated umbilical arteries. When the vessel cannot be endoscopically visualized, its position can be deduced by following the external iliac toward the inguinal canal, which is marked by the insertion of the round ligaments. The inferior epigastric artery arises right at this site.

Laceration of inferior epigastric vessels is usually preventable if an avascular midline site is selected for auxiliary trocar insertion.[1] Trocar insertion sites lateral to the external edge of the rectus muscle or the round ligament insertion at the inguinal ring are generally safe. This is generally 6 to 7 cm from the midline in average-size women.[18] Proceeding laterally, however, increases the risk of injury to the external iliac vessels, so the surgeon must be careful.

If laceration of the inferior epigastric artery or vein is identified during laparoscopy, full-thickness sutures should be placed 1 to 2 cm above and below the trocar insertion site to ligate lacerated and retracted vessels. These sutures should be placed under laparoscopic guidance whenever possible, so as to avoid trauma to intraabdominal structures.[1] A large urologic curved needle or specially designed needles for laparoscopic use can be used to secure the lacerated vessel (Fig. 25.2). On occasion the bleeding vessel can be visualized lap-

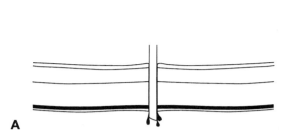

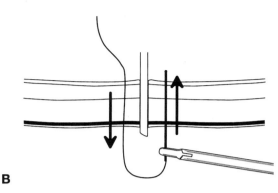

FIGURE 25.2. Lacerated inferior epigastric vessels (**A**) can be secured by passing a Keith straight needle into the peritoneal cavity on one side of the vessel and out on the other side with the aid of a laparoscopic needle holder (**B**). The bleeding vessel should be secured 1–2 cm above and below the injury to compensate for retraction of the cut vessel ends. The bleeding can be tamponaded temporarily with an inflated Foley bulb (see Fig. 25.3).

aroscopically and bipolar cautery can be used to secure hemostasis. Alternately, a no. 12 Foley catheter can be passed down the 5-mm sleeve into the abdomen, where the balloon is inflated with 5 to 10 ml of water. The sleeve is removed and the Foley balloon is pulled tightly up against the abdominal wall to occlude the vessel (Fig. 25.3). A hemostat or Kelly clamp is applied to the catheter as it exits the abdomen to maintain pressure on the vessel. If these measures fail to secure hemostasis, the skin incision should be enlarged and dissection

performed to isolate and ligate the bleeding vessel.[19]

Inferior epigastric artery laceration is more likely to occur when large laterally placed trocars are used, such as the 12-mm sleeves for endoscopic staplers during laparoscopic-assisted vaginal hysterectomy. Specially designed 2- to 3-mm access devices with radially expandable sleeves (Step, InnerDyne, Sunnyvale, CA) potentially allow for a safer and more controlled entry when large sleeves are needed (Fig. 25.4).

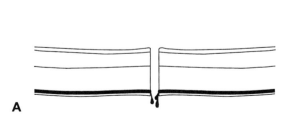

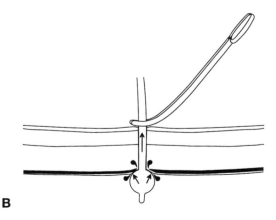

FIGURE 25.3. Inferior epigastric vessels that have been lacerated (**A**) may be tamponaded by passing a Foley catheter through the auxiliary sleeve into the abdomen, inflating the Foley balloon with sterile water, and pulling the balloon up against the abdominal wall (**B**). A clamp can be used to maintain pressure on the Foley balloon.

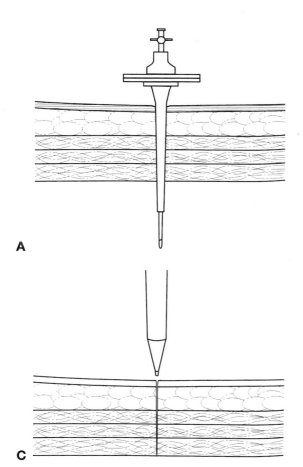

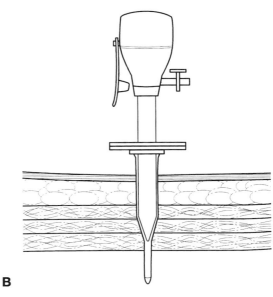

FIGURE 25.4. **A:** Radially expandable sleeves are placed through 3-mm skin incisions into the abdominal cavity. **B:** A tapered blunt dilator is inserted that expands the sleeve and creates a tissue tract by splitting tissue layers along paths of least resistance. **C:** After the cannula is removed the layers of abdominal wall muscles contract, leaving a series of nonoverlapping slits resembling a gridiron incision. Wound sizes are smaller than for comparable 10-mm to 12-mm trocars, and there is potentially less risk of abdominal wall blood vessel injury and incisional hernias.

At times laceration of the inferior epigastric artery may be diagnosed only postoperatively. Large preperitoneal hematomas can accumulate whose only symptom may be excessive incisional pain in the area of an auxiliary trocar. Palpation of a large unilateral paramedian mass on the abdominal wall or a significant decline in hematocrit suggests the diagnosis. An ultrasound of the abdominal wall is sometimes helpful. After diagnosis, the wound should be explored, the hematoma drained, and the artery or vein ligated proximal and distal to the laceration.[1] Unfortunately the site of bleeding may not always be identified, having clotted off by the time the exploration is performed. After the repair is complete, the patient should be admitted and observed overnight for signs or laboratory evidence of resumed bleeding.

Major Retroperitoneal Vessels

Injury to a major retroperitoneal vessel with massive hemorrhage is one of the most catastrophic complications of laparoscopy. The vessels generally involved are the aorta, vena cava, and right and left common iliac arteries and veins.[6] Every laparoscopist must be trained in the prevention, identification, and management of this complication.

The umbilicus is variably located, from directly over to 2 to 3 cm below the lower end of the aorta in the dorsosupine patient. The lower end of the aorta rotates upward in the Trendelenburg position, bringing the common iliac vessels and their branches closer to the horizontal plane. Furthermore, the umbilicus will be displaced upward, particularly in obese patients. As a result, the distance between the umbilicus and the aorta is reduced, and there is an increased risk of injury to retroperitoneal vessels if the laparoscopist fails to adjust for these positional changes.[1] To minimize the risk, the Veress needle and umbilical trocar should be directed toward the hollow of the sacrum, away from the sacral promontory, above which the aorta bifurcates.[1] The insertion of the auxiliary trocars should be directed downward, toward the fundus of the uterus, and not toward the sacrum or the side walls.

Although the majority of penetrating injuries to major retroperitoneal vessels occur during insertion of the Veress needle or laparoscopic trocar, the aorta can also be injured by the scalpel used to incise the intraumbilical or subumbilical region of the abdominal wall. The umbilical skin should always be elevated before a skin incision; deep incisions without adequate elevation or fixation of the skin can facilitate injury to deeper structures (Fig. 25.5). In very thin patients the anterior abdominal wall may be within 2 to 3 cm of the aorta, and in all patients, regardless of size or weight, the umbilicus itself is only several centimeters thick.[1]

Major retroperitoneal vessel injury caused by the Veress needle may be identified at the time it occurs by the aspiration test.[1] If diagnosis is made at this time, the Veress needle is left in place and laparotomy is performed through a midline inferior skin incision. After entering the abdomen, the aorta should be compressed. Leaving the Veress needle in place serves to obstruct the hemorrhage somewhat and to guide the vascular surgeon to the injured vessel. Because large retroperitoneal hematomas may conceal the site of injury, the Veress needle can help localize the injury. Care must be taken in performing the laparotomy not to move the Veress needle too much for fear of extending the vascular injury. If the Veress needle cannot remain relatively stationary as the result of operating conditions, it should be removed. The Veress needle is not necessary for localization of the injured area, and in–out injuries to both arteries and veins can become hemostatic through mechanisms of local spasm or tamponade of the injury.

If a laparoscopist should insert a Veress needle and hit the bony sacrum, the needle should be removed and laparoscopy quickly performed. An optical trocar (Visiport, US Surgical) allows for very rapid direct entry into the abdomen to assess the need for immediate laparotomy. Vascular injuries caused by the laparoscopic or auxiliary trocars are larger than those caused by the Veress needle, cause profuse hemorrhage, and usually result from im-

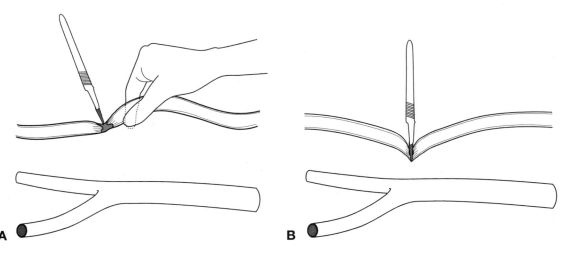

FIGURE 25.5.   Method for making initial skin incision at the umbilicus. **A:** The intraumbilical tissue should be elevated to minimize the risk of inadvertently damaging underlying structures such as bowel or major blood vessels (**B**).

proper technique. The auxiliary trocars usually produce common or external iliac vessel injury because the instrument deviates from the midline at the time of insertion; this contrasts with the uncontrolled thrust usually associated with primary trocar injuries.[1]

Immediate midline laparotomy should be performed whenever a vascular injury is strongly suspected.[1] On entering the abdomen, the laparoscopist should compress the aorta below the level of the renal arteries. This will reduce hemorrhage until the vascular surgeon arrives.[1] On occasion, the diagnosis is delayed because retroperitoneal bleeding has occurred instead of intraperitoneal bleeding. Cardiovascular collapse in the absence of overt intraabdominal hemorrhage may be caused by retroperitoneal bleeding or anesthetic complications. The retroperitoneal space should be immediately and thoroughly inspected for evidence of concealed hemorrhage. Because the venous system is under relatively low pressure, the intraabdominal pressure of insufflated CO_2 (usually 12–16 mmHg) may be sufficient to temporarily tamponade a puncture site even in large veins. This may allow time for natural hemostatic mechanisms to work. Nevertheless, gas should be suctioned out of the abdomen and inspection performed for bleeding while the abdomen slowly reinsufflates under low pressure.

Cardiovascular collapse in the recovery room following laparoscopy should be treated as retroperitoneal hemorrhage and hypovolemic shock unless proven otherwise.[1]

Mesosalpingeal and Meso-ovarian Bleeding

Mesosalpingeal and meso-ovarian hemorrhage is the most frequent vascular injury associated with operative laparoscopy. Injury to mesosalpingeal vessels usually results from dissection, laceration, or transection at the time of tubal surgery. These vessels may also be damaged by the Veress needle or various trocars.[1] Hemostasis can usually be obtained laparoscopically with bipolar electrocoagulation, microfibrillar collagen (Avitene), endocoagulation, endoclip application, silicone band ligature (Falope ring), or various intraabdominal sutures. However, these methods require that the site of bleeding be identified to be effective and may further damage the tube or

ovary. Although bleeding from the mesosalpingeal vasculature may initially seem profuse, the application of pressure to the bleeding site with an atraumatic grasper (e.g., Kleppinger bipolar paddles or adhesion grasper [Karl Storz Endoscopy—America, Inc., Culver City, CA]) for 3 to 5 min may suffice. The adnexa should be observed closely for hematoma formation, especially before removal of the laparoscope. An additional auxiliary puncture site frequently is useful to facilitate exposure and compression of the injury. The laparoscopist should avoid hemostatic techniques that might compromise ovarian circulation, and should certainly avoid the infundibulopelvic vessels. Laparotomy is seldom needed to secure hemostasis.[1,5]

Miscellaneous Vascular Injuries

A variety of vascular injuries may complicate operative laparoscopy. Perforation of omental vessels is usually diagnosed by visualizing the lacerated vessels. Broad ligament and mesosalpingeal vessels may be damaged by overly vigorous manipulation of the uterus or adnexa. Biopsy site hemorrhage can occur, regardless of the size of the specimen. Hemorrhage can occur during adhesiolysis, ovarian cystectomy, and uterosacral ligament ablation. Laparoscopic myomectomy sites may also bleed.[1,7]

The laparoscopist must make every effort to avoid hemorrhage. Vascular adhesions should be endocoagulated, electrocoagulated, or sutured before adhesiolysis.[7] Uterosacral ligament or posterior broad ligament bleeding must be handled carefully because of the proximity of the ureter.[1] Coagulation of most bleeding sites can be achieved laparoscopically.

Gastrointestinal Injuries

Clinically evident gastrointestinal tract injury is a serious complication, with an incidence of as many as 3 per 1000 operative procedures. However, the true incidence is believed to be higher because many small, self-limited injuries may go undiagnosed.[1]

Gastrointestinal injuries are caused by either lacerations or burns (electrocoagulation, laser).[1] Lacerating injuries can be produced at the time of insertion of the Veress needle, laparoscopic trocar, or auxiliary trocars. Previous abdominal surgery, bowel distension, inflammatory bowel disease, and unsuspected intraabdominal disease are risk factors.[1] However, more than half of gastrointestinal injuries occur in patients without risk factors.[20] Lacerating injuries are frequently diagnosed at the time of laparoscopy. In contrast, thermal injury is usually diagnosed postoperatively, after a seemingly uncomplicated laparoscopy.[1]

Stomach Injury

Gastric distension is the major risk factor for perforating injury to the stomach. Distension may occur before anesthesia as a result of aerophagia in an anxious patient. More often, however, gastric distension has occurred during preoxygenation before induction of anesthesia. The lower edge of the stomach may extend below the umbilicus in as many as 25% of horizontally positioned women.[1]

Gastric perforation by the Veress needle is suspected when gastric juice is obtained during the aspiration test. If the aspiration test is not performed and gas is insufflated, eructation or stomach borborygmi is very suspicious for intragastric location of the Veress needle. A nasogastric tube should be placed to decompress the stomach if gastric perforation is suspected. Removal and reinsertion of a new Veress needle is then performed. During laparoscopy, it is important to identify the site of gastric perforation and to assess the extent of damage and bleeding. If there is no bleeding, the gastric musculature will usually seal off the perforation spontaneously. A nasogastric tube is left in place; it facilitates healing by minimizing stomach distension and leakage of gastrointestinal fluid into the peritoneal cavity.[1]

A sharp trocar injury to the stomach is usually larger than that caused by the Veress needle. Injuries less than 5 mm in diameter may be managed conservatively, as they are no larger than those produced by a gastrostomy tube. Larger lacerations require laparotomy and primary closure.[1]

Small Bowel Injury

Perforation of the small intestine by the Veress needle can be recognized when greenish intestinal fluid is recovered during the aspiration test. Small intestinal fluid is almost sterile. Through-and-through perforations of the intestine may occur if the bowel is adherent to the anterior abdominal wall at the site of Veress needle insertion, or if the bowel is inadvertently grasped while elevating the abdominal wall (Fig. 25.6). These injuries may escape detection by the aspiration test. Perforations of the small intestine with the Veress needle usually heal spontaneously. The musculature of the bowel wall generally seals off the perforation and prevents intraperitoneal leakage of intestinal fluid.[1]

If intestinal fluid is obtained, the Veress needle should be removed; laparoscopy can be completed by insertion of a new needle at a different angle. Every effort should be made to identify the site of perforation. Although serious complications seldom follow a Veress needle perforation of the intestine, there may be a lacerated blood vessel in the bowel wall or mesentery. In this case, the degree of bleeding or hematoma formation is ascertained. Evidence of active bleeding or continued enlargement of a hematoma requires laparotomy to secure hemostasis. If bleeding is minimal or the hematoma is stable, hospitalization for observation is recommended. Even in the absence of vascular trauma, any patient who has sustained a small bowel perforation should be hospitalized for 24 to 48 hr of observation.[1]

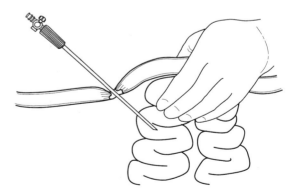

FIGURE 25.6. Care must be taken when manually elevating the abdominal wall to avoid grasping the intestines inadvertently, which can contribute to intestinal injury.

On occasion, gas will be insufflated into the lumen of the bowel because the aspiration step was not accurate.[1] Intraintestinal pressure may be similar to intraperitoneal opening pressure. Several liters of gas may be insufflated into the intestinal lumen without raising the insufflating pressure. The passage of gas from the rectum may signal intraluminal insufflation into the large bowel. This obviously increases the risk of subsequent trocar injury to the intestine.[1] Uncommonly, the Veress needle partially penetrates the intestinal wall. Serious complication seldom follows unless the abnormal location is not recognized and gas is insufflated, causing bullous distension of the intestinal wall. Insufflation pressure will rapidly rise in this event. Diagnosis of bullous distension requires hospitalization for observation because the intestinal wall occasionally ruptures. The gas is usually reabsorbed without sequelae.[1]

Injuries caused by sharp trocars may be more serious.[1] Superficial lacerations limited to the intestinal serosa do not need repair if the site is hemostatic; patients can be discharged without overnight hospitalization. Deeper lesions to the intestinal wall require careful evaluation. Lacerations that are narrower than the diameter of a Veress needle can be managed conservatively by observation, nothing by mouth, and prophylactic antibiotic coverage for anaerobes and enterobacteria. Larger lacerations of the intestinal wall or small lacerations that have spilled intestinal fluid into the peritoneal cavity require laparotomy for repair. Clean-edged lesions can be repaired in layers.[1,21] Ragged lacerations, or lacerated bowel that has been avulsed from the mesentery, require segmental bowel resection and reanastomosis.[1,21]

Gastrointestinal injuries during laparoscopic adhesiolysis may occur during blunt separation of bowel loops. This is more likely to occur in patients with endometriosis, pelvic inflammatory disease, or prior laparotomy. Sharp dissection is preferred over blunt dissection when adhesions are dense or tissue planes are obscured.[21]

Thermal injury usually results from the use of electrocautery devices, although lasers can produce similar injuries.[1,21-23] Thermal injuries are usually not recognized or suspected at the time of surgery. Unsuspected injury can occur by inadvertent direct contact of a monopolar electrode to the bowel, intraperitoneal transmission of sparks from an active monopolar electrode across to a nearby loop of bowel, or electrical discharge from an operative laparoscope through which a unipolar instrument has been placed (see Chapter 5). Alternatively, heat may be transmitted from the cauterized organ to a neighbor.[21] Thermal damage can also occur if the bowel wall is directly electrocoagulated to achieve hemostasis during adhesiolysis or to fulgurate endometriosis. Lasers such as the KTP (potassium-titanyl-phosphate) and Nd:YAG (neodymium:yttrium aluminum garnet) can produce thermal injury mimicking electrocautery lesions. Also, the heat from the endoscopic light can cause injury if the laparoscope is inadvertently allowed to rest on the bowel.

Patients with thermal bowel injuries may remain asymptomatic for as long as 3 days postoperatively.[1,21] Vague complaints of abdominal discomfort are replaced by early signs of peritonitis: nausea, vomiting, anorexia, fever, and abdominal pain. The time-course of symptoms cannot be used to reliably distinguish thermal from lacerating injuries.[22,23] Bowel lacerations usually become symptomatic within 12 to 48 hr, but sometimes the onset of symptoms is delayed for more than a week. In contrast, thermal injuries can become symptomatic before 48 hr postoperatively. Gross and microscopic analysis of the area of injury, however, reliably differentiates the cause of intestinal trauma. An intravenous pyelogram (IVP) should also be performed to diagnose a ureteral injury that may present similarly to bowel injuries. Microscopically, thermal injury demonstrates an area of coagulative necrosis, absence of capillary ingrowth and fibromuscular coat reconstruction, and absence of white blood cell infiltration except at the borders of the lesions.[22,23] Grossly, bipolar thermal injuries demonstrate blanched serosa and minimal necrosis, in contrast to unipolar thermal and lacerating injuries, which demonstrate large perforations and prominent exudate within 4 days of injury.[22,23]

The possibility of small bowel injury should be suspected when a patient complains of increasing abdominal pain or peritonitis symptoms after laparoscopy.[1,23] These patients should be readmitted for observation and conservative therapy including antibiotics. If the patient fails to respond within 24 hr, laparoscopy should be repeated or laparotomy performed to search for a perforation site.[1,23] If the area of thermal damage is superficial and 5 mm or less, expectant management is appropriate.[24] Larger or deeper thermal injuries are treated with wide resection and reanastomosis. The resection should extend 3 to 5 cm into healthy tissue on either side of the bowel injury because of the extensive, delayed coagulation necrosis and inflammatory reaction that occur after monopolar, bipolar, and laser injuries.[21]

Large Bowel Injuries

Traumatic injury of the large intestine during insertion of the Veress needle is a rare event but can be serious because of the bacterial growth present in large bowel contents. It may be recognized by the recovery of fecally stained fluid during the aspiration test. The Veress needle should be withdrawn and discarded and pneumoperitoneum established by using another Veress needle. The perforated area must be identified at the time of laparoscopy. Peritoneal fluid should be aspirated for bacterial culture.[1] Entry of even small amounts of fecal contamination into the peritoneal cavity is serious. Perforating colonic injuries are usually treated by layered primary closure, copious peritoneal lavage, and broad-spectrum antibiotic coverage.[1,21] Veress needle injuries may need minimal closure or full thickness depending on the length of the injury.

Injuries to the large bowel caused by a trocar are more serious than Veress needle injuries and require laparotomy. Small 1- to 2-cm lacerations may be treated by primary closure.[1,21] More significant trauma to the ascending colon is generally managed by resection of the lacerated segment of bowel. Primary anastomosis can be performed, but more commonly the anastomosis follows a period of fecal diversion by ileostomy.[1] Major injuries to the de-

scending colon, sigmoid colon, or rectum are usually treated by proximal diverting colostomy, resection of the injured segment of bowel, and delayed reanastomosis.[1,21] A proximal colostomy is generally indicated if the injury is large, the blood supply to the damaged bowel is compromised, the closure is under tension, or the bowel was inadequately prepared. Adjunctive measures involve copious peritoneal lavage, closed-suction drainage, nasogastric suction, and antibiotic coverage.[21]

Thermal injuries and lacerations to the colon can occur during difficult adhesiolysis or during attempts to secure hemostasis. Thermal injuries are generally diagnosed postoperatively in patients presenting with peritonitis. Primary closure of the defect is generally not recommended because the area of damage extends lateral to the visible trauma. Resection, proximal colostomy, and delayed reanastomosis are usually indicated.[21]

Small Bowel Incarceration

Incarceration of small bowel through a laparoscopic, usually the umbilical, incision is a very rare event, fewer than 1 occurrence per 5000 cases (Fig. 25.7).[25] Asymptomatic herniation or pinching of small bowel probably occurs equally infrequently. Nausea, vomiting, anorexia, and abdominal distension generally begin 3 to 7 days postoperatively, but onset of symptoms has been observed in the immediate postoperative period.[26] The umbilical region becomes indurated and tender. Abdominal x-rays demonstrate multiple air/fluid levels, dilated small bowel loops, and absence of air in the rectum. Laparotomy, resection of any nonviable intestinal segment, and primary anastomosis are the usual treatment. Expectant management in cases of symptomatic incarceration of intestine or omentum is inappropriate because spontaneous resolution seldom occurs. Delaying laparotomy increases the risk that the herniated bowel segment will be nonviable and will require resection.[1,26]

The majority of incisional hernias involve 10-mm or 12-mm umbilical or auxiliary trocar sites. A variety of preventive measures have been advised to avoid herniation: (1) use of smaller trocars whenever possible; (2) use of

FIGURE 25.7. Herniation of the small intestine at the site of the umbilical trocar may be prevented by withdrawing the laparoscope while observing closure of the peritoneum and suturing the fascia closed.

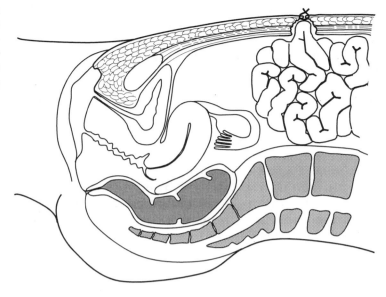

radially expanding sleeves if possible; (3) direct visualization during removal of auxiliary sleeves; (4) use of a Z-track method to introduce trocars (Fig. 25.8); (5) closure of the fascia at the trocar site; and (6) removal of the umbilical sleeve and the laparoscope together while visualizing closure of the peritoneum as they are withdrawn. Excess CO_2 should be suctioned out of the abdomen under direct visualization or be allowed to escape through open valves before removal of the umbilical sleeve and laparoscope, and excess abdominal pressure (including the patient's coughing or heaving) should be minimized during their removal.[1,25-27]

Postoperative Ileus

Adynamic ileus may occur after laparoscopic lysis of bowel adhesions. Abdominal distension, nausea, vomiting, and constipation typically occur within the first 48 hr after surgery. Pain, fever, and peritoneal signs are minimal. Bowel sounds will be minimal to absent. Flat plate and upright abdominal X-rays will show dilated small and large intestines, scattered air/fluid levels, and some residual gas from the pneumoperitoneum. Treatment is conservative. Na-

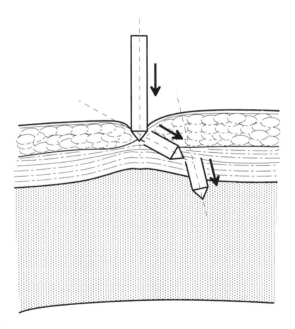

FIGURE 25.8. The Z-track technique for inserting a conical umbilical trocar (*arrows*). The skin is penetrated in a perpendicular manner, and the trocar is directed caudally to perforate muscle and fascia, then perpendicularly to pass through the peritoneum. When the trocar sleeve is withdrawn at the conclusion of the procedure, the defect closes to minimize the risk of intestinal herniation.

sogastric suction removes swallowed air, prevents further gastric distension, and relieves nausea. Intravenous fluids are administered until intestinal function spontaneously recovers.[21]

Open Laparoscopy

Open laparoscopy has been suggested as a useful technique to reduce the risk of intestinal injury. However, bowel injuries seem to occur with a similar frequency with both open and closed laparoscopy technique.[15,28] In spite of this, open laparoscopy or optical trocars should be considered for patients who are at increased risk for bowel injury.

Urinary Tract Injuries

The incidence of urinary tract injury during laparoscopy is approximately 1 to 2 per 1000 procedures.[3,4]

Bladder Injury

Injury to the urinary bladder is most likely when the bladder has not been catheterized before or during laparoscopy and in women with distorted anatomy (Fig. 25.9). Previous abdominal pelvic surgery may cause the bladder to be drawn upward, increasing the risk of bladder injury. However, the most common factor increasing the risk of bladder injury is a

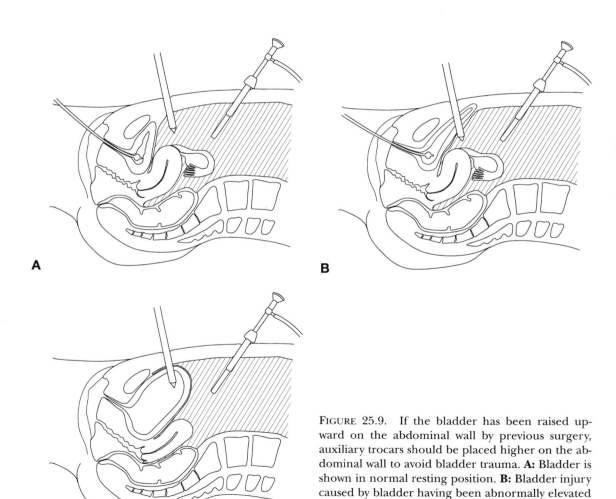

A

B

C

FIGURE 25.9.   If the bladder has been raised upward on the abdominal wall by previous surgery, auxiliary trocars should be placed higher on the abdominal wall to avoid bladder trauma. **A:** Bladder is shown in normal resting position. **B:** Bladder injury caused by bladder having been abnormally elevated on the abdominal wall. **C:** Injury caused by failure to catheterize the bladder.

distended bladder. As little as 100 ml of urine exposes the bladder to an increased risk of trauma.[1] Therefore, the bladder should be catheterized before all laparoscopies, and an indwelling catheter is recommended for every operative laparoscopy.[1]

The bladder can be damaged by the Veress needle, sharp trocars, or any auxiliary instrument used during laparoscopic surgery. Veress needle injuries usually occur because the bladder was not emptied before surgery or because of a misdirected needle insertion. Short patients, children, and young teenagers have smaller umbilicopubic distances, and small amounts of urine may raise the risk of bladder injury.[1] The aspiration test will usually yield urine if the bladder has been perforated. Insufflation of small amounts of gas will cause a rapid rise in insufflation pressure, suggesting that the needle is within a closed space, and gas may leak from the urethra. If the bladder has been perforated, the Veress needle is withdrawn and a new one inserted. The muscular bladder wall seals off this injury, facilitating spontaneous healing. Postoperative catheterization is maintained for 1 to 3 days. If gas has been insufflated into the bladder, it should be allowed to escape through the Veress needle before withdrawing the needle. If the needle has already been removed, catheterization will usually deflate the bladder.[1]

Trocar injuries to the bladder occur as frequently as Veress needle injuries; about 50% of trocar injuries are caused by the laparoscopic trocar and 50% by auxiliary trocars.[15] If the bladder has been raised and fixed by prior surgery, the site of trauma is usually at the site of attachment to the anterior abdominal wall (see Fig. 25.9). If an abnormal location of the bladder is suspected, auxiliary trocars should be placed higher on the abdominal wall. The bladder can also be filled retrograde with sterile saline to identify its upper boundary.[29] The trocars can be placed while directly visualizing the upper limits of the full bladder. Trocar trauma to the bladder can also result from an uncontrolled thrust.[1]

If the bladder has been filled retrograde, care must be taken not to injure it if the peritoneum tents over the trocar tip or a safety shield that snapped into place after the fascia was penetrated. Skim the trocar and sleeve along the anterior abdominal wall and into the laparoscopic sleeve (withdraw the laparoscope into the sleeve at this time); the peritoneum will usually retract as you do this. As with Veress needle injuries, a distended bladder is most at risk, but even a catheterized bladder can be injured if poor technique is used in placing the laparoscopic or auxiliary trocars because abnormal adherence of the bladder to the abdominal wall is not observed. When the bladder lumen has been entered by a trocar, the size of the laceration generally dictates therapy. Continuous postoperative drainage for 4 to 5 days is usually sufficient to allow 5-mm or smaller lacerations to heal. Larger lacerations will usually require primary closure in layers and transurethral or suprapubic drainage for 7 to 10 days.[1,29,30] Closure of the bladder may be performed laparoscopically.

The bladder can also be damaged during the course of laparoscopic surgery. Blunt trauma may occur if excessive force is used to try to mobilize the bladder or adhesions. Adhesions between the bladder and the anterior uterine wall should be dissected sharply.[1] Electrocoagulating instruments and lasers can damage the bladder, and days may elapse before the onset of symptoms.

Trocar and other injuries to the bladder may be seen or suspected during the course of the laparoscopic procedure. The urine output may become bloody or reduced, urine may be seen leaking into the pelvis, or the trocar may be seen traversing an area that is close to the bladder's location onto the anterior abdominal wall. If injury is suspected, the bladder can be filled retrograde with sterile milk or dilute methylene blue through the Foley catheter and observed for leakage. Alternately, 5 ml of IV indigo carmine or methylene blue may be injected and the bladder observed for leakage, or a cystoscopy performed to visualize a trocar traversing the bladder. If an injury is suspected but not confirmed by these methods, retrograde cystography can be performed. In general, small bladder injuries diagnosed during the course of laparoscopy heal with continuous Foley drainage, and large injuries diagnosed at the time are repaired by laparotomy.[1,29,30]

Bladder injuries that are overlooked at the time of surgery and electrosurgical or laser injuries to the bladder have several characteristic symptoms. Decreased urine output, bloody urine, suprapubic pain, and fullness all suggest bladder injury; blood urea nitrogen may be markedly elevated because of reabsorption of urine from the peritoneal cavity. The usual symptoms are the inability to void spontaneously and failure to obtain urine by catheterization. The bladder perforation may allow urine to extravasate into the peritoneal cavity or into the space of Retzius, where large amounts of urine can accumulate asymptomatically. Suprapubic pain will eventually occur with extraperitoneal accumulations.[1] Retrograde cystograms confirm the diagnosis by visualizing the extravasation of contrast material. Transabdominal repair will usually be necessary for those injuries caused by laser or electrocoagulation instruments and for most large trocar injuries diagnosed postoperatively. Smaller injuries may heal with prolonged catheter drainage.[1,29,30]

Urachal Cysts and Vesicourethral Diverticula

Urachal cysts and vesicourethral diverticula may be perforated during laparoscopy with resultant hematoma formation, leakage of urine from incisions, or intraperitoneal spillage of urine. A voiding cystourethrogram or IVP are usually diagnostic. Prolonged catheterization of the bladder may facilitate spontaneous healing of small punctures. Larger lacerations may require surgical resection of the urachal defect.[1,31]

Ureteral Injury

The ureter is less commonly injured than the bladder.[1] Ureteral injury usually manifests symptoms within 5 days of surgery, but these may be delayed for 2 to 3 weeks. Presenting symptoms usually include fever, peritonitis, pelvic mass, hematuria, and leukocytosis.[32,33] The ureter is most commonly injured 2 to 3 cm from the ureterovesical junction or at the pelvic brim. It is particularly susceptible to injury

when cautery is used in the area of the uterosacral ligaments to control bleeding or fulgurate endometriosis, and when endoscopic linear staplers are used in the vicinity of the ureter.[34] Ureteral damage localized to the pelvic brim is usually associated with laparoscopic sterilization procedures.[32] The technique of displacing the uterus to put the adnexa under tension stretches the infundibulopelvic ligament and displaces the ureter medially, closer to the site of cautery. In these instances, the cautery forceps probably inadvertently touches the pelvic side wall. The ureter is also susceptible to injury in difficult endometriosis cases, particularly those in which the ovary is adherent to the lateral pelvic side wall.[32]

Several methods to protect the ureter from injury have been described.[33] Hydrodissection has been recommended to displace the ureter laterally, but this is unlikely to afford significant protection as it often remains firmly attached to the medial leaf of the peritoneum. Adding indigo carmine to the 150 to 200 ml of fluid infused for hydrodissection, however, helps to outline the course of the ureter at the point before it enters the cardinal ligament.[33] The ureter may be mobilized laterally by sharp dissection through a peritoneal incision.[35] Adhesions and inflammation may make this type of dissection difficult, if not impossible. The surgeon considering placing ureteral stents cystoscopically before an operative laparoscopy procedure is likely to encounter conditions distorting the course of the ureter or the ability of the laparoscopist to follow its course. A clear understanding of the course of the ureter within the pelvis is essential for the safe use of electrocautery or laser.[32,33]

Ureteral injury is usually diagnosed by an IVP. However, a repeat laparoscopy may be used to diagnose the injury. Because symptoms overlap with those of bowel injury, an IVP should be performed to exclude ureteral injury when a bowel injury is suspected.[32] Ureteral injuries will be treated surgically depending on the location and extent of injury. Uretero–ureteral reanastomosis, ureteroneocystostomy, and transverse ureteroureterostomy are usually required; however, placement of a ureteral stent may suffice in some situations.[32,33]

Infectious Complications

Laparoscopy is considered a clean-contaminated operation. Although breaks in aseptic technique are unavoidable during operative laparoscopy, infectious morbidity is rare and may range from mild superficial incisional infection to life-threatening peritonitis.[1]

Wound infections occur in 0.8% to 1.3% of cases. Mild infections develop within 48 to 72 hr after the procedure. Erythema occurs early and may be replaced by suppuration. Sutures should be removed and the wound cleaned. Antibiotic coverage for *Staphylococcus aureus* and hemolytic streptococcus should be initiated and the wound allowed to heal by secondary intention.[1]

Flare-up of clinically silent or chronic salpingitis may lead to pelvic inflammatory disease and peritonitis. Pelvic infection, however, rarely occurs as a result of laparoscopy unless inadvertent gastrointestinal injury has occurred.[1] Transcervical chromotubation may carry vaginal organisms into the peritoneal cavity; however, the level of contamination is low.[36] Dye should not be injected transcervically if active pelvic infection is present or suspected. If tubal patency needs to be assessed in patient with apparent chronic salpingitis, antibiotic prophylaxis should be administered.[36]

Neurologic Complications

Nerve injury complicated 0.5 per 1000 operative laparoscopies in two consecutive AAGL membership surveys.[4,5] Brachial palsy has been observed in patients maintained in a steep Trendelenburg position for an extended period of time, and use of shoulder braces appears to increase this risk. Ample padding, abducting the patient's arms to her side, and minimizing the duration of the procedure may reduce the risk of a brachial plexus injury. Hyperextension of the arm must be avoided, and the surgeon and assistant should not lean on the extended arm.[1]

Sciatic or peroneal nerve injury may occur because the patient is in the lithotomy or semilithotomy position. Sciatic nerve injury has occurred after as little as 35 min in the semilitho-

tomy position. Stretching of the nerve presumably causes the injury.[1] Sciatic nerve injury sustained during laparoscopy is usually self-limited. Motor and sensory deficits usually appear immediately after surgery, progress for several weeks, and resolve over the following 3 to 9 months.[1] Peroneal nerve injury results in classic footdrop. Suggestions to prevent sciatic/peroneal nerve injury include (1) the use of knee- and foot-supporting stirrups; (2) raising and lowering both legs simultaneously to place them in stirrups while carefully extending the hip and knee joints; (3) flexing the knees before flexing the hips; (4) limiting external hip rotation; and (5) avoiding undue pressure on the inner aspect of the thigh.[1]

Nerve stretch is the most common type of injury associated with laparoscopy. Problems occasionally seen that can also cause postoperative neurologic symptoms include herniated disc, multiple sclerosis, strokes, and hysterical paralysis.

Summary

Complications are an inevitable part of a surgeon's career. Therefore, every gynecologist must be familiar with laparoscopic complications. Refining personal operative technique is critically important,[37] and knowing your limits is equally important to minimizing complications. Many complications are caused by momentary attention lapses; some are inevitable, and some are the result of poor judgment. Although our goal is to prevent and avoid complications, we must be ready to recognize them when they occur and be prepared to treat them as well.

References

1. Borten M. *Laparoscopic Complications: Prevention and Management.* Philadelphia: BC Decker; 1980.
2. Corfman RS, Diamond MP, DeCherney A, eds. *Complications of Laparoscopy and Hysteroscopy.* Cambridge: Blackwell Scientific; 1993.
3. Hulka JF, Soderstrom RM, Corson SL, et al. Complications Committee of the American Association of Gynecological Laparoscopists: first annual report. *J Reprod Med.* 1975;10:301–306.

4. Peterson HB, Hulka JF, Phillips JM. American Association of Gynecologic Laparoscopists' 1988 membership survey on operative laparoscopy. *J Reprod Med.* 1990;35:590–591.

5. Hulka JF, Peterson HB, Phillips JM, Surrey MW. Operative laparoscopy—American Association of Gynecologic Laparoscopists 1991 membership survey. *J Reprod Med.* 1993;38:569–571.

6. Ohlgisser M, Sorokin Y, Heifetz, M. Gynecologic laparoscopy: a review article. *Obstet Gynecol Surv.* 1985;40:385–396.

7. Semm K. *Operative Manual for Endoscopic Abdominal Surgery.* Chicago: Year Book Medical Publishers; 1987.

8. Erickson LD. Insufflation needle insertion techniques: management of perforation of bowel and bladder. In: Corfman RS, Diamond MP, DeCherney A, eds. *Complications of Laparoscopy and Hysteroscopy.* Cambridge: Blackwell Scientific Publications; 1993:22–29.

9. Nordestgaard AG, Bodily KC, Osborne RW, Buttorff JD. Major vascular injuries during laparoscopic procedures. *Am J Surg.* 1995;169:543–545.

10. Poindexter AN, Ritter M, Fahim A, et al. Trocar introduction performed during laparoscopy of the obese patient. *Surg Gynecol Obstet.* 1987;165:57–59.

11. Kaali SG, Bartfai G. Direct insertion of the laparoscopic trocar after an earlier laparotomy. *J Reprod Med.* 1988;33:739–740.

12. Byron JW, Fujiyoshi CA, Miyazawa K. Evaluation of the direct trocar insertion technique at laparoscopy. *Obstet Gynecol.* 1989;74:423–425.

13. Mlyncek M, Truska A, Garay J. Laparoscopy without use of the veress needle: results in a series of 1,600 procedures. *Mayo Clin Proc.* 1994; 69:1146–1148.

14. Holtz G. Insufflation of the obese patient. In: Corfman RS, Diamond MP, DeCherney A, eds. *Complications of Laparoscopy and Hysteroscopy.* Cambridge: Blackwell Scientific Publications; 1993:42–45.

15. Yuzpe AA. Pneumoperitoneum needle and trocar injuries in laparoscopy: a survey on possible contributing factors and prevention. *J Reprod Med.* 1990;35:485–490.

16. Corson SL, Batzer FR, Gocial B, et al. Measurement of the force necessary for laparoscopic trocar entry. *J Reprod Med.* 1989;34:282–284.

17. Mintz M. Risks and prophylaxis in laparoscopy: a survey of 100,000 cases. *J Reprod Med.* 1977; 18:269–272.

18. Pring DW. Inferior epigastric hemorrhage, an avoidable complication of laparoscopic clip sterilization. *Br J Obstet Gynecol.* 1983;90: 480–482.

19. Johns DA. Perforation of the inferior epigastric vessels. In: Corfman RS, Diamond MP, DeCherney A, eds. *Complications of Laparoscopy and Hysteroscopy.* Cambridge: Blackwell Scientific Publications; 1993:38–41.

20. Kaali SG, Barad DH. Incidence of bowel injury due to dense adhesions at the site of direct trocar insertion. *J Reprod Med.* 1992;37:617–618.

21. Alvarez RD. Gastrointestinal complications in gynecologic surgery: a review for the general gynecologist. *Obstet Gynecol.* 1988;72:533–540.

22. Levy BS, Soderstrom RM, Dail DH. Bowel injuries during laparoscopy: gross anatomy and histology. *J Reprod Med.* 1985;30:168–172.

23. Soderstrom RM, Levy BS. Bowel injuries during laparoscopy: causes and medicolegal questions. *Contemp Obstet Gynecol.* 1986;31:41–45.

24. Thompson BH, Wheeless CR. Gastrointestinal complications of laparoscopy sterilization. *Obstet Gynecol.* 1973;41:669–676.

25. Montz FJ, Holschneider CH, Munro MG. Incisional hernia following laparoscopy: a survey of the American Association of Gynecologic Laparoscopists. *Obstet Gynecol.* 1994;84:881–884.

26. Thomas AG, McLymont F, Moshipur J. Incarcerated hernia after laparoscopic sterilization: a case report. *J Reprod Med.* 1990;35:639–640.

27. Kadar N, Reich H, Liu CY, Manko GF, Gimpelson R. Incisional hernias after major laparoscopic gynecologic procedures. *Am J Obstet Gynecol.* 1993;168:1493–1495.

28. Brill AI, Nezhat F, Nezhat CH, Nezhat C. The incidence of adhesions after prior laparotomy: a laparoscopic appraisal. *Obstet Gynecol.* 1995; 85:269–272.

29. Martin DC. Trocar injuries to the bladder. In: Corfman RS, Diamond MP, DeCherney A, eds. *Complications of Laparoscopy and Hysteroscopy.* Cambridge: Blackwell Scientific Publications; 1993:56–59.

30. Schiff SF. Bladder injuries during laparoscopic surgery. In: Corfman RS, Diamond MP, DeCherney A, eds. *Complications of Laparoscopy and Hysteroscopy.* Cambridge: Blackwell Scientific Publications; 1993:78–80.

31. McLucas B, March C. Urachal sinus perforation during laparoscopy: a case report. *J Reprod Med.* 1990;35:573–574.

32. Grainger DA, Soderstrom RM, Schiff SF, et al. Ureteral injuries at laparoscopy: insights into

diagnosis, management, and prevention. *Obstet Gynecol.* 1990;75:839–843.

33. Grainger DA. Ureteral damage associated with transection of the uterosacral ligaments. In: Corfman RS, Diamond MP, DeCherney A, eds. *Complications of Laparoscopy and Hysteroscopy.* Cambridge: Blackwell Scientific Publications; 1993:87–90.

34. Woodland MB. Ureteral injury during laparoscopy-assisted vaginal hysterectomy with the endoscopic linear stapler. *Am J Obstet Gynecol.* 1992;167:756–757.

35. Kadar N. Dissecting the pelvic retroperitoneum and identifying the ureters: a laparoscopic technique. *J Reprod Med.* 1995;40:116–122.

36. Pyper RJD, Ahmet Z, Houang ET. Bacteriological contamination during laparoscopy with dye injection. *Br J Obstet Gynaecol.* 1988;95:367–371.

37. See WA, Cooper CS, Fisher RJ. Predictors of laparoscopic complications after formal training in laparoscopic surgery. *JAMA.* 1993;270:2689–2692.

Part III
Operative Hysteroscopic Procedures

26

General Techniques and Instrumentation of Operative Hysteroscopy

Yolanda R. Smith, Denise Murray, and Howard A. Zacur

Hysteroscopy is a term derived from the Greek words to view (skopeo) and uterus (hystera). As a procedure it was first successfully performed in a living human subject in 1869 by Pantaleoni, who used a tube with an external light source to detect "vegetations within the uterine cavity."[1] No attempt was made by Pantaleoni at that time to distend the uterine cavity during this procedure. Over the past 100 years developments in optics, fiberoptics, instruments, and distending media have resulted in equipment and techniques that now allow us to diagnose and treat intrauterine disorders using hysteroscopy. The purpose of this chapter is to review these instruments and their accessories, as well as the distending media, lighting, indications, contraindications, and preoperative preparation for this procedure.

Instruments

In general, hysteroscopes may be classified as rigid or flexible; designed for diagnostic or operative use; and possessing fixed or variable focusing. Key specifications of the hysteroscope are its scope diameter, lens offset, sheath diameter, and ability to be used with a variety of distending media.

Rigid Hysteroscopes

Rigid hysteroscopes, currently the most commonly used, are usually preferred for operative procedures as they contain one or more channels within the sheath through which to pass instruments. The hysteroscope is composed of an endoscope that is usually enclosed in a

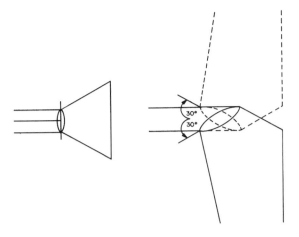

FIGURE 26.1.   *Left:* A 60° field of view lens centered at 0° to axis of scope (i.e., 0° viewing angle). *Right:* A 60° field of view when viewing angle is 30° (*solid line*). When the endoscope is rotated 180° (*dashed line*), the potential field of view is much greater than that of the 0° telescope. (Prescott R. Optical principles of endoscopy. *J Med Primatol.* 1976;5:133–147 and S. Karger, AG Publishers, Basel.)

metal tube or "sheath" through which distending media or instruments may pass. Sheath diameters may be as small as 3.3 mm (10 Fr.) for diagnostic use or as large as 8 mm (24 Fr.) for operative use. Recent improvements in hysteroscopic equipment include the development of sheaths that can convert any hysteroscope (including diagnostic) into a continuous flow system.

Optics of Rigid Hysteroscopes

The lens system employed in rigid endoscopes may be divided into three types: classical, Hopkins, and graded index lens system (GRIN)[2] (see Fig. 4.3). In the classical system, the width of the lenses is far less than the length of the telescope and the distance between lenses is relatively large. Using the Hopkins rod system, the lenses are large in diameter and the separation between lenses is small; in fact, most of the telescope is occupied by lenses. In the graded lens system (GRIN), the entire telescope is occupied by a slender rod of glass (see Chapter 4).

The image through the hysteroscope is affected by the degree of field of view allowed by

the outer lens of the hysteroscope, as well as by the angle of this lens to the central axis of the telescope. Most hysteroscopes possess an outer lens that will provide a 60° to 90° field of view, depending on the distending medium. This view will be wider in gaseous than aqueous media because the refractive index is better. The outer lens of the hysteroscope may be centered along the axis of the endoscope so that a 360° rotation of the telescope will not result in a change in view. This is called a 0° scope (Fig. 26.1). Alternatively, the lens may be offset (fore-oblique) by 25° to 30° to the axis of the telescope. When the telescope is rotated 360°, an expanded field of view is seen (Fig. 26.1).

Last, the lens system may focus only when the telescope is in contact with the object to be viewed (e.g., contact hysteroscope), or it may provide a magnified or reduced image of the object to be viewed depending on whether the endoscope is brought closer to or taken further away from the object to be viewed. Under these latter conditions, the hysteroscope view is described as "panoramic."

Operative Hysteroscopes

Two operative hysteroscopic setups are generally available. One relies on operative sheaths through which the diagnostic hysteroscope (generally 4 mm in diameter) is placed; the other consists of a hysteroscope constructed with an offset eyepiece and a straight operating channel. The first type of hysteroscopic setup usually uses hysteroscopes with a 30° angle of view and a 3- to 4-mm-diameter lens system.

There are several types of operative sheaths. The first has a single channel designed for the insertion of flexible 7-Fr. instruments (Figs. 26.2 and 26.3). The disadvantage of this setup is the relatively small size of the instrument jaws and the loss of cutting power from the flexibility of the scissor shaft. Another type of operative sheath consists of a fixed rigid instrument tip (i.e., scissors, biopsy forceps, or foreign-body forceps) attached to the dorsal aspect of the distal end of the sleeve, such that the instrument tip is in full endoscopic view. The disadvantage of this instrumentation is that the sheath must be changed to vary the tips used, which requires that the entire hyster-

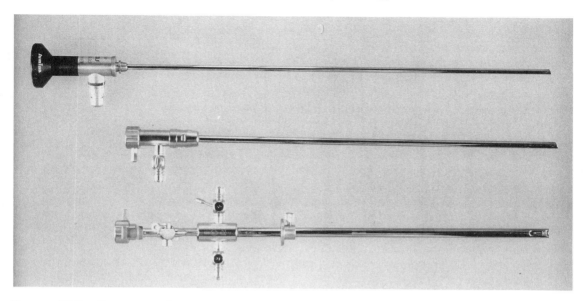

FIGURE 26.2.   From *top* to *bottom:* 25° hysteroscope, 4 mm in diameter; 7-mm diagnostic sheath; and 7-mm operative sheath for the placement of flexible 7-Fr. instruments (Richard Wolf Medical Instruments Corp. Rosemont, IL).

oscope be removed. Furthermore, because the tip is fixed to the sheath which in turn is fixed to the hysteroscope, the entire endoscopic unit must be moved when the instrument tip needs to be advanced or withdrawn, reducing the viewing field or illumination.

Finally, a resectoscope (Fig. 26.4) may be used. This instrument consists of an endoscope

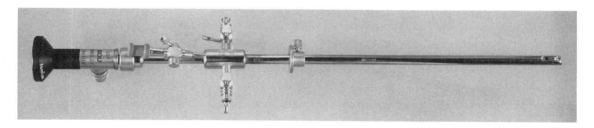

FIGURE 26.3.   Hysteroscope within operative sheath for flexible instruments.

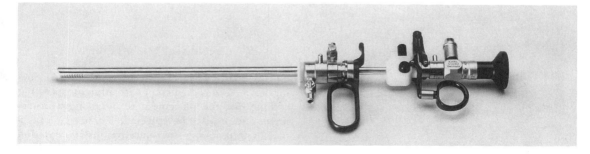

FIGURE 26.4.   Resectoscope assembled (courtesy of Karl Storz Endoscopy, Culver City, CA).

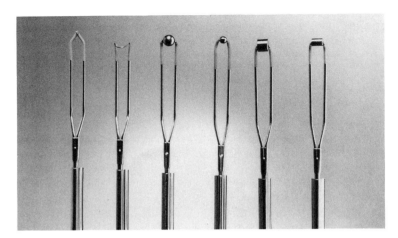

FIGURE 26.5. Various roller ball and wire loop instruments (courtesy of Karl Storz Endoscopy, Culver City, CA).

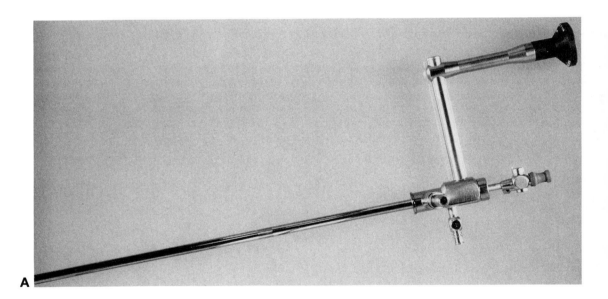

A

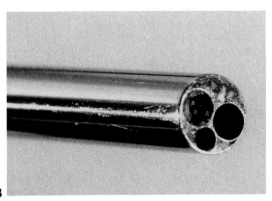

B

FIGURE 26.6. **A:** Operative hysteroscope (0° viewing angle, 7-mm diameter) with straight operating channel for the placement of 3-mm rigid instruments and displaced eyepiece. **B:** Tip of rigid operative hysteroscope with operative instrumentation (*larger*) and insufflation (*smaller*) ports. (Richard Wolf Medical Instruments Corp., Rosemont, IL.)

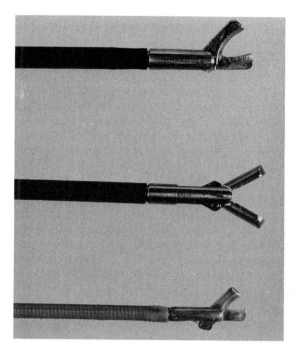

FIGURE 26.7. Close-up of jaws of 3-mm rigid scissors (*top*) and biopsy forceps (*middle*), and 7-Fr. (2.1-mm) flexible scissors (*bottom*). Note the much larger jaws of the 3-mm scissors. (Richard Wolf Medical Instruments Corp., Rosemont, IL.)

placed through an operative sheath that allows for the continuous circulation of nonviscous media to distend the uterine cavity, while also permitting the placement of a wire loop or roller ball accessory (Fig. 26.5).

The operating right-angle hysteroscope has a single operative channel through which 3-mm instruments can be placed (Fig. 26.6). Because the lens system has only a 10° angle of view, it may be somewhat more difficult to visualize the tubal ostia. Furthermore, the diameter of the lens is smaller, resulting in less light transmission and a smaller image. However, the instruments are significantly larger and stronger than the flexible ones previously described (Fig. 26.7).

Contact Hysteroscopes

Contact hysteroscopes rely on GRIN lens for their optics and do not require either a distending medium or fiberoptic light for illumination and visualization. These endoscopes require a light-collecting chamber located near the eyepiece that will transmit light down the endoscope glass guide toward the object of interest. To be viewed, the endoscope must either be touching or almost touching the surface of interest. Light is transmitted down the glass guide of the endoscope toward the surface, which will reflect the light back toward the eyepiece of the endoscope. Because of the rigid glass guide, there is no distortion from transmitted images, and these may be magnified 1.6 times without the need for special lenses. Greater magnification, to 100×, is possible depending on the eyepiece used.

Contact hysteroscopes are sometimes used for colpohysteroscopy to evaluate cervical atypia. Major advantages to the contact hysteroscope include no need for a special light source, excellent visualization even in the presence of bleeding, and no need for use of a distending medium. Major disadvantages of the contact hysteroscope include lack of a panoramic view, which increases the chance that a lesion may be missed, and inability to operate through the scope (e.g., take a directed biopsy).

Flexible Hysteroscopes

Flexible endoscopic equipment had previously been used only for the diagnosis of gastrointestinal disorders. Flexible hysteroscopes of extremely small diameters have recently been introduced with outer tip diameters of only 2.5 mm, making these instruments potentially ideal for office diagnostic procedures. These scopes may be used for diagnostic or operative indications and do not require an outer "sheath" (Fig. 26.8).

Drawbacks to the use of flexible hysteroscopes include the fact that only a gaseous distending medium is recommended and that resolution is reduced because fiberoptics are employed both for visualization and for lighting. The ground substance (adhesive) between the glass fibers results in a grainier image.

The Distending Media

Hysteroscopic visualization of the uterine cavity without a contact hysteroscope will require a means of expanding the uterine cavity for

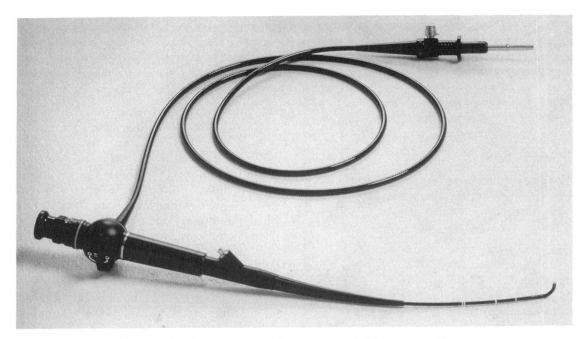

FIGURE 26.8.   Flexible operating hysteroscope (Olympus Corp., Lake Success, NY).

panoramic viewing with rigid or flexible hysteroscopes. Lack of suitable distending medium delayed the early development of the hysteroscope. One explanation for the failure to use distending media earlier were the beliefs by investigators at the time that the medium could either contaminate the uterine environment with vaginal pathogens or that the uterus as a muscular organ would not be distendable by the medium.

It was not until 1925, when Dr. I.C. Rubin used CO_2 gas to distend the uterine cavity for hysteroscopic viewing, that the successful use of a distending medium was reported.[3] In his early studies Dr. Rubin found that the procedure produced the best results when performed during the early follicular phase of the menstrual cycle. Traumatic bleeding during the procedure was further minimized by coating the hysteroscope sheath with epinephrine. Despite Dr. Rubin's early success with this method, bleeding still obscured vision, preventing others from easily using this procedure until the technique was improved in the 1960s. In 1949 Norment used an air-filled transparent balloon attached to the tip of the hysteroscope to distend

the cavity.[4] Visibility was limited, however. Silander in 1963 modified this approach by using saline instead of air to fill the balloon. Improved visibility was reported, but the field of view was limited and abnormal structures such as small polyps were not recognized because of compression by the balloon.[5] Distending media for hysteroscopy may be divided into three general classes: (1) liquid, nonviscous; (2) liquid, viscous; and (3) gaseous.

Liquid Nonviscous Media

Liquid medium (water or saline) for uterine distension was initially proposed by Heineberg in 1914, who used a water irrigation system to clean the hysteroscope of blood and mucus as well as distend the uterine cavity.[6] Water irrigation systems were later used to rinse the hysteroscope lens, but bleeding still obscured the view.

To allay fears that fluids passing into the uterine cavity could be passed in turn into the abdominal pelvic cavity, Schroeder in 1934 measured intrauterine pressures to determine the conditions under which fluid would pass from the uterus into the abdomen.[7] He found that intrauterine pressures exceeding 55 mmHg allowed liquid to pass into the fallopian tubes. He also noted that suspending a reservoir containing the fluid for uterine distension 650 mm above the patient resulted in an intrauterine pressure of 25 to 30 mmHg, and placement at 950 mm above the patient resulted in an intrauterine pressure of 35 mmHg. Under these conditions, fluid would remain within the uterine cavity.

Although water or saline were the first nonviscous liquids used as a distending media for hysteroscopy, other fluids were and are being tried. In 1970 use of a 5% dextrose solution was proposed; however, large volumes of fluid were required and visualization was difficult in the presence of bleeding. More recently, use of Ringer's lactate, 1.5% glycine, or 3.3% sorbitol solutions have become popular as alternative media for uterine distension. These solutions are frequently used as irrigants for urological procedures, for example, at transurethral prostatectomy.

Glycine is an amino acid that is mixed with water as a 1.5% solution for hysteroscopic use. The glycine solution is electrolyte free and can therefore be used in procedures requiring electrosurgery. It is hypoosmolar (200 mOsm/liter) and can cause hypoosmolar hyponatremia if significant intravascular absorption occurs.[8] In addition, glycine is metabolized to ammonia and may result in encephalopathic symptoms and changes in visual acuity.[9]

Solutions of sorbitol, or sorbitol and mannitol (2.7% sorbitol and 0.54% mannitol; Sorbitol-Mannitol Irrigation, Abbott Laboratories, Abbott Park, IL), are also used for hysteroscopic procedures. Sorbitol and mannitol are hexitol ($C_6H_{14}O_6$) isomers and are nonelectrolytes. These solutions are also slightly hypotonic, and the addition of mannitol provides an osmotic diuresis. Sorbitol is metabolized to fructose and glucose, while mannitol is inert.[8]

Advantages of the liquid nonviscous distending media include their availability, low cost, and ease of use. Unfortunately, crystalloid solutions are miscible with blood and extensive flushing is required to provide a clear field of view. When use of electrosurgical instruments is anticipated, normal saline should *not* be used because of its conductive nature.

Liquid Viscous Media

In 1968, Menken utilized a viscous material, polyvinylpyrrolidone, to distend the uterine cavity.[10] Although it was inert and nonconductive, it was yellowish in color and not biogradable, attributes that limited its usefulness. In 1970, Edstrom and Fernstrom described the use of 32% dextran-70 in 10% dextrose in water as a distending medium for hysteroscopy.[11] This solution was quite viscous, but it was clear and allowed the hysteroscope to be used for diagnostic as well as therapeutic use.

Dextran is a polysaccharide first isolated from beet sugar, where it is formed by the action of the bacteria *Leuconostoc mesenteroides*. Hundreds of glucose molecules make up the polysaccharide molecule, and these molecules are bound together through 1:6 and 1:4 glucosidic linkages. Two forms of dextran exist, one of 70,000 and the other of 40,000 kilodaltons (kDa). Hyskon®, which is currently available and approved for hysteroscopic use, is a 32% solution of the 70,000-kDa form in 10% glucose. This fluid is clear, sterile, electrolyte free and nonconductive, and not easily miscible with blood. Instruments must be thoroughly cleaned to prevent crystallization of this viscous material, which will occlude channels and valves.

Gaseous Media

Renewed interest in use of CO_2 for hysteroscopy followed the work of Lindemann in 1971, who designed special equipment for its administration.[12] The problem of gas leakage from the cervix was solved by using a metal doughnut bell that fit snugly around and into the cervix by means of suction induced by a small vacuum pump. The hysteroscope could then be passed through a rubber O-ring placed in the center of the bell (Fig. 26.9). A distinctive risk of using gaseous agents as distending media is gas embolism. This risk was almost completely eliminated by the development of an insufflating apparatus designed to limit gas

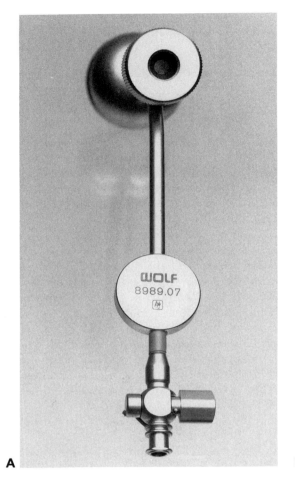

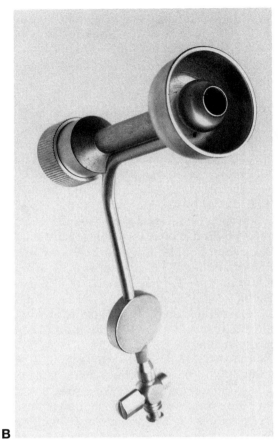

A   **B**

FIGURE 26.9.   A 7-mm operative portio adapter. **A:** Portion that faces the hysteroscope. **B:** The side of the portio adapter that faces the cervix. (Richard Wolf Medical Instruments Corp., Rosemont, IL.)

flow to no more than 100 ml CO_2 per minute while keeping the intrauterine pressure at values less than 200 mmHg. These limits were identified by Lindemann from earlier animal and human studies when the electrocardiogram, $PaCO_2$, and blood pH were monitored.[13]

Use of other gaseous agents to perform hysteroscopy is limited by the risk of embolism. For example, use of nitrous oxide (N_2O) as a distending medium was reported by Hulf et al. in 1979.[14] In this study N_2O was compared to CO_2, and a rise in $PaCO_2$ was seen only when N_2O was used. This rise was believed to result from the "dead space" induced by N_2O molecules as a result of their inability to solubilize in blood. Gas media that do not solubilize well in blood thus increase the risk for embolism. Fortunately, CO_2 does solubilize well in blood.

Administration of CO_2 during hysteroscopy should only be provided by insufflators designed specifically for this purpose. For example, laparoscopy insufflators result in CO_2 flow rates 10 to 20 times greater (1–2 liters per minute) than hysteroscopic insufflators (0.1 liter per minute). Increased flow rates also increase the risk of gas embolism as the increased gas volume will be more difficult to solubilize.

Bleeding and bubbling, which reduce visualization, still limit the effectiveness of CO_2 as a distending medium. However, CO_2 is easy to use and it is clean. It also has a refractive index of 1.0, allowing it to present a nonmagnified and wider field of view to the operator than either Hyskon® (with a refractive index of 1.39) or saline (refractive index, 1.37). Other advantages include its ready availability, rapid absorption, and relative safety.

Choice and Administration of Liquid Distending Media

All types of distending media may be utilized for diagnostic hysteroscopy and hysteroscopic biopsies, lysis of adhesions, or resections. However, accumulation of blood may make visualization difficult when CO_2 or liquid nonviscous

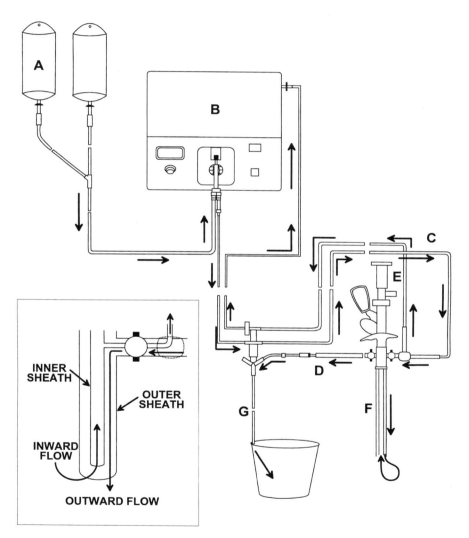

FIGURE 26.10. Continuous flow hysteroscopy system. The reservoir of intravenous solutions (A) is connected with a Y-tubing to the pump (B). The inflow tubing (C) is connected to the hysteroscope sheath. The pressure tubing (E) is connected to an outer sheath. The outflow tubing (D) is connected to an inner hysteroscope sheath. The outflow tubing and relief valve tubing (G) are connected to the fluid-collection system (see *inset*). (Redrawn with permission from Shirk GJ, Gimpelson RJ. Control of intrauterine fluid pressure during operative hysteroscopy. *J Am Assoc Gynecol Laparosc.* 1994;1: 229–233.)

media are used. Procedures using electro-surgery usually require liquid viscous nonconductive media. If lasers are used, nonviscous media are preferred because the laser may carmelize the viscous dextran medium.

Early methods of administering low-viscosity solutions such as water or saline into the uterine cavity relied primarily on raising a fluid-filled reservoir to a predetermined height above the patient to create a specific intrauterine pressure. This technique remains in effect today but has been modified by use of a blood pressure cuff. In brief, uterine distending solutions made available in soft plastic bags (e.g., 5% dextrose in water solution) are elevated above the patient and enwrapped by a blood pressure cuff inflated to produce 150 mmHg pressure. This technique will allow flow of distending medium at rates suitable for performing hysteroscopy. More recently, fluid pumps designed especially for hysteroscopic use have become commercially available (e.g., Continuous Flow Resectosurge Pump, ACMI, Stanford, CT; or the Controlled Distention Irrigation System, Zimmer, Dover, OH). Continuous-flow pumps allow the operator to set the intrauterine pressure between 0 and 80 mmHg. A closed-feedback loop constantly monitors the cavity pressure and automatically regulates the flow to maintain the set target pressure (Fig. 26.10).[15]

High-viscosity solutions (e.g., dextran-70) are generally administered by manual injection through a 50-cc syringe connected by intravenous tubing to the hysteroscope. This technique has led to great variations in intrauterine pressure and volume of dextran used. Most often manual injection results in greater amounts of media being used than is necessary. Use of a Harvard infusion pump to compress the syringe plunger was described by Lavy et al. to provide additional control over the administration of the dextran.[16] This apparatus was then modified to allow the pump motor to disengage when infusion pressures exceed 150 to 175 cmH_2O (approximately 110–130 mmHg). More recently, the pump has been further modified and made available commercially (e.g., DeCherney Pump, Cabot Medical Corp., Longhorne, PA). Instead of a motor drive to create pressure, these new infusion pumps use CO_2 to force dextran into the uterine cavity at preset flow and pressure rates. Use of reduced volumes of dextran to perform diagnostic and operative hysteroscopy has been the result of this technological advance.

Maintenance Versus Continuous Flow of Distending Media

Mention should be made of the difference between operative hysteroscopy procedures that rely on a continuous flow of distending media versus those that do not. In brief, when a viscous medium such as dextran is used the fluid may be introduced slowly into the uterine cavity through the hysteroscope. Once the cavity has been distended, only small amounts of additional viscous media need be added to maintain uterine distension. This is not viewed as a continuous-flow system because excess fluid usually is lost through the cervical os, leaking around the hysteroscope sheath. Nonetheless, only small volumes of dextran are usually required to complete most procedures. The major advantage to this system is that the outer diameter of the operating hysteroscope may be kept relatively small.

In contrast, when less viscous media are used constant flushing of the cavity is required to maintain a clear operating field. This requires a continuous-flow endoscopic sheath. These instruments contain an inner sheath that transmits the fluid into the uterine cavity and an outer sheath through which media flows from the uterine cavity (Fig. 26.10, inset). The major disadvantage of this system is the size of the outer sheath that must be used, 5.5 mm to 9 mm.

Lighting

Development of fiberoptic lighting systems has revolutionized endoscopic procedures by providing high-intensity light from halogen or xenon lamps at power outputs of 100 to 300 W. Heat from these lamps is minimized by filtering out the infrared spectrum. This allows sufficient "cold light" to be transmitted along light-emitting fibers so that endoscopic diagnostic and therapeutic procedures can be performed. Light cords may transmit light through fibers or liquid. Fiber-filled cords are less expensive but may transmit less light than liquid-filled cords. Modern-day light generators also can provide brief flashes of brilliant light for still photography (see Chapters 4 and 7).

Accessory Instruments

In addition to the hysteroscopes, other accessory instruments are required for performing intrauterine surgery. These instruments may be passed through the operating channel of the hysteroscope or passed in parallel to the endoscope to aid in diagnosis or therapy. These accessory instruments include biopsy forceps, grasping forceps, scissors, wire cautery loop, roller ball cautery, laser, and fine wire and balloon uterotubal cannulae.

Biopsy forceps may be rigid or flexible, and may pass within the operating channel of the hysteroscope or alongside it. Tissue samples from the uterine cavity may be taken with these forceps under direct vision. Similarly, flexible or rigid scissors may be positioned in the uterine cavity and used to lyse adhesions or septa. Wire cautery loops passed through appropriately insulated hysteroscopes may also be used to lyse adhesions or resect septa and submucous fibroids. The wire loop or roller ball may also be employed to electrocoagulate and ablate the uterine endometrium. Such procedures are currently being used to treat some patients with menorrhagia (see Chapter 29).

A neodymium:yttrium-aluminum-garnet (Nd:YAG) laser using a 0.6-mm quartz optical fiber may also be passed through the operating channel of the hysteroscope. Once inside the uterine cavity, 40 to 60 W of power may be applied to destroy the uterine endometrium. Alternatively, a radiofrequency thermal probe may be passed through the operating channel of the hysteroscope and into the uterine cavity to accomplish the same task. It must be energized at 27.12 MHz with an incident power level of 550 W to thermally ablate the endometrium.

Tubal cannulation devices are available that can pass through the operating channel of the hysteroscope and into the interstitial portion of the fallopian tube to alleviate obstruction. These cannulae may be used either with a small guidewire probe alone, or as a guidewire surrounded by a balloon, which may be inflated once passed into the interstitial portion of the fallopian tube (see Chapter 31).

Video Imaging

The invention of miniaturized cameras that rely upon charge-coupled device (CCD) chips has resulted in extremely small ($1 \times 1 \times 1.5$ in.) and lightweight (1.6-oz) cameras that are sterilizable, making them ideal for endoscopic use. Using currently available light sources, these cameras may be connected to the hysteroscope and to a video monitor to allow both surgeons and assistants to visualize endoscopic procedures. This may be extremely important for some operative hysteroscopic procedures in which technical assistance is required and the assistant must be aware of what the primary surgeon is attempting to accomplish. Using this equipment the operative procedure may be recorded on video tape and replayed later for the patient or other physicians (see Chapter 7).

Indications and Contraindications to Hysteroscopy

The indications can be classified into a few general headings (Table 26.1). In essence, hysteroscopy is indicated when any form of intrauterine pathology is suspected and diagnosis and therapy are required. An extensive discussion of indications, contraindications, preparation, and technical procedures for hysteroscopy can be found in Dr. Robert Neuwirth's excellent monograph on hysteroscopy.[17]

Contraindications are few, and usually relative. Hysteroscopy is not recommended in pa-

TABLE 26.1. Indications for hysteroscopy.

Abnormal uterine bleeding
  A. Diagnosis
    1. Premenopausal patient
    2. Postmenopausal patient
  B. Therapy
    1. Biopsy and/or directed curettage
    2. Polyp removal
    3. Excision of submucous fibroid
    4. Ablation
Foreign bodies
  A. Diagnosis
    1. Identification
    2. Localization
  B. Therapy
    1. Removal of IUD (intrauterine device)
    2. Removal of suction catheter tip
    3. Removal of ossified products of conception
    4. Removal of laminaria
Infertility/recurrent abortions
  A. Diagnosis
    1. Uterine synechiae
    2. Uterine malformation
    3. Interstitial tubal occlusion
  B. Therapy
    1. Lysis of synechiae
    2. Resection of uterine septum
    3. Removal of interstitial tubal block
    4. Potential for intratubal insemination
Prenatal diagnosis
  A. Fetoscopy
  B. Directed chorionic villus sampling
Contraceptive therapy
  A. Blockage of uterotubo ostium with plugs
  B. Destruction of uterotubal ostium

tients with acute or chronic uterotubal infection, nor is it usually advised in patients who are actively bleeding or menstruating. However, removal of an IUD (intrauterine device) causing infection or a polyp causing bleeding *are* indications for the procedure. Certainly, unintentional instrumentation of the gravid uterus with a hysteroscope is not desirable, although the hysteroscope under planned conditions may serve as a fetoscope.

Preoperative Preparation for Hysteroscopic Surgery

Hysteroscopy is usually performed during the early follicular phase of the menstrual cycle to enhance visibility because the endometrium is thinner and less vascular at this time. This may be the only preparation required when hysteroscopy is performed primarily as a diagnostic procedure.

When hysteroscopic surgery is planned, specialized preoperative and postoperative care may be required. For example, removal of large intrauterine polyps or resection of submucous fibroids may be facilitated by preoperative hormonal therapy with danocrine (400–800 mg/day) or gonadotropin-releasing hormone analog (GnRH analog) for 1 to 3 months before the procedure. Although not currently approved by the Federal Drug Administration (FDA) for these indications, use of these medications will usually result in decreased size and vascularity of the uterine polyp or fibroid to be removed. Use of danocrine or GnRH analog therapy has also been recommended before proceeding with endometrial ablation because these medications will diminish the thickness of the endometrium, ensuring a greater likelihood that the lining will be completely destroyed.

For certain operative hysteroscopic procedures, concomitant laparoscopy or its availability is recommended. This may be of advantage in some cases in which lysis of uterine synechiae, excision of uterine septum, removal of fibroids, ablation of the endometrium, or removal of a uterotubal occlusion is required. Laparoscopic visualization under these conditions could potentially prevent or minimize the complication of perforation, as well as monitor successful cannulation of a previously proximally obstructed fallopian tube. In some cases of severe uterine adhesions, laparoscopy may also be used to allow transfundal injection of methylene blue into the scarred uterine cavity to assist the hysteroscopist in identifying the limits of the uterine cavity.

Specialized postoperative therapy may also be required in certain circumstances. Correction of severe uterine synechiae may necessitate temporary intrauterine insertion of an inert foreign body to prevent uterine wall readherence (e.g., an IUD or Foley catheter) while also providing exogenous estrogen therapy (e.g., conjugated estrogens given in daily doses of 0.625 or 1.25 mg for 25–30 days). Postoperative estrogen therapy without insertion of a foreign body may also be useful following lysis of a uterine septum, as recent studies have shown that estrogen given under these conditions stimulates more rapid reepithelization of the endometrium. Preoperative and postoperative broad-spectrum antibiotic coverage may also be desirable. Intra- and postoperative antibiotics may be employed when previously unsuspected or undiagnosed intrauterine infection is discovered, or the procedure is long and operative contamination is suspected.

Removal of large submucous fibroids may result in excessive uterine bleeding. Blood loss in this situation may be controlled by placing a large Foley catheter balloon within the uterine cavity and keeping the balloon expanded for as long as 24 hr.

Finally, special preoperative therapy may be required to lyse severe uterine synechiae through a severely stenotic cervix. In this circumstance, cervical dilatation with laminaria and use of intraoperative ultrasonography to guide the hysteroscope may be of help.

References

1. Pantaleoni DC. An endoscopic examination of the cavity of the womb. *Med Press Circular (London)*. 1869;8:26–27.
2. Prescott R. Optical principles of endoscopy. *J Med Primatol*. 1976;5:133–147.
3. Rubin IC. Uterine endoscopy, endometroscopy with the aid of uterine insufflation. *Am J Obstet Gynecol*. 1925;10:313–327.
4. Norment WB. Improved instruments for the diagnosis of pelvic lesions by the hysterogram and water hysteroscope. *N C Med J*. 1949;10:646–649.
5. Silander T. Hysteroscopy through a transparent rubber balloon in patients with carcinoma of the uterine endometrium. *Acta Obstet Gynecol Scand*. 1963;42:284–299.
6. Heineberg A. Uterine endoscopy: an aid to precision in the diagnosis of intra-uterine disease. *Surg Gynecol Obstet*. 1914;18:513–515.
7. Schroeder C. Uber den ausbau und die leistungen der hysteroskopie. *Arch Gynaekol*. 1934;156:407–419.
8. Witz CA, Silverberg KM, Burns WN, Schenken RS, Olive DL. Complications associated with the absorption of hysteroscopic fluid media. *Fertil Steril*. 1993;5:745–756.
9. Mizutani AR, Parker J, Katz J, Schmidt J. Visual disturbances, serum glycine levels and transurethral resection of the prostate. *J Urol*. 1990;144:697–699.
10. Menken FC. Endoscopic observations of endocrine processes and hormonal changes. In: *Simposio Esteriodes Sexuales*, Bogata, 1968, pp 24–26.
11. Edstrom K, Fernstrom I. The diagnostic possibilities of a modified hysteroscopic technique. *Acta Obstet Gynecol Scand*. 1970;49:327–330.
12. Lindemann HJ. CO_2—Hysteroscopy today. *Endoscopy*. 1979;2:94–100.
13. Lindemann JH, Mohr J. CO_2 hysteroscopy: diagnosis and treatment. *Am J Obstet Gynecol*. 1976;124:129–133.
14. Hulf JA, Corall IM, Knights KM, et al. Blood carbon dioxide tension changes during hysteroscopy. *Fertil Steril*. 1979;32:193–196.
15. Shirk GJ, Gimpelson RJ. Control of intrauterine fluid pressure during operative hysteroscopy. *J Am Assoc Gynecol Laparosc*. 1994;1:229–233.
16. Lavy G, Diamond MP, Shapiro B, et al. A new device to facilitate intrauterine instillation of dextran 70 for hysteroscopy. *Obstet Gynecol*. 1987;70:955–957.
17. Neuwrith R. Hysteroscopy. In: Friedman EA, ed. *Major Problems in Obstetrics and Gynecology*. Vol. 8. Philadelphia: WB Saunders; 1975:1–116.

27

Operative Hysteroscopic Procedures

Eric S. Knochenhauer and Richard E. Blackwell

Although the operative cystoscope was modified for intrauterine surgery in 1927, it was not until 1970 that Erstrom and Fernstrom utilized dextran as the distending medium, permitting hysteroscopists to perform complex transcervical surgery. The union of the modern operative hysteroscope with appropriate distending medium has made possible the precise localization of various intrauterine pathologies and their treatment with a variety of operative techniques, including sharp dissection, electrocautery, and laser.

Following are discussed the operative hysteroscopic treatment of patients with abnormal uterine bleeding, with an abnormal uterine contour on hysterosalpingography, with suspected Asherman's, or requiring removal of an intrauterine foreign body or evaluation of a suspected uterine perforation. In addition to these indications, operative hysteroscopy is used for the resection of submucous leiomyomata (Chapter 28), ablation of the endometrium (Chapter 29), treatment of congenital uterine abnormalities (Chapter 30), and transcervical recanalization of the fallopian tubes (Chapter 31), as discussed elsewhere in this volume.

Indications and Patient Selection

Abnormal Uterine Bleeding

In the past, patients with abnormal uterine bleeding unresponsive to hormonal manipulation underwent dilation and curettage (D&C) to rule out malignancy and as treatment. Unfortunately, this blind technique resulted in failure to render a diagnosis or adequately treat a significant number of cases.[1] Removal of intrauterine polyps or submuceous fibroids often requires direct visualization. The diagnosis of adenomyosis, although requiring a myometrial biopsy for conformation, is made with greater assurance following a negative hysteroscopic examination.

Abnormal Uterine Contour on Hysterogram

In couples with reproductive failure, the hysterosalpingogram (HSG) defines the size and structure of the uterine cavity and the patency of the fallopian tubes, and often suggests the presence of adhesions or other pathology. When the HSG is properly performed under fluoroscopic control, small polyps, fibroids, and intrauterine adhesions may be diagnosed with considerable precision. In addition, congenital uterine malformations and tubal occlusion may be detected. In patients with a normal HSG there probably is little indication for hysteroscopy. Alternatively, most intrauterine filling defects are best investigated and treated by transcervical hysteroscopic surgery.

Suspected Asherman's Syndrome

The patient with secondary amenorrhea who has a history of intrauterine trauma should undergo evaluation to rule out Asherman's syndrome. However, Asherman's syndrome presents most frequently with infertility or habitual pregnancy loss, not amenorrhea. Asherman's syndrome (partial or complete obliteration of the endometrial cavity by synechiae) almost always occurs in the presence of uterine trauma or manipulation associated with infection or hypoestrogenemia, such as following D&C for miscarriage, removal of an infected intrauterine device (IUD), or retained products of conception. Patients with a negative history for such events should be investigated for hypo- or hypergonadotropism, resulting in the development of hypoestrogenemia and amenorrhea. In the patient with suspected Asherman's syndrome an HSG should be attempted before hysteroscopy to clearly define the lesion. Oftentimes, however, fusion of the lower uterine segment will render the procedure impossible on an outpatient basis.

Suspected Intrauterine Foreign Body

The operative hysteroscope is extremely useful in the localization of a lost IUD. Most frequently, these are buried in either the anterior or posterior fundal wall, in a uterus that is either markedly ante- or retroflexed. In addition, other intrauterine foreign bodies may be located and removed hysteroscopically. Further, patients who undergo a spontaneous abortion and develop secondary amenorrhea may be found to have retained products of conception, even 6 months after the miscarriage. Removal of the retained tissue generally results in restoration of menstruation.

Evaluation of the Perforated Uterus

Some surgeons consider perforation of the uterus to be a contraindication to hysteroscopy, while others have suggested that this technique permits confirmation of the surgical accident and assessment of damage. Once a perforation is confirmed, tamponade of the uterine cavity, or laparoscopy with electrocautery of the injury, can be used to control bleeding. In rare occasions hysteroscopy and transcervical cauterization have been used to locate and coagulate intrauterine bleeding following transabdominal myomectomy.

Equipment

Operative hysteroscopy can be performed using three distending media: carbon dioxide (CO_2), 5% dextrose in water (D_5W), and 32% dextran-70 (Hyskon). Electrolyte solutions (e.g., normal saline or lactate Ringer's solution) should not generally be used for operative work because these media are electrically conductive. Each of these respective media has their proponents. The authors usually prefer to use a 32% dextran-70 solution (Hyskon, Pharmacia, Inc., Columbus, OH). Dextran-70 has an excellent index of refraction, is immiscible with blood, is highly suitable for operative procedures, and is relatively safe[2] (see Chapter 26). It should be noted, however, that both pulmonary edema and anaphylactic reactions have been reported with the use of Hyskon, although no such reactions have been seen at our institution during the past 20 years. Dextran-70 has the disadvantage of damaging operative instruments if the medium is allowed to dry on their surfaces or various orifices. Therefore, instruments should be cleaned in very hot water immediately following procedures using Hyskon.

Operative hysteroscopes contain single or multiple channels, which allow insertion of either rigid or flexible grasping forceps, biopsy forceps, scissors, coagulating electrodes, and laser fibers. Operative hysteroscopes may consist of a fore-oblique diagnostic hysteroscope (generally 4 mm in diameter) with a 6- to 7-mm operative sheath with operative ports for flexible operative 7-Fr. instruments (see Fig. 26.1), or a dorsal fixed instrument tip, resembling a cystoscope. Alternatively, the authors prefer a 7-mm operating hysteroscope with an offset right-angle eyepiece and a 10° field of vision (Richard Wolf Corp., Rosemont, IL). This endoscope contains a single operative channel, allowing the introduction of rigid 3-mm operative instruments (see Fig. 26.2). These instruments are generally insulated for use as unipolar electrosurgical tips. The smaller 7-Fr. flexible instruments used with some operative hysteroscopes are less powerful (see Fig. 26.3), and may increase the operative time and the amount of distension required to complete the procedure.

Pediatric or adult urologic resectoscopes have been modified for use in the resection of intrauterine fibroids, septae, and endometrial ablation. These are generally used in conjunction with a distending medium, such as sorbitol or glycine, and an electrosurgical generator set at 60 to 120 W. The depth of burn with these instruments is usually not greater than 2 mm. Modification of these rectoscopes utilizing a roller ball can be employed to ablate the endometrium (see Chapter 28).

Many types of fiber-transmitted lasers, including argon, Nd:YAG, and KTP, have been employed through the operative hysteroscope.[3] However, in our opinion none of these lasers is as efficient or user friendly as the more conventional equipment just described. For additional discussion of hysteroscopic instrumentation, refer to Chapter 26.

Specific Techniques

Operative hysteroscopy is best performed during the early to midfollicular phase because of the reduced risk of an unsuspected pregnancy, reduced endometrial thickening, and clearest view of the tubal ostium. Furthermore, a corpus luteum will generally be absent if simultaneous operative laparoscopy is required.

Resection of an Endometrial Polyp

Endometrial polyps are simple to remove via operative hysteroscopy. Once located with the diagnostic hysteroscope, polyp forceps can be used to rapidly extract them, after which a repeat hysteroscopy will confirm the absence of any additional lesions. Occasionally, polyps that are difficult to extract are removed following transection of their stalk with operative scissors (Fig. 27.1). Little or no bleeding occurs with resection of these polyps.

Removal of Submucous Myomas

Various types of fibroids may be treated with the operative hysteroscope.[4] The fibroid that is the

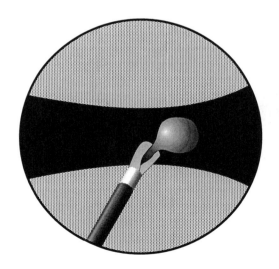

FIGURE 27.1. An intrauterine polyp may be removed using polyp forceps after being located by hysteroscopy. Alternatively, some polyps require that their stalk be transected (*depicted*) before extraction.

simplest to handle is the pedunculated type that protrudes into the uterine cavity, only attached to the endometrial wall via a thin stalk. These lesions, once identified, can frequently be grasped with polyp forceps, crushed, and removed in small pieces. This type of myomectomy usually progresses very rapidly, and twisting the stalk will minimize blood loss.

Some fibroids, the sessile submucous type, partially protrude into the cavity. A few of these lesions may be extracted with polyp forceps, producing a defect that may or may not re-

quire hemostasis with either transhysteroscopic electrocautery or the placement of a distended Foley catheter balloon. More commonly, these lesions are approached with the resectoscope, which is used to "shave" the myoma to its endometrial base.[5] This technique can be carried out alone or in combination with laparoscopy. Postoperatively, a silastic balloon catheter is placed within the uterine cavity and conjugated estrogens 1.25 mg twice daily are administered for a month to facilitate endometrial regeneration.

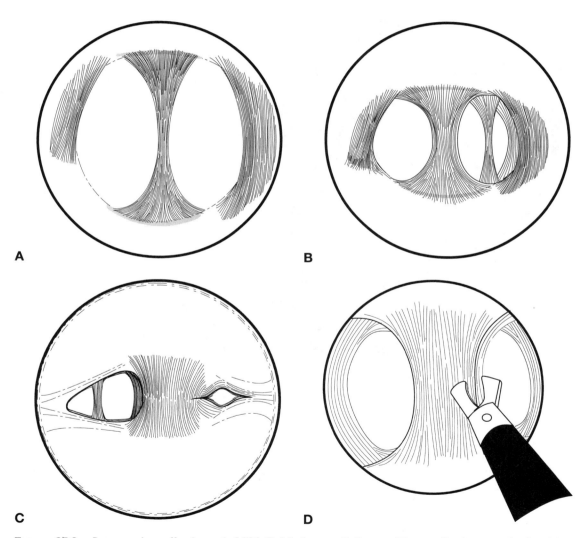

FIGURE 27.2. Intrauterine adhesions. **A:** Mild. **B:** Moderate. **C:** Severe. These adhesions can be lysed hysteroscopically using 3-mm scissors (**D**).

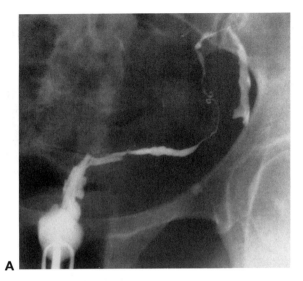

A

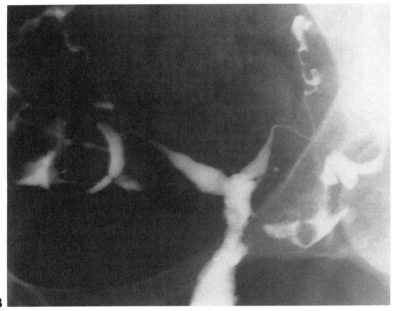

B

FIGURE 27.3. **A:** Hysterosalpinogram of patient with Asherman's syndrome following a D&C for placenta accreta. Note thin sliver of endometrial cavity. **B:** Same patient after hysteroscopic resection of intrauterine adhesions. Both fallopian tubes are now visualized. Although a small amount of residual synechiae is observed, these were not treated. The patient subsequently conceived and delivered at term. (Courtesy of Dr. Ricardo Azziz.)

Three months of preoperative administration of a long-acting gonadotropin-releasing hormone (GnRH) analog may result in a 40% to 50% reduction in myoma size and a decrease in tumor vascularity,[6] facilitating hysteroscopic removal. Furthermore, because GnRH analog suppression produces an even more marked reduction in uterine wall thickness, a sessile submucous fibroid may become pedunculated. See Chapter 28 for a more in-depth discussion of hysteroscopic myomectomy.

Removal of Intrauterine Synechiae and Adhesions

Intrauterine adhesions are perhaps the most common lesions encountered by the operative hysteroscopist.[7] Once these are diagnosed by HSG, a blind D&C can often be carried out to break up minimal intrauterine adhesions, followed by reinvestigation with the hysteroscope. More substantial adhesive disease is best treated with hysteroscopy. Some adhesions disappear during dilation of the cervix, and others can be simply lysed with operative scissors (Fig. 27.2). However, on occasion extensive intrauterine dissection is required to restore the normal uterine contour (Fig. 27.3).

In severe Asherman's syndrome, careful creation of a neouterine space with Hanks dilators under direct laparoscopic vision, followed by hysteroscopic dissection of both lower uterine segment and fundus, is required. It is extremely important that the operator follow the curvature of the uterine cavity (Fig. 27.4) when incising adhesions; otherwise, either an anterior (if the uterus is acutely retroflexed) or a posterior (with anteverted uteri) perforation will occur. Only in patients with extensive dissection and denudation of the endometrial lining are IUDs or balloon catheters inserted into the uterine cavity postoperatively to prevent approximation of the opposing walls. Postoperatively, 2.5 mg of conjugated estrogens is administered daily for 1 month. It is also suggested, with extensive intrauterine manipula-tion, that broad-spectrum oral antibiotics be employed for 5 to 7 days.

Removal of a Retained IUD

The most common foreign body that gynecologists are asked to remove from the uterine cavity is a retained IUD, although these occasions are becoming interesting less frequent. Marked anteflexion or retroflexion of the uterus generally makes the cavity more difficult to explore blindly. The location of the lost IUD may be established preoperatively by transvaginal sonography or an HSG. Once localized, extraction is performed using an IUD hook or other appropriate instrument. In general, those IUDs that cannot be retrieved in the office with either a Novak curette, an IUD hook, or office hysteroscopy require operative hysteroscopy.

At hysteroscopy the IUD will generally be found embedded in the anterior or posterior uterine wall near the fundus. Most IUDs may be extracted by simply locating them with a diagnostic hysteroscope and subsequently removing them with a sharp serrated curette (e.g., Novak), using slow, sustained traction. Adhe-

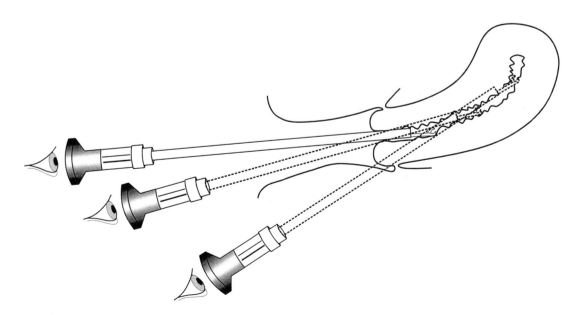

FIGURE 27.4. It is extremely important that the operator follow the curvature of the uterine cavity when incising adhesions to avoid either an anterior (if the uterus is acutely retroflexed) or a posterior (with anteverted uteri) perforation.

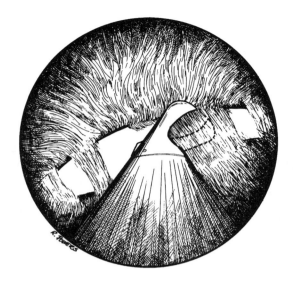

FIGURE 27.5.   Hysteroscopic lysis of intrauterine adhesions surrounding an embedded IUD with rigid 3-mm scissors.

sions covering the IUD may have to be initially lysed with operative scissors (Fig. 27.5). If this maneuver fails to remove the IUD, polyp forceps may be inserted into the uterine cavity, after removal of the hysteroscope, and the object grasped and extracted. However, occasionally the IUD will break in two with this maneuver. Occasionally an IUD will perforate the uterine wall and extend under the serosa. The IUD can be pulled back through the uterine wall with hysteroscopic biopsy forceps or may be extracted transabdominally with the laparoscope. Infrequently, an IUD will be so firmly lodged in the myometrium that the device must be cut in two with rigid operative scissors and each half extracted with combined laparoscopy/hysteroscopy. Any bleeding may be coagulated via laparoscopy, with the bipolar cautery forceps inserted into the perforation tract.

Results

Hysteroscopy has proven to be very useful in the diagnosis and treatment of abnormal uterine bleeding. When diagnostic hysteroscopy was compared to blind D&C in 342 patients, both techniques gave similar results in 271,

while hysteroscopy provided a more accurate diagnosis in 60 patients and D&C provided a more accurate diagnosis in 11 patients.[8] Review of the literature for gestational outcome after treatment of intrauterine adhesions supports the use of hysteroscopy.[9] Blind interruption of adhesions in 69 patients collected from the literature resulted in a 40% term pregnancy rate. Alternatively, in one study, 62 patients treated hysteroscopically demonstrated an 87% pregnancy rate.[9]

The results for hysteroscopic myomectomy have been slightly less favorable. In one study, approximately 83.9% of patients had normal menses after resection of the fibroids and only 19% (18 of 94 patients) had a subsequent term pregnancy.[10] Pregnancy rates of women undergoing hysteroscopic myomectomy reported in several studies are not consistent. The pregnancy rate can vary depending on the population studied and whether a history of infertility, either primary or secondary, is present. It is a rare exception when IUDs cannot be extracted either hysteroscopically or by combined hysteroscopic/laparoscopic technique.

References

1. Gimpleson RJ. Panoramic hysteroscopy with directed biopsies versus dilatation and curettage for accurate diagnosis. *J Reprod Med.* 1989;29: 575–578.
2. Carson SA, Hubert GD, Schriock ED, et al. Hyperglycemia and hyponatremia during operative hysteroscopy with 5% dextrose in water distension. *Fertil Steril.* 1989;51:341–343.
3. Baggish MS, Baltoyannis P. New techniques for laser ablation of the endometrium in high-risk patients. *Am J Obstet Gynecol.* 1988;159:287–292.
4. DeCherney AH, Polan ML. Hysteroscopic management of intrauterine lesions and intractable uterine bleeding. *Obstet Gynecol.* 1983;61: 391–397.
5. Neuwirth RS. Hysteroscopic management of symptomatic submucous fibroids. *Obstet Gynecol.* 1983;62:509–511.
6. Friedman AJ, Barbieri RL, Doubilet PM, et al. A randomized, double-blind trial of gonadotropin-releasing hormone agonist (leuprolide) with or without medroxyprogesterone acetate in the treatment of leiomyomata uteri. *Fertil Steril.* 1988;49:404–409.

7. March CM, Israel R, March AD. Hysteroscopic management of intrauterine adhesions. *Am J Obstet Gynecol.* 1978;130:653–657.

8. Gimpelson RJ, Rappold HO. A comparative study between panoramic hysteroscopy with directed biopsies and dilatation and curettage. *Am J Obstet Gynecol.* 1988;158:489–492.

9. March CM, Israel R. Gestational outcome following hysteroscopic lysis of adhesions. *Fertil Steril.* 1981;36:455–459.

10. Derman SG, Rehnstrom J, Neuwirth R. The long-term effectiveness of hysteroscopic treatment of menorrhagia and leiomyomas. *Obstet Gynecol.* 1991;77:591–594.

28

Hysteroscopic Myomectomy

Stefanie Schupp Christian and William D. Schlaff

In 1976, Neuwirth and Amin[1] described the first reported hysteroscopic myomectomy using a urologic resectoscope. With subsequent modification of equipment and technique, hysteroscopic resection of submucous myomata is now a well-established procedure in the gynecologic armamentarium. Hysteroscopic myomectomy offers many advantages over hysterectomy or abdominal myomectomy. The procedure is usually performed in an ambulatory surgical setting. Laparotomy is avoided, thereby significantly reducing the postoperative recovery period. Furthermore, a hysterotomy incision is avoided, which eliminates the need for future cesarean sections in most instances. Finally, results are comparable to traditional abdominal approaches.

Preoperative Evaluation, Indications, and Patient Selection

Any patient with a symptomatic submucosal myoma may be considered a candidate for hys-

teroscopic resection. These patients frequently present with menorrhagia and metrorrhagia, anemia resulting from abnormal bleeding, pelvic pressure, pelvic pain including dysmenorrhea, infertility, or fetal wastage during the first or second trimester.[2]

Before considering hysteroscopic myomectomy, a thorough preoperative evaluation is required. Endometrial sampling should be performed when indicated. Hysterosalpingography (HSG) or diagnostic hysteroscopy are the most common studies used to confirm the presence of a submucosal myoma.[3] In some cases, ultrasound or magnetic resonance imaging (MRI) may also be useful. HSG has the potential advantage of allowing assessment of tubal patency and may demonstrate multiple channels in the tumor mass that communicate with the uterine cavity thus suggesting a diagnosis of adenomyosis (Fig. 28.1). Therefore, preoperative HSG, often in addition to a sonogram, are recommended to assist the surgeon in developing a three-dimensional sense of the myoma before attempting myomectomy. Hysteroscopy alone may not provide adequate information regarding depth and size of the myoma or about the location of the involved tubal ostia, particularly if the myoma precedes the ostium.

Fluid contrast ultrasound (sonohysterography) is a new technique that promises to be very useful in the diagnosis of intrauterine lesions and may eventually supplant both HSG and diagnostic hysteroscopy in the preoperative detection of submucosal myomata. This procedure is performed by injecting a small amount of sterile saline into the uterine cavity through a pediatric Foley catheter or feeding tube and using the fluid contrast to identify myomas, polyps, or other pathology.

When preparing a patient for hysteroscopic myomectomy, the procedure should be scheduled during the proliferative phase of the cycle. In women with large myomata, 3 cm or more, strong consideration should be given to preoperative hormonal suppression. Preoperative gonadotropin-releasing hormone (GnRH) analog therapy has been demonstrated to reduce myoma volume by 30% to 35%.[4,5] An additional advantage of preoperative treatment with a GnRH analog is the decrease in endometrial proliferation and vascularization, resulting in better visualization and decreased fluid resorption, which theoretically decreases the risk of fluid overload. However, the use of GnRH analogs can cause heavy, irregular bleeding during the first month of therapy, and persistent bleeding that could exacerbate a preexisting anemia is common in women with intracavitary myomata. The first dose of GnRH analog should be given at the time of menses, a second dose should be given 4 weeks later, and surgery should be scheduled 2 to 4 weeks after the second injection. Danazol given at a dose of 400 to 800 mg/day for 6 weeks is an alternative approach to a GnRH analog. A variety of progestins and oral contraceptive pills have also been used preoperatively. However, these medications cause endometrial decidualization rather than atrophy and are not as effective for myoma shrinkage as are the GnRH analogs and danazol.

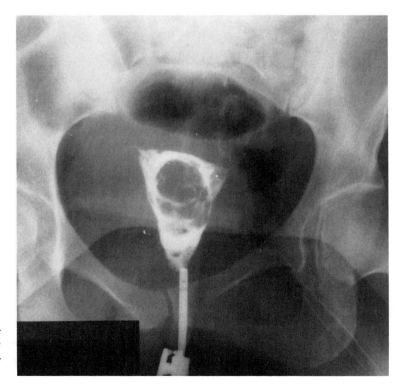

FIGURE 28.1. Hysterosalpingogram with large intrauterine filling defect caused by a submucous myoma.

Instrumentation and Technique

Several electrodes are available for hysteroscopic myomectomy. A monopolar cautery wire loop may be used to shave the myoma. A loop of 0.015-in. gauge wire is recommended, as finer wire may bend or break.[6] Additional electrodes include a roller ball or roller cylinder for coagulation and a pointed tip for cutting or coagulation. Alternatively, a neodymium:yttrium-aluminum-garnet (Nd:YAG) laser with a sapphire tip may be used through the operative channel of the hysteroscope for myomectomy.[7] An operating hysteroscope with rigid or semirigid scissors can sometimes be used for pedunculated submucous myomas.

Several distending media are available. Hyskon (32% dextran-70) offers the advantage of high viscosity, which permits distension of the endometrial cavity with little spillage back through the cervix. Use of more than 500 ml of Hyskon is discouraged because of the risk of pulmonary edema.[8] Hyskon® is immiscible with blood, and bleeding points may be identified easily. However, the immiscibility and high viscosity prevent rapid flow of Hyskon® and may result in poor visualization of the operative field when there is a significant amount of blood, mucous, or shed endometrium.

In the presence of brisk bleeding, alternatives to Hyskon®, such as normal saline, lactated Ringer's solution, 1.5% glycine solution, or sorbitol may be preferable. The use of these lower viscosity solutions allows rapid clearance of blood and myomatous fragments. However, electrical current is dissipated in ionized media such as normal saline. Therefore, if the operator plans to use electrosurgery, sorbitol or glycine would be a more appropriate low-viscosity distension solution.

For best visualization, a pump system should be used to deliver distending media. Large-bore tubing (either urologic or arthroscopic) allows rapid flow into and through the inflow channel. Inflow pressure should not exceed 80 to 100 mmHg. Connecting the outflow port of the resectoscope to suction bottles with low suction (100 mmHg) is recommended. This technique allows the surgeon to increase turnover of distension medium by increasing outflow rather than by increasing the inflow head of pressure, which would theoretically cause a greater risk of intravascular intravasation.[9] This technique also permits the operating team to monitor the volume of distension fluid that has been absorbed by the patient.

Careful preoperative preparation is critical. Anemia should be corrected before surgery, and autologous blood should be banked or a cross-match obtained preoperatively. If the patient is nulliparous or if the cervical os is relatively small, dilating the cervix with laminaria or other hydrophilic adjuncts placed the evening before surgery should be considered. This step will increase the likelihood of an easy and atraumatic insertion of the large hysteroscopic resectoscope instruments. The laminaria may be removed and replaced the morning of surgery to maximize cervical dilatation. The cervix should be dilated sufficiently to allow insertion of the hysteroscopic instruments, but not so much that the seal between the cervix and the hysteroscope is lost. Prophylactic antibiotics may be considered, but there are no definitive data to support their use.

Pedunculated Submucous Myomas

Pedunculated submucosal myomas can be excised using a resectoscope (Fig. 28.2) or with hysteroscopic scissors. Sometimes the vascular stalk can be coagulated before removing the myoma to reduce blood loss. The line of resection follows the endometrial surface. This technique is most suitable for pedunculated myomas in the center of the endometrial cavity. The myoma should be removed with the resectoscope, or with graspers, and sent for histologic examination. In uncommon cases, the myoma cannot be removed and may be left in place to degenerate within the uterus or be expelled during the first menstruation following the procedure.[3]

Sessile Submucous Myomas

Some submucous myomas have a wide base and may be practically intramural. The resectoscope may be used to shave the myoma to the

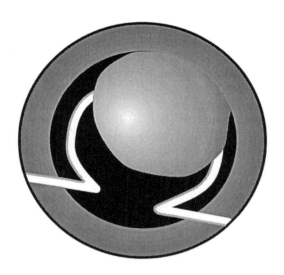

FIGURE 28.2.   90° Loop electrode behind a pedunculated intracavitary myoma.

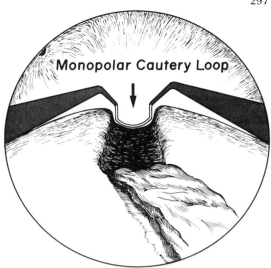

FIGURE 28.4.   Technique for resectoscopic shaving of submucous myoma.

level of the adjacent endometrium. The myoma is progressively shaved toward the lower uterine segment using a flat or a 90° loop electrode and pure cutting current with a setting of 70 to 120 W (Figs. 28.3 and 28.4). The power setting should be low initially and adjusted upward until a smooth, unimpeded motion of the loop through the myoma is achieved. Adjusting the power as indicated by ease of movement of the loop, rather than using a fixed power, may reduce the risk of fracturing the loop.[10] To cut through tissue cleanly with minimum drag, the surgeon should use the highest power with which he or she is comfortable, up to 120 W. The current should be activated only when adequate visualization is achieved.

Fragments of tissue that remain in the intrauterine cavity during the procedure can be removed by turning off the fluid inflow and withdrawing them through the outer resectoscope sheath. This technique has the advantage of minimizing the number of times the sheath is withdrawn from the uterus and cervix. Alternately, ovum forceps, myoma graspers, or suction curettage can be used to remove pieces of myoma. Bleeding points can be fulgurated with either a wire loop, roller ball, or roller cylinder.

Some surgeons utilize the Nd:YAG laser to resect submucosal myomas. However, deaths from air embolization have been reported when carbon dioxide (CO_2) has been used to cool the Nd:YAG laser during endometrial ablation. Therefore, fluid should always be used to cool the sapphire tip if the Nd:YAG laser is

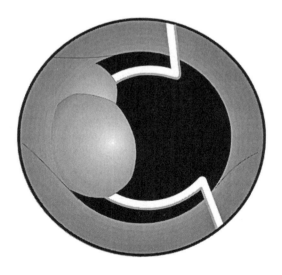

FIGURE 28.3.   A loop electrode behind multiple sessile submucous myomas.

used. No studies have compared the resecto-scope to the Nd:YAG laser for hysteroscopic myomectomy.

Prophylactic postoperative estrogen therapy has been used for patients desiring the potential of fertility.[11] This therapy has been advocated to accelerate endometrial healing and prevent adhesion formation, particularly in those cases in which a large denuded surface remains, or in patients who are hypoestrogenic as a result of preoperative GnRH analog therapy. Although the incidence of endometrial adhesions following hysteroscopic myomectomy is unknown, it appears to be quite low, and the use of estrogen in this setting has not been established as beneficial.

Ablation of the endometrium has been demonstrated to be an effective adjunct to myomectomy in the treatment of patients with a history of heavy uterine bleeding who no longer desire to maintain their fertility (see Chapter 29).[11] Endometrial ablation can be accomplished using either roller ball electrocautery or the Nd:YAG laser. Once again, no studies have compared results obtained using these two techniques. Adenomyosis or cryptic endometrial adenocarcinoma are theoretical risks of uterine ablation.

The surgeon should exercise caution in both patient selection and operative technique when contemplating any operative hysteroscopic procedure for the treatment of leiomyomata. If visibility is poor or if the patient is at significant risk of complications, the procedure should be abandoned and abdominal myomectomy should be performed.

Results

Short-term results reveal control of excessive bleeding in more than 90% of patients treated with either resection alone or resection with ablation.[12] In long-term follow-up of surgeries performed with the resectoscope, 22.3% of patients treated with submucous resection alone had recurrent abnormal bleeding and 16.1% required further surgery. In contrast, 22.5% of patients who underwent myomectomy and endometrial ablation had recurrent abnormal uterine bleeding, but only 8.1% required further surgery.[11] In a 2-year follow-up of single myomectomies with or without endometrial ablation performed with Nd:YAG laser, menorrhagia/metrorrhagia recurred in 2% to 4% of patients.[13] In cases of multiple submucosal and intramural myomata, the rate of recurrence was 25%. If future fertility is not desired by such patients, definitive therapy, that is, hysterectomy, should be considered. Fertility rates following hysteroscopic myomectomy are varied and difficult to compare. Delivery rates of greater than 50% have been reported for hysteroscopic, resectoscopic, and laser resection of submucosal myomas.[3,14–17]

Large Myomata

Several authors have specifically addressed the issue of hysteroscopic myomectomy for large myomata. Loffer[15] performed resectoscopic myomectomies on 43 patients, each of whom had at least one myoma that measured more than 1.5 cm or weighed more than 8 g after resection, and each of whom had been treated with 2 months of danazol or leuprolide. The myomas were initially shaved to the level of the endometrial cavity leaving a portion of intramural fibroid flush with the endometrial wall. The author noted that at the end of the procedure while tissue fragments were being removed from the endometrial cavity, the uterus contracted, causing a portion of the remaining intramural myoma to be extruded into the cavity. Further resection was necessary to avoid prolapse of the extruded portion.

Based on subsequent hysterectomy or repeat hysteroscopy in some of his patients, the author speculated that the incompletely resected intramural portion of sessile fibroids either becomes necrotic or covered by endometrium. After more than 12 months of follow-up, he noted that in 75% to 93% of patients their excessive bleeding was controlled without further therapy, and 58% of the patients with infertility delivered live-born infants.[14]

Donnez reported using the Nd:YAG laser to resect myomata as large as 15.4 cm[2] in 60 women following pretreatment with a GnRH analog.[3] He resected as much of the myoma as possible and drilled the remainder of the myoma with the laser to destroy its vascularity. GnRH suppression was continued for an additional 8 weeks, followed by another resection of the remainder of the myoma, which was by then protruding well into the uterine cavity. The resected myoma was left in the uterine cavity at the end of this second procedure. No concomitant laparoscopy was performed; however, the author recommends simultaneous laparoscopy in some cases. Follow-up hysteroscopy, performed 2 to 3 months later, revealed resolution of the myomata and restoration of normal menstrual flow in all patients. Of those patients desiring conception, 16 of 24 (67%) became pregnant and all had full-term, live-born deliveries.

Risks and Complications

The most common complications of hysteroscopic resection of myomata include hemorrhage, uterine perforation, electrolyte abnormalities, and vascular coagulation disturbances. Heavy bleeding can be managed either by efforts to tamponade the bleeding with an intrauterine balloon or Foley catheter, or by local vasoconstriction using a dilute vasopressin-soaked pack placed into the uterus.[18]

Uterine perforation is the most frequent complication of operative hysteroscopy.[19] Uterine perforation can be further complicated by associated injury to other pelvic or abdominal viscera.[20] Laparoscopic surveillance performed at the time of operative hysteroscopy may allow the surgical assistant to warn the operator if the hysteroscopic dissection is nearing the uterine serosa. Additionally, laparoscopy may also allow immediate diagnosis of perforation. Therefore, diagnostic laparoscopy should be considered at the time of hysteroscopic resection of a large submucosal myoma, when the surgery is performed by a less experienced operative hysteroscopist, or whenever there is a high risk for perforation.

Known complications of Hyskon® in hysteroscopic surgery include fluid overload, pulmonary edema, coagulation defects, anaphylaxis, and spurious laboratory results including falsely elevated blood glucose levels, unreliable total protein and bilirubin assays, and erroneous cross-matching of blood.[2] Dilutional hyponatremia, pulmonary congestion, and possibly pulmonary edema have been reported when other crystalloid fluids are used. In addition to routine preoperative laboratory studies, the surgeon may want to consider obtaining a coagulation panel, electrolytes, liver function studies, and blood type and screen before selected difficult cases, to establish a reliable baseline before the induction of potentially spurious laboratory results.

Intraoperatively, the volumes of distension medium infused and recovered must be meticulously recorded, and manufacturers' stated volume limits should be strictly observed. For instance, the package instructions for Hyskon® include a volume limit of 500 ml per patient. This volume limit refers to the total amount infused, not the amount absorbed by the patient. The patient should be monitored carefully for any evidence of intravascular overload. If regional anesthesia is used, mental status change may be a finding associated with progressive hyponatremia. Operative time should be kept to a minimum, and if necessary, the case should be terminated and completed as a two-step procedure. The surgeon, operating room team, and anesthesia personnel must work together closely in an attempt to prevent these complications. Preoperatively, treatment with a GnRH analog can decrease myoma volume, thus reducing operative time and decreasing the size of the raw denuded surface.

Alternative Techniques

Expectant management of leiomyomata should be elected for patients with minimal symptoms unless the fibroids either grow rapidly or obscure the adnexa.[21] Symptoms caused by myomata may improve after a course of GnRH analog therapy, and symptomatic relief may persist even after regrowth of fibroids.[8] Endometrial ablation may be an effective but temporary modality to control bleeding in a patient with a myomatous uterus.[22] Abdominal myomectomy remains the preferred technique for the removal of symptomatic intramural and subserosal myomata in patients who desire preservation of fertility. Hysterectomy is the procedure of choice for patients who have symptomatic fibroids and no longer desire fertility.

Conclusions

In the carefully selected patient, hysteroscopic resection of a submucous myoma is cost effective and has excellent results both in the management of irregular bleeding and as a fertility-promoting procedure. Long-term control of menometrorrhagia is 80% to 95%. Fertility rates are more than 60% in patients trying to conceive postoperatively, and pregnancy wastage is markedly reduced. Studies are needed to compare the results of hysteroscopic myomectomy performed with Nd:YAG laser with those obtained with a resectoscope.

References

1. Neuwirth RS, Amin HK. Excision of submucous fibroids with hysteroscopic control. *Am J Obstet Gynecol.* 1976;126:95–99.
2. Buttram VC Jr, Reiter RC. Uterine leiomyomata: etiology, symptomatology, and management. *Fertil Steril.* 1981;36:433–445.
3. March CM. Uterine surgical approaches to reduce prematurity. *Clin Perinatol.* 1992;19:319–331.
4. Schlaff WD, Zerhouni EA, Huth JA, Chen J, Damewood MD, Rock JA. A placebo-controlled trial of a depot gonadotropin-releasing hormone analogue (Leuprolide) in the treatment of uterine leiomyomata. *Obstet Gynecol.* 1989;74:856–862.
5. Donnez J, Nisolle M, Grandjean P, Gillerot S, Clercks F. The place of GnRH agonists in the treatment of endometriosis and fibroids by advanced endoscopic techniques. *Br J Obstet Gynaecol.* 1992;999:31–33.
6. McLucas B. Intrauterine applications of the resectoscope. *Surg Gynecol Obstet.* 1991;172:425–430.
7. Donnez J, Gillerot S, Bourgonjon D, Clercks F, Nisolle M. Neodymium:YAG laser hysteroscopy

in large submucous fibroids. *Fertil Steril.* 1990;54:999–1003.
8. Zbella EA, Moise J, Carson SA. Noncardiogenic pulmonary edema secondary to intrauterine instillation of 32% dextran 70. *Fertil Steril.* 1985;43:479–480.
9. Brooks PG. Hysteroscopic surgery using the resectoscope: myomas, ablation, septae and synechiae. Does pre-operative medication help? *Clin Obstet Gynecol.* 1992;35:249–255.
10. Letterie GS. Loop fracture during intrauterine surgery with a gynecologic resectoscope (letter). *Am J Obstet Gynecol.* 1994;170:1839–1840.
11. Derman SG, Rehnstrom J, Neuwirth RS. The long-term effectiveness of hysteroscopic treatment of menorrhagia and leiomyomas. *Obstet Gynecol.* 1991;77:591–594.
12. Serden SP, Brooks PG. Treatment of abnormal uterine bleeding with the gynecologic resectoscope. *J Reprod Med.* 1991;36:697–699.
13. Donnez J, Nisolle M, Clercks F, Casavas-Roux F, Sausroy P, Gillerot S. Advanced endoscopic techniques used in dysfunctional bleeding, fibroids, and endometriosis, and the role of gonadotropin-releasing hormone agonist treatment. *Br J Obstet Gynaecol.* 1994;101:2–9.
14. Valle RF. Hysteroscopic removal of submucous leiomyomas. *J Gynecol Surg.* 1990;6:89.
15. Loffer FD. Removal of large symptomatic intrauterine growths by the hysteroscopic resectoscope. *Obstet Gynecol.* 1990;76:836–840.
16. Corson SL, Brooks PG. Resectoscopic myomectomy. *Fertil Steril.* 1991;55:1041.
17. Hallez JP. Single-stage total hysteroscopic myomectomies: indications, techniques, and results. *Fertil Steril.* 1995;63:703–708.
18. Townsend DE. Vasopressin pack for treatment of bleeding after myoma resection. *Am J Obstet Gynecol.* 1991;165:1405–1407.
19. Peterson HB, Hulka JF, Phillips JM. American Association of Gynecologic Laparoscopists 1988 membership survey on operative hysteroscopy. *J Reprod Med.* 1990;35:590–591.
20. Sullivan B, Kenney P, Seibel M. Hysteroscopic resection of fibroid with thermal injury to sigmoid. *Obstet Gynecol.* 1992;80:546–547.
21. Entman SS. Uterine leiomyoma and adenomyoses. In: Jones HW, III, Wentz AC, Burnett LS, eds. *Novak's Textbook of Gynecology.* 11th ed. Baltimore: Williams & Wilkins; 1988:443–454.
22. Lomano J. Endometrial ablation for the treatment of menorrhagia: a comparison of patients with normal, enlarged, and fibroid uteri. *Lasers Surg Med.* 1991;11:8–12.

29

Endometrial Ablation

James F. Daniell

Abnormal uterine bleeding is a major health problem in women today. In the past, when hormonal therapy failed, this was treated primarily by hysterectomy. Over the last decade, hysteroscopic techniques of endometrial destruction have been developed that allow some of these women with bothersome bleeding to avoid a hysterectomy or the need for hormonal therapy while controlling their abnormal bleeding. This chapter reviews two FDA-approved (U.S. Federal Drug Administration) techniques for destroying the endometrium, including neodymium:yttrium-aluminum-garnet (Nd:YAG) laser and the resectoscope, using both the wire loop electrode and the rolling ball or barrel electrode.

X-Ray therapy had been used in the past to produce premature menopause with cessation of menses in women. Unfortunately, this also destroyed ovarian function and often had serious sequelae. Sclerosing agents have been investigated for intrauterine instillation to destroy the endometrium, but these have not met with success in large trials. Failure of therapy or accidental intraperitoneal spill with catastrophic consequences severely limits the use of these therapies. Goldrath et al. initially reported on the use of the Nd:YAG laser for destruction of the endometrium.[1] The laser energy was introduced via a flexible fiber simplifying hysteroscopic delivery. During the past decade, this technique has been shown to be efficacious and of benefit to most women who meet the proper criteria for having the procedure performed.[2,3]

More recently, a modified urological resectoscope using a wire loop or a rolling ball (roller ball) electrode has allowed electrocoagulation to be used as an alternative to laser for destroying the endometrium.[4-8] The advantages of both laser and electrosurgery for endometrial ablation are that the patient can avoid major surgery, will maintain ovarian function, and may have a permanent reduction or elimination of menstrual bleeding.

Indications and Patient Selection

The indications for endometrial ablation are very clear today. They include significant menorrhagia that is bothersome to the patient and failure of the patient to respond to standard therapy, including hormone manipulation and dilation and curettage (D&C). In addition, the patient should have a cavity free of pathology including fibroids or polyps that may be inducing the abnormal bleeding. The patient should be through with childbearing and have a benign endometrium with no hyperplasia or premalignant lesions.

Careful preoperative counseling and selection of patients is critically important, both for proper fulfillment of expectations and for understanding of the outcome by the patient. This counseling should include a discussion of the fact that the procedure may not eliminate bleeding, but hopefully will reduce flow significantly and thereby reduce the patient's symptomatology. Patients who have intrauterine pathology, however, might opt for more definitive therapy such as hysterectomy because of the potential for recurrence of fibroids or polyps. The patient should be warned about the possibility of pregnancy, because the procedure does not sterilize.[9] Incidental laparoscopic tubal sterilization should be offered to patients who are at risk for pregnancy.

The younger patient should be aware that preoperative suppression of the endometrium is critical for successful destruction of the endometrium down to the basalis. This can be accomplished either with medroxyprogesterone acetate (Provera®), GnRH analogs (Lupron® or Synarel®), or danazol (Danocrine®) administration. All these drugs should be administered for a minimum of 1 month preoperatively, and probably postoperatively as well to the younger patient.

Preoperative screening of the endometrial cavity should be performed by endometrial biopsy, preferably combined with an office hysteroscopy. This will minimize the risk of missing intrauterine pathology, which may occur with a blind D&C. We have found polyps and submucosal fibroids in patients having had multiple D&Cs and a purportedly "normal uterine cavity." It is important to note, however, that at the time of endometrial ablation small fibroids and polyps can be resected and removed. Proper diagnosis and treatment may eliminate the metromenorrhagia without need for an ablative procedure.

Thus, our preoperative evaluation includes counseling, office hysteroscopy, and directed endometrial biopsy. Hormonal suppression to produce a hypoestrogenic state and a thin endometrium is then begun. Recent data suggest that older women have satisfactory results following endometrial ablation, even without preoperative suppressive therapy.[10] Thus, to avoid additional costs, we perform a suction D&C followed by endometrial ablation without preoperative suppression in patients more than 45 years of age. Our success rates have been unchanged by this approach, employed over the past 2 years. In patients who are anemic, preoperative suppression allows time for correction of the hematocrit through the induction of temporary amenorrhea.

Patients with known uterine fibroids should be counseled about the potential for persistent growth of these leading to the need for subsequent hysterectomy, even though the abnormal bleeding may be controlled by the ablation. Some authors, however, report good results with endometrial ablation in the presence of fibroids.[11] In addition, patients with significant pain associated with their uterine bleeding may have adenomyosis or other pelvic pathology that could later require a hysterectomy. Patients need to understand these possibilities before undergoing hysteroscopic endometrial ablation. Certainly a concomitant laparoscopy can be offered to obtain a more definitive diagnosis if pain is a significant factor. Laparoscopic treatment of endometriosis or transection of the uterosacral ligaments may be offered to patients with dysmenorrhea should pathology be found. If indicated, subserosal fibroids can be removed through the laparoscope at the time of the hysteroscopic ablation.

Patients with medical problems should be evaluated preoperatively. Patients at high risk for complication at hysterectomy are commonly referred for endometrial ablation and can benefit most from this procedure. However, appropriate medical and anesthetic consultation can minimize the risks. Fluid overload secondary to absorption of the distending media used during the hysteroscopic ablation is a significant risk,[12] particularly for patients with cardiac compromise. Other potential risks include uterine perforation with possible bowel injury.

Instrumentation

The prerequisites for hysteroscopic endometrial ablation include adequate training of the physician in both diagnostic and operative hysteroscopy and a thorough understanding of laser or electrosurgery physics, depending on the ablation technique of choice. Appropriate informed consent should be well documented.

A typical room setup is seen in Fig. 29.1. Certainly a laser safety officer and laser-certified operating room circulating personnel should maintain the Nd:YAG laser and ensure that proper safety precautions for protecting the eyes of the operator and others in the room are being followed. Fluid monitoring and fluid

infusion rates are critical and should be well understood and controlled by the circulating nurse.

Instrumentation includes a good light source, a video camera, with either a direct coupler or beam splitter, depending on the preference of the operator, and a fluid infusion system. Our distension medium of choice is glycine (1.5% solution), so that either electrosurgery or laser can be used. Hyskon® (32% Dextran-70) can also be used, particularly if bleeding is a problem. If Hyskon® is used, total volumes of more than 300 ml should not be instilled, except in rare circumstances and only after consultation with the anesthesiologist because of the risks of fluid overload and pulmonary edema. Careful monitoring of the patient's circulatory and pulmonary status during the procedure is an important safety measure.

For endometrial ablation with the Nd:YAG laser, a three-channel hysteroscope is preferred (Fig. 29.2). This allows for constant infusion of the distending medium and constant drainage of excess fluid. A third channel is used to introduce the 600-μm Nd:YAG fiber. With the Nd:YAG laser, an eye filter should be used at

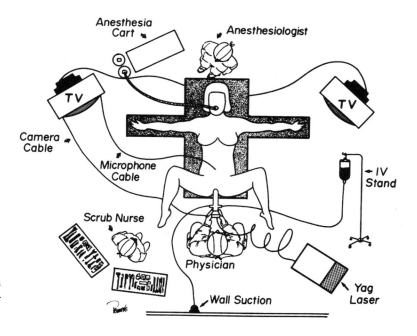

FIGURE 29.1. Operating room setup for operative hysteroscopy.

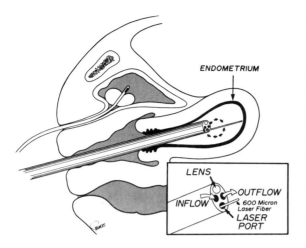

FIGURE 29.2. Endometrial ablation using the Nd:Yag laser is best performed with a three-channel hysteroscope with a 25° optic.

suring all the fluid used for uterine distention must be used (Fig. 29.3). We use 3-liter containers of glycine, and use a continuous-flow system with both the Nd:YAG laser and the resectoscope. After 3 liters of glycine have been infused, we measure the volume that has been recovered from the inflow port and the catch basin then accurately estimate the volume of medium absorbed by the patient before continuing with the case. Intravenous diuretics can be given after consultation with the anesthesiologist, either electively before surgery or intraoperatively if fluid absorption is noted to be greater than 1000 ml. Postoperative central venous pressure (CVP) monitoring can be used as indicated, based on the recommendations of the anesthesiologist or internal medicine consultants.

Technique

Nd:YAG Technique

As shown in Fig. 29.2, under direct hysteroscopic view, the 600-μm Nd:YAG fiber is used to photocoagulate around each tubal ostium. Following this, the fiber is used to photocoagulate the endometrium, being careful to treat each contiguous area adequately. We use a

all times to protect the operator. Concomitant laparoscopy is probably a wise option when beginning to perform endometrial ablation procedures, but it is not routinely required unless patients have an indication for laparoscopy or desire elective sterilization.

Bladder drainage is mandatory in all cases, and a system for accurately capturing and mea-

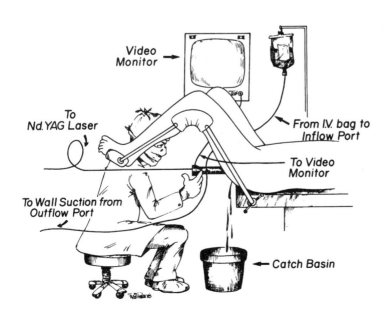

FIGURE 29.3. Operating room setup for accurately capturing all the fluid used for uterine cavity distension during operative hysteroscopy.

combination of airbrushing, a no-touch technique in which the fiber is held just off the uterine wall, with gentle touching of the fiber to the uterine wall (stippling or pointillism) (Fig. 29.4). Finally, furrowing is accomplished by dragging the fiber away from the fundus in consecutive grooves along the lateral, anterior, and posterior uterine walls. Under continuous high flow of glycine, all endometrial surfaces are treated under direct vision.

If visibility is obscured because of bleeding, the intrauterine pressure can be raised by temporarily blocking off the outflow of the glycine or by increasing pressure on the infusion bag. The goal is to have the intrauterine pressure equal the vascular pressure of the myometrium, so that blood flow is stopped in the basalis layer of the endometrium. In cases in which bleeding becomes a significant problem, we stop the infusion with glycine and gently instill one ampule of pitressin, diluted with 20 ml of saline, into the uterine cavity; after waiting a minute to allow absorption into the endometrium, the excess is then withdrawn. This temporarily constricts the uterine vessels. Following this, immediate coagulation of visible bleeders with the Nd:YAG laser usually effectively controls bothersome bleeding. One should avoid digging deep furrows into the uterine wall and lasering deeply along the cer-

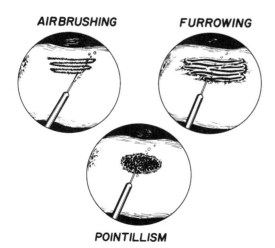

FIGURE 29.4. Nd:YAG laser techniques used to photocoagulate the intrauterine walls.

vical sidewalls because this may lacerate the cervical branch of the uterine artery. After treating all contiguous areas, the hysteroscope is removed. The total volume absorbed and the amount of energy used for the procedure are calculated and recorded.

Resectoscopic Technique

The setup and technique for the resectoscope are similar to that with the laser. The only difference is that the cervix usually has to be dilated a bit more because of the larger diameter of our resectoscope. Our operative hysteroscope with a port for the Nd:YAG laser fiber is 6.2 mm in diameter versus one that is 8 mm in diameter for our resectoscope. It is important to use a continuous-flow resectoscope that has both an inflow and an outflow port to allow continuous circulation of the distending medium. Most urological resectoscopes do not have this feature, but endoscope manufacturers have now developed special hysteroscopic resectoscopes that have an inflow channel for the distending media around the optics of the system with outflow through the outer channel of the hysteroscope. This provides continuous inflow of clean distending media in front of the lens and outflow of media from the uterine cavity away from the lens. A lens with a 30° angle of view is preferred for most of these procedures to obtain good lateral vision of each cornu.

If the wire loop resectoscope is being used, it is mandatory that beginner surgeons have a laparoscope in the abdominal cavity to visualize the external uterine surface as there may be difficulty accurately judging the depth of endometrial penetration with this electrode. Alternatively, if the roller ball or barrel is used, a laparoscopy is not routinely required because these electrodes do not penetrate deeply into the myometrium, merely rolling over the surface of the endometrium.

The author prefers the 4-mm roller ball technique. A power setting of 100 W adequately treats the endometrium to the basalis and spares the deeper myometrium. The ablation is begun by gently pushing the ball electrode into each cornua. This is the most dangerous part of the procedure, because too much upward pressure can lead to uterine perforation or transmural bowel injury, even without perforation. The anterior uterine wall is treated next, because bubbling can occur with use of electrical current. These bubbles can be removed from the cavity by occasionally pushing the scope up against the fundus so that the bubbles will pass out through the outflow ports on the outside of the hysteroscope. Because the outflow ports are at least 1 cm back from the tip of the scope, when the hysteroscope is pulled back into the cervical canal obstruction of the outflow channels may occur and reduce visibility. Intermittently pushing the scope forward to permit the outflow of fluid is helpful. This problem usually occurs only when the uterine cavity is small or when treating the lower portions of the cavity.

The electrode is rolled gently along the wall of the endometrial cavity, treating each contiguous area so that there is blanching and ablation of the endometrium down to the basalis (Fig. 29.5). This can be visually determined by the whiteness that occurs on the floor of the treated area of the endometrial cavity, which suggests that myometrium has been reached. The ball electrode must be cleaned occasionally to remove tissue debris. The operator can either remove the electrode to physically clean it or switch to the pure coagulation mode at 100 W and carefully roll the electrode along

the lower walls of the cavity to burn off the tissue. A clean electrode will transmit energy more effectively. If bleeding is encountered, the same techniques previously described for Nd:YAG are used. If intrauterine pathology is encountered, a polypectomy or myomectomy may be performed.

Alternative Techniques

Several new methods for destruction of the endometrium transcervically without direct vision are currently under investigation but as of this writing have not received FDA approval. Experimentally, microwave heating of the endometrial cavity via placement of a catheter inside the uterine cavity with several microwave-receiving antennae attached to the catheter has been shown to achieve endometrial temperatures to 60°C. A similar system is in clinical trials for treatment of prostatic hypertrophy but has not yet been used in human uterine studies. Three other methods for thermal ablation of the endometrial cavity are under clinical trials now in America: a radiofrequency probe device, a balloon that allows circulation of hot fluid, and an inflatable bag fitted with rectangular electrodes.

All four of these new systems are designed to produce controlled thermal damage to the endometrial cavity that it is hoped will perma-

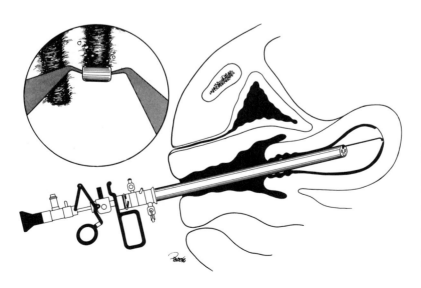

FIGURE 29.5. The roller ball technique consists of gently rolling the ball along the wall of the endometrial cavity and treating each contiguous area to the point of blanching the endometrium and thus achieving ablation down to the basalis.

nently destroy enough endometrial tissue to stop or reduce uterine bleeding. Early reports from outside the United States suggest that success rates of 80% for treatment of menorrhagia may be obtainable but that retreatment may be necessary to obtain higher amenorrhea rates. Clearly, if safe effective endometrial destruction can be obtained without hysteroscopic control, it should become more economical and easier to manage menorrhagia in an office setting.

The two techniques for endometrial ablation that have acquired the most acceptance in America are the Nd:YAG laser ablation and the roller ball electrode. The alternative technique, favored by Europeans, is the resectoscope wire electrode. The problem with this technique, in our opinion, is that it may cut deeply into the myometrium and thus must be performed concomitant with laparoscopy by inexperienced surgeons. Increased bleeding is a major risk. Because of this, only skilled hysteroscopists should use the wire electrode, and then often only under laparoscopic visualization.

It is at present unclear which technique has the greatest advantage for long-term control of menometrorrhagia. The Nd:YAG laser technique has a greater length of patient follow-up time, as it has been used for at least 15 years. In the author's practice, endometrial ablation was begun in 1983 and the Nd:YAG laser was used exclusively until the late fall of 1988. Between the fall of 1988 and the following year, we used a combination of both Nd:YAG laser and resectoscope, using the Nd:YAG laser initially around the ostia and fundus while using the roller ball electrode for the lateral side walls. Beginning in 1990, we have used the roller ball exclusively for this procedure.

Our reasons for changing from endometrial ablation with the Nd:YAG laser to resectoscope include the following:

1. Our operating time for endometrial ablation with the Nd:YAG laser averaged 45 min. Our operating time with the roller ball currently is approximately 20 min in women with normal uterine cavities, representing a significant reduction in patient anesthesia time.

2. In addition, the risk to the operator is less with cautery than with the Nd:YAG laser. There is no risk to the surgeon's eyes with cautery, while that risk always exists with Nd:YAG laser endometrial ablation.
3. The use of the fiber is more tedious and can lead to more bleeding problems because the fiber digs into the wall of the endometrium and larger vessels can be entered accidentally but are not occluded. The ball electrode does not present this problem, as it rolls along the surface of the endometrium without trauma so that a uniform depth of destruction is obtained.
4. The Nd:YAG laser fiber diameter is 600 μm, while the barrel electrode that we routinely use is 4 mm in diameter. This gives us a much greater surface area contact, which accounts for the rapidity with which we can accomplish this procedure of endometrial destruction using the ball electrode.
5. There is a major difference in the cost of the equipment; a Nd:YAG laser costs approximately $100,000 but the equipment for endometrial ablation with the resectoscope costs no more than $6,000.

Unfortunately, neither technique is yet taught in many residency programs, so interested gynecologists who have no experience in hysteroscopy with endometrial ablation must undertake special training. This is now easily available, as many workshops are occurring in various sites around the United States today that offer training in endometrial ablation both with the Nd:YAG laser and with the resectoscope. Nonetheless, as noted in Chapter 2, training is only completed after a 12-month period of preceptorship and supervised surgery.

Results

Results for endometrial ablation with the Nd:YAG laser now span 15 years, with several reports including large numbers of patients. A recent British study reported 600 cases with no significant complications, a 90% satisfaction rate, and a 6.8% subsequent hysterectomy rate. The initial success rate reported by Goldrath[1] was as high as 90%, although other investiga-

TABLE 29.1.   Results of Nd:YAG laser hysteroscopic endometrial ablation.[21]

Author	Distending media	n	Satisfactory	Failure	Complication
Goldrath et al.	Dextrose	216	96%	6%	7 hematometria
					1 perforation
					1 postoperative hemorrhage
					1 pulmonary edema
					1 hyponatremia
Petrucco and Gillespie	Normal saline	34	87%	13%	1 perforation
					1 bowel injury
Lomano	Normal saline	10	100%		None
Daniell et al	Normal saline	144	84%	16%	1 perforation
					2 bleeding
					1 pulmonary edema
Baggish and Baltoyannis	Hyskon	14	93%	7%	1 pulmonary edema
Davis	Normal saline	25	52%	48%	1 pulmonary edema
Bent and Ostergard	Normal saline	42	81%	19%	3 pulmonary edema
Garry et al.	Normal saline	600	83%	17%	None
Loffer	Normal saline	100	83%	17%	None
Donnez	Normal saline	153	92%	8%	None
Total:		1338			

tors have not been able to achieve this, which probably reflects the fact that Dr. Goldrath used greater power densities and more vigorous application of Nd:YAG laser energy than is currently used. Table 29.1 lists some reported results over the past decade for endometrial ablation by various investigators using the Nd:YAG laser.

Endometrial ablation using the resectoscope has a shorter history, and thus fewer reports have been published. Those that have appeared note similar success rates to those obtained with Nd:YAG endometrial ablation (Table 29.2). Our personal results are listed in Table 29.3 for initial cases of endometrial ablation with the Nd:YAG laser alone, and Table

TABLE 29.2.   Reported results of endometrial ablation with resectoscope.[21]

Author	Distending media	Number	Patients Satisfied (%)	Failure (%)	Complications	Current Used
DeCherney and Polan (1987)	Hyskon	21 wire loop excisions	95	5	None	—
Vancaillie (1989)	Hyskon	14 ball ablations	93	7	None	40–70 W coagulation
Townsend et al. (1990)	Sorbitol	50 ball ablations	90	10	1 fluid overload hyponatremia	90–100 W
Maher and Hill (1990)	Glycine	350 part resections/ part ablations	95	5	NS	50 W coagulation fundus; 100 W cutting side walls
Magos et al. (1991)	Glycine	250 wire loop resections (22 partial only)	90	10	4 perforation 1 hemorrhage	100–125 W blended cutting
Serden and Brooks (1991)	Glycine	96 ball ablations	97	7	1 fluid overload 1 perforation	
Daniell et al. (1992)	Glycine	61 ball ablations	80	20	1 perforation in patient with prior Nd:YAG ablation	100 W blended cutting to fundus; 75 W coagulation to side walls
Loffer (1995)	Glycine	147 ball ablations	80	20	None	NS
Pooley et al. (1995)	Glycine	359 resections	82	18	None	NS
Nelson (1995)	Glycine	450 resections	90	10	1 pregnancy	NS

TABLE 29.3. Results of Nd:YAG laser ablation: West Side Hospital, June 1984 to December 1988[a]

Age (yr)	Patients (n)	Results		
		Good (amenorrhea)	Fair (light flow)	Poor (persistent AUB)[b]
16–35	23	10 (43%)	3 (12%)	10(43%)
36–45	68	31 (46%)	29 (43%)	8(11%)
46–76	53	40 (75%)	9 (17%)	4(8%)
Totals:	144	81 (56%)	41 (28%)	22(16%)

[a]Minimum 3-month follow-up of 144 cases during 54-month study period, or 2.7 cases/month.
[b]AUB, Abnormal uterine bleeding.

TABLE 29.4. Results of resectoscope endometrial ablation: West Side Hospital, January 1990 to June 1991[a]

Age (yr)	Patients (n)	Results		
		Good (amenorrhea)	Fair (light flow)	Poor (persistent AUB)[b]
14–35	4	2 (50%)	1 (25%)	1 (25%)
36–45	30	16 (53%)	11 (37%)	3 (10%)
46–60	6	5 (83%)	1 (17%)	0
Totals:	40	23 (58%)	13 (32%)	4 (10%)

[a]Minimum 3-month follow-up.
[b]AUB, Abnormal uterine bleeding.

29.4 lists our initial results with the resectoscope only. Note that the results are very similar for both techniques and improve with the age of the patient.

Long-term results are just becoming available for endometrial ablation with the resectoscope. Loffer studied 147 patients treated with the resectoscope with follow-up as long as 3 years, and 77% of patients reported excellent results.[13] Subsequent hysterectomy was performed for persistence of bleeding in 13%. Loffer's success is similar to the results reported by Donnez in a 4-year follow-up of 153 women treated with the Nd:YAG laser. Of these patients, only 8% required further treatment, with 11 hysterectomies and 4 repeat procedures.[14] In our practice, 3 patients developed recurrent bleeding after more than a year of amenorrhea, suggesting that some remaining endometrial tissue may slowly regrow. All these patients were under 40 years of age, and subsequent office hysteroscopy and biopsy revealed isolated small reddish areas of viable normal endometrium.

In a recent comparison of endometrial ablation to abdominal hysterectomy, there was a more rapid recovery, less pain, and lower complication rates.[5] In addition, the global costs of therapy for dysfunctional uterine bleeding were much less with endometrial ablation than hysterectomy in a 1993 British study.[6] Another recent retrospective review compared both vaginal and abdominal hysterectomy to endometrial ablation and found total direct and indirect cost per case to be significantly less. This savings even persisted when the costs of failures were considered.[15]

Safety of Endometrial Ablation

The safety of endometrial ablation has been well documented. However, there are reports in the literature documenting bowel complications related to the use of both the Nd:YAG laser and the resectoscope.[16,17] Either Nd:YAG laser or electrocautery can be very dangerous if not used appropriately and proper safety precautions are not followed, with death occurring. The operator must at all times be able to visualize either the tip of the fiber, the roller ball, or the wire electrode. It is risky to work in visibility that is less than good and no one should operate without having proper training or equipment.

Accidental perforation with the hysteroscope can never be entirely avoided. Special caution should be exercised when using the resectoscope or laser, as the penetrating ability of these instruments is great. Clearly, there is a high risk of organ damage beyond the uterus if perforation occurs. Scientific investigation of the effects of electrosurgery on the myometrium have begun, but no clear safe guidelines are yet available.[18] To maximize safety, power to the instruments should only be activated when the tip is in clear view and while it is being drawn back toward the operator.

Other complications of hysteroscopic endometrial ablation have been reported or postulated. Goldrath described seven patients with hematometria discovered postoperatively because of cervical stenosis; thus he now recommends routine sounding of the uterus at the 6-week postoperative visit. Gas embolism has occurred in two cases of laser ablation with fatal results.[19] This disastrous complication arose from the inappropriate use of a gaseous medium to cool the tip of the fiber during Nd:YAG laser firing. Masking cancer of the endometrium because of subsequent adhesion formation has also been postulated as a long-term complication of endometrial ablation. This is particularly worrisome in patients treated with the Nd:YAG laser, because cervical stenosis may occur and subsequent external bleeding may not signal subsequent disease. Although hidden malignancy is unlikely in a population without any previous atypical changes, only long-term follow-up can determine this risk.

It must be remembered that endometrial ablation is not a sterilizing procedure. Patients at risk for pregnancy should be aware of this and possibly offered a concomitant tubal ligation. Reports of pregnancy after endometrial ablation include a term birth by cesarean delivery with no problems with placental removal,[9] and an elective abortion with laparoscopic tubal ligation without complication in a patient who conceived after being amenorrheic for 18 to 20 months.[20] In our own practice, eight months following endometrial ablations, a patient conceived unexpectedly. She then suffered a spontaneous miscarriage at 3 months gestation, with severe postabortal hemmorhage secondary to retained placental fragments. After a first suction curettage, she was transfused and underwent a second operation under hysteroscopic guidance to remove the retained fragments. A simultaneous tubal ligation was performed.

The credentialing process for endometrial ablation should include these three steps.

1. Obtain privileges for the basic hysteroscopy procedures.
2. After adequate training in hysteroscopy, attend a course that offers hands-on training in use of the type of energy one wishes to use for endometrial ablation, either laser or electrocautery.
3. As the final step, complete a preceptorship with an acknowledged expert in the procedure.

In our opinion, no one should attempt the procedure until these three steps are taken. One must obtain some hands-on experience in the operating room, both observing, and serving and participating, in a case under the direction of an experienced hysteroscopist. Certainly, expertise with the Nd:YAG laser does not imply expertise with the roller ball and vice versa. Each technique has subtle differences, and adequate training and hands-on experience are necessary before attempting this procedure on patients. For more discussion of training and credentialing in operative endoscopy, see Chapters 2 and 3.

Conclusions

With the advent of the much simpler, less expensive, and more rapid technique of roller ball endometrial ablation, many surgeons who were discouraged from this procedure because of concern about the use of the Nd:YAG laser or with the costs of the procedure may now begin to explore its potential. There are two basic groups of patients who seek out endometrial ablation. The first are patients with surgical or medical problems and significant menorrhagia refractory to hormonal therapy, in whom the risk of hysterectomy is high. These women are clearly good candidates for the procedure. The second group of patients are those who have read about the procedure or heard about it and seek it out because it is a new technology. These patients often have minimal menorrhagia, and are often not good candidates for the procedure because they are younger, with higher endogenous estrogen levels and more lush endometrium.

There is great risk for abuse of the procedure, particularly as it becomes simpler to perform. Some physicians are already promoting the procedure through television ads and local media publicity. The goal of all health care providers should be to provide excellent health care while minimizing costs and risks to the patients. Certainly, endometrial ablation in the properly selected and counseled patient meets this goal by eliminating the bothersome problem of metromenorrhagia while offering a simple, rapid outpatient procedure that, if properly performed, can be very safe and effective with long-term benefits to the patient.

As more and more gynecologists become competent in hysteroscopy and become familiar with these techniques, there will probably be a significant increase in the number of women undergoing endometrial ablation. Twenty-five percent of hysterectomies performed in North America today are for metromenorrhagia only, with benign endometrium. Most of these patients in the next decade could become candidates for this simple outpatient procedure that could replace the more complicated, expensive, and risky hysterectomy. Proper education of both patients and physicians is critical so that all can benefit from this new technology.

References

1. Goldrath MH, Fuller TA, Segal S. Laser photo-vaporization of the endometrium for the treatment of menorrhagia. *Am J Obstet Gynecol.* 1981;140:14–18.
2. Daniell J, Tosh R, Meisels S. Photodynamic ablation of the endometrium with the Nd:YAG laser hysteroscopically as a treatment of menorrhagia. *Colposcopy Gynecol Laser Surg.* 1988;2: 43–47.
3. Garry R, Shelley-Jones D, Mooney P, Phillips G. Six hundred endometrial laser ablations. *Obstet Gynecol.* 1995;85:24.
4. Vancaillie TG. Electrocoagulation of the endometrium with the ball-end resectoscope. *Obstet Gynecol.* 1989;74:425–429.
5. Pinion SB, Parkin DE, Abramovich DR, et al. Randomised trial of hysterectomy, endometrial laser ablation and transcervical endometrial resection for dysfunctional uterine bleeding. *Br Med J.* 1994;309:979.
6. Schulper MJ, Bryan S, Dwyer N, Hutton J, Stirrat GM. An economic evaluation of transcervical endometrial resection v. abdominal hysterectomy in the treatment of menorrhagia. *Br J Obstet Gynecol.* 1993;100:244.
7. Magos AL, Baumann R, Lockwood GM, Turnbull AC. Experience with the first 250 endometrial resections for menorrhagia. *Lancet.* 1991; 337:1074–1078.
8. Daniell JF, Kurtz BR, Ke RW. Hysteroscopic endometrial ablation using the rollerball electrode. *Obstet Gynecol.* 1992;80:329–332.
9. Hill DJ, Maher PJ. Pregnancy following endometrial ablation: A case review. *Gynaecol Endosc.* 1992;1:47–49.
10. Lefler HT, Sullivan GH, Hulka JF. Modified endometrial ablation: electrocoagulation with vasopressin and suction curettage preparation. *Obstet Gynecol.* 1991;77:949–953.
11. Lomano J. Endometrial ablation for the treatment of menorrhagia: a comparison of patients with normal, enlarged, and fibroid uteri. *Lasers Surg Med.* 1991;11:8–12.
12. Feinberg BI, Gimpelson RI, Godier RN. Pulmonary edema after photocoagulation of the endometrium with the Nd:YAG laser: a case report. *J Reprod Med.* 1989;34:431–434.
13. Loffer FD. Long term follow-up of patients undergoing endometrial ablation with the Nd:YAG laser or the resectoscope. Abstract presented at the 4th biennial meeting of the International Society for Gynecologic Endoscopy, April 26–29, 1995, London, England.
14. Downes E, Tyack A. Long term follow-up after endometrial laser ablation. A retrospective study of 124 patients. Abstract presented at the 4th biennial meeting of the International Society for Gynecologic Endoscopy, April 26–29, 1995, London, England.
15. Brumsted JR, Blackman JA, Badger GJ, Riddick DH. Hysteroscopy versus hysterectomy for the treatment of abnormal uterine bleeding: a

comparison of cost. *Fertil Steril.* 1996;65:310–316.

16. Perry CP, Daniell JF, Gimpelson RJ. Bowel injury from Nd:YAG endometrial ablation. *J Gynecol Surg.* 1990;6:199–203.

17. Kivnick S. Kanter MH. Bowel injury from rollerball ablation of the endometrium. *Obstet Gynecol.* 1992;79:833–835.

18. Duffy S, Reid PC, Smith JHF, Sharp F. In vitro studies of uterine electrosurgery. *Obstet Gynecol.* 1991;78:213–220.

19. Baggish MS, Daniell JF. Catastrophic injury secondary to the use of coaxial gas-cooled fibers and artificial sapphire tips for intrauterine surgery: a report of five cases. *Lasers Surg Med.* 989;9:581–584.

20. Mongelli JM, Evans AJ. Pregnancy after transcervical endometrial resection (letter to the Editor). *Lancet.* 1991;338:110.

21. Daniell JF. Endometrial ablation as an alternative to hysterectomy. In: Diamond MP, Daniell JF, Jones HW, eds. *Hysterectomy.* Cambridge, MA: Blackwell Science; 1995:167–180.

30

Hysteroscopic Treatment of Congenital Uterine Anomalies

Scott M. Slayden and J. Benjamin Younger

Congenital anomalies of the mullerian system are estimated to occur in approximately 0.1% to 1.5% of females in the general population.[1] These anomalies are collectively associated with a 20% reproductive failure rate most frequently seen as recurrent spontaneous abortion or premature delivery.[2] Of women with preterm fetal wastage, the incidence of mullerian anomalies is estimated to vary between 1% and 12%. Approximately 90% of these anomalies involve the uterus, and the majority (80%) are septate uterus.[3] These malformations are often noted incidentally; in other cases the diagnosis is made during the workup of infertility or repeated fetal wastage.

There are three general types of mullerian anomalies: mullerian agenesis, disorders of vertical fusion (e.g., transverse vaginal septa), and abnormalities of lateral fusion (e.g., uterus didelphis, bicornuate uterus, septate uterus). Pregnancy wastage has been associated with disorders of lateral uterine fusion that are either asymmetric or symmetric. Asymmetric anomalies are anatomically diverse and are most commonly seen as the unicornuate uterus. Symmetric anomalies of lateral fusion include the didelphic, bicornuate, and septate uteri, which are often collectively referred to as a "double uterus." Of all uterine anomalies, the septate uterus is the only one amenable to operative hysteroscopic treatment and thus receives the majority of attention in this chapter. In general, other uterine anomalies are not amenable to hysteroscopic revision.

The septate uterus is thought to occur when the mullerian ducts fuse properly but canalization is incomplete. The appearance of the remaining septum is highly variable and has been classified[4] as broad- (>3 cm) or narrow based, thin, or thick. The septum can protrude from the fundus downward only a short way (subseptate or incomplete uterine septum) or descend all the way through the cervix, giving the appearance of a "double cervix." Most commonly, the septum terminates near the level of the internal cervical os.

Septate uteri are associated with a higher incidence of fetal wastage than either the bicornuate or didelphic types, as high as 85% in some reports.[3] Various theories have been proposed to explain the increased fetal loss. The septum may be less vascular and more fibrous than normal myometrium, impeding proper implantation. This may also cause the endometrium covering the septum to be less responsive to hormonal stimuli. The septum may impede proper placental growth with associated early fetal loss or, rarely, development of intrauterine growth retardation (IUGR) if pregnancy continues. Finally, preterm labor and delivery as well as malpresentation occur at a higher frequency in pregnancies complicated by the septate uterus.

For the majority of the twentieth century the standard approach to correcting a septate uterus was by transabdominal surgery, employing either the Jones or Tompkins metroplasty technique. This approach was abandoned during the 1980s because of increasing evidence in favor of an equally successful hysteroscopic technique. This evidence has been validated in several large studies finding the hysteroscopic technique to be highly cost effective and of significantly less morbidity.[5,6] It can be performed in an outpatient setting and obviates the need for subsequent delivery by cesarean section. Finally, it does not carry the risk of postoperative pelvic adhesions, as do abdominal procedures, which may impede subsequent fertility.

The transcervical route for removal of a uterine septum is not new. In 1882 Schroder performed the transvaginal division of a septum in a patient with a history of pregnancy wastage. He blindly introduced two long stomach clamps into the uterine cavity, placing one anteriorly and the other posteriorly across the septum. The septum between the clamps was then divided with scissors. The clamps were left in place for 24 hr and then removed with minimal bleeding. Postoperatively the patient conceived within 1 month and carried a normal pregnancy. A number of other investigators subsequently reported removing uterine septa in a similar fashion.

Several recent case studies have proposed a hysteroscopic approach to mullerian anomalies other than the septate uterus. For example, a preliminary report of eight patients with malformations related to diethylstilbestrol (DES) exposure suggested selected patients may have an improved reproductive outcome after hysteroscopic revision of the uterine cavity.[7] Another report demonstrated the feasibility of managing symptomatic noncommunicating hematometria in three patients using hysteroscopic endometrial ablation of the rudimentary horn. In a 3-year follow-up, the patients remained symptom free without recurrence of hematometria or dysmenorrhea.[8] Although these initial reports involve only a few patients, they represent possible areas of expansion in the hysteroscopic management of uterine abnormalities.

Patient Selection and Diagnosis

Most septa are discovered during workup for a history of recurrent miscarriages, infertility, premature deliveries, or malpresentations. Occasionally, a septum is noted at the time of delivery, particularly during cesarean section or at dilation and curettage (D&C) for incomplete abortion. Less frequently, a particularly lengthy septum is noted on observing a divided cervix on pelvic exam or is detected in conjunction with a longitudinal vaginal septum. Importantly, the mere presence of a uterine septum in the absence of reproductive tract complaints does not warrant surgical intervention. It is also important to note that a septate uterus itself rarely causes difficulty in conceiving, and patients who complain of infertility should undergo a complete evaluation for other factors affecting fertility before undertaking corrective surgery.

The most important study in detecting these uterine malformations is the hysterosalpingogram (HSG). Unfortunately, the HSG cannot differentiate a bicornuate (Fig. 30.1) from a septate uterus (Fig. 30.2) because the difference between the two is in the shape of the fundus, which is not discernible with this radiographic study.

Generally, differentiation of septate versus bicornuate uterus is made during direct visualization of the uterine fundus with laparoscopy. Surgical correction then follows with the indicated hysteroscopic or abdominal procedure.

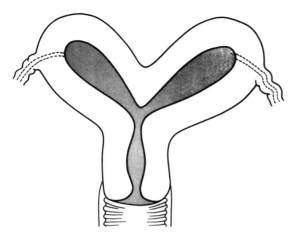

FIGURE 30.1. A bicornuate uterus, whose hysterosalpingogram (HSG) appearance is similar to that of the septate uterus (see Fig. 30.2). Laparoscopic examination of the uterine fundus is usually necessary to differentiate the two types of uterine malformations. Hysteroscopic surgery of a bicornuate uterus would quickly lead to fundal perforation without correcting the defect.

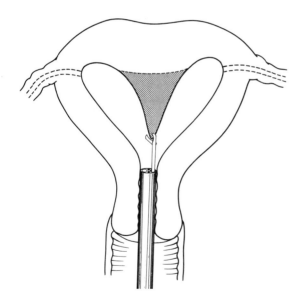

FIGURE 30.2. A typical subseptate uterus. The uterine fundus viewed laparoscopically is broad and may have an external "notch," giving it a slight bicornuate appearance. The septum is thin in its lower portion and widens near the fundus. This type of septum is easy to visualize and divide hysteroscopically. The hysteroscope is kept in the lower uterus to increase the field of vision, and the scissors are advanced as the division progresses.

More recently, sonographic or magnetic resonance imaging (MRI) studies have been used to establish the diagnosis preoperatively. Although adding to the overall diagnostic cost, particularly in the case of MRI, these studies are highly accurate (90% with ultrasound and 99% with MRI) and may provide important information necessary for preoperative counseling and surgical planning.[9,10]

Preoperative Evaluation

A preoperative HSG should always be obtained, even in those instances in which the septum has been diagnosed by prior hysteroscopy/laparoscopy. The HSG should be made available to the operator during surgery, because it provides a clear depiction of the length and thickness of the septum; this is particularly important as hysteroscopy is associated with a somewhat impaired depth perception. The HSG is especially useful when one uterine cavity is much smaller, or when the septum extends all the way through the cervix. Finally, an HSG provides a permanent record of the anomaly, establishing a baseline with which to assess adequacy of surgery.

Presurgical treatment of patients with danazol or a gonadotropin-releasing hormone (GnRH) agonist does not seem to be indicated given the relative avascularity of the uterine septum. A randomized study of 193 patients undergoing hysteroscopic metroplasty failed to demonstrate any difference in operative blood loss or reproductive outcome in patients treated with leuprolide acetate when compared to a similar untreated control group.[11]

As patients with mullerian fusion defects are at increased risk of also having congenital anomalies of the urinary tract, a preoperative intravenous pyelogram (IVP) is recommended. This study may reveal renal or collecting system anomalies in 10% to 20% of patients with septate uterus compared to a maximum of 50% to 65% in patients with more severe anomalies such as uterine agenesis, didelphis, or unicornuate uterus. Candidates for corrective surgery should be in good general health and exhibit no coagulopathy. They should discontinue oral contraceptives, aspirin, or other nonsteroidal antiinflammatory drugs at least 2 weeks before surgery. Patients undergoing this operation should have the desire to conceive and have a reproductively healthy male partner. There should be no other insurmountable or untreated cause of infertility present. All patients complaining of habitual losses must undergo a full evaluation of coexisting factors before surgical therapy.

Instrumentation

Although the following description of the technique of operative hysteroscopic metroplasty focuses on the use of scissors, either lasers or resectoscopes can be used to accomplish this division. Current studies have found no appreciable difference in outcome when comparing these instruments. Operator experience seems to be the most significant variable. These authors prefer to use 3-mm rigid scissors, through a large right-angle operating hysteroscope with 170° field of vision (Richard Wolf Company of Rosemont IL, 8931.31). These scissors do a better job of dividing the thicker septum encountered at the uterine fundus and in puncturing or cutting a hole in a complete septum when necessary (see following). The smaller 7-Fr. flexible scissors may be used for thinner septa. If the resectoscope is used, it is important to incise the septum and avoid creating a large defect by "shaving" the septal tissue as in a hysteroscopic myomectomy.

There are several choices of distending media for operative hysteroscopy (Chapter 26). This surgeon prefers Hyskon® (32% dextran-70, Pharmacia Laboratories, Piscataway, NJ) as it is not miscible with blood and has a good refractive index, providing excellent visualization. However, this medium has some drawbacks (Chapters 26 and 32). It may make handling of instruments difficult, and it is imperative that all equipment that comes in contact with Hyskon® be cleaned in hot soapy water immediately after use. The use of Hyskon® in gynecology has been associated with bleeding coagulopathy, adult respiratory distress syndrome, pulmonary edema, and allergic reactions including anaphylactic shock. Nonetheless, most adverse reactions have been associated with prolonged operating time and the use of large volumes of medium. It is recommended that the total volume of Hyskon® used be less than 300 ml per patient, regardless of operating time. Instruments that generate heat (e.g., resectoscopes and lasers) tend to carmelize the dextran-70.

Carbon dioxide (CO_2) as a distension medium is also quite popular, particularly in Europe, but visualization in the presence of bleeding may be inadequate. Fortunately, most septa are thin and relatively avascular. CO_2 is the appropriate distending medium when employing the CO_2 laser because its beam will not penetrate liquid. However, a significant complication of CO_2 distension may be rapid intravenous absorption, which can lead to air embolization and death, particularly when CO_2 is used to cool laser fibers. See Chapter 26 for a more in-depth discussion of distension media.

Solutions less viscous than Hyskon® can also be used as they provide reasonably good visualization and are easier to handle and administer. Solutions containing dextrose do not mix with blood quite as easy as those that do not. Larger volumes can be absorbed, and hyperglycemia and hyponatremia have been reported when using 5% dextrose and water.

Technique

The operation should be scheduled for the early follicular phase of the menstrual cycle, when the risk of pregnancy is minimal and endometrial visualization is optimal. In many instances a preoperative distinction between a bicornuate uterus and a septate uterus has not clearly been made. Laparoscopy, along with examination of the preoperative HSG, will establish the diagnosis and identify other pathology of the reproductive tract. Once the diagnosis of a septate uterus is confirmed, the laparoscope is left in place to monitor the hysteroscopic operation and to reduce the risk of perforation. Nonetheless, it is usually not necessary to perform the procedure under laparoscopic guidance unless the surgeon has limited experience. A speculum is then inserted into the vagina, and the cervix is exposed and grasped with a tenaculum.

Careful cervical dilation is extremely important to avoid bleeding that may obscure the operative field. A dilute vasopressin solution may be injected paracervically for hemostasis. The cervix should be dilated only enough to allow the insertion of the hysteroscope into the cavity, maintaining a tight fit around the instrument shaft, for good containment of the distending media. If there is not a snug fit, a double-tooth tenaculum or two single-tooth tenaculums, one on each side of the cervix, may be used. Alternatively, a pursestring suture may be placed around the cervix, to snug it around the hysteroscope and to serve for traction.

It is extremely important to maintain traction on the cervix throughout the procedure, keeping the long axis of the uterus parallel to the patient's sacrum. A flexed uterus is more likely to be perforated and is also associated with decreased visibility with rigid hysteroscopes. Once the hysteroscope is placed within the uterus, a full inspection of the cavities is performed, visualizing each tubal ostium for proper orientation. The inferior margin of the septum is then identified and divided transversely using rigid scissors (see Fig. 30.2). Successive bites of the septum are progressively taken upward, moving the hysteroscope from side to side (ostium to ostium). If the uterus is sharply anteverted or retroverted, care should be taken to follow the curve of the uterus. Otherwise, posterior or anterior perforation, respectively, is likely. There is no need to actually resect the septum or remove any tissue. Once the septum is divided in its midportion, the cut fibromuscular tissue retracts into the contiguous uterine wall.

Septal tissue is generally quite fibrous and avascular; as division approaches the fundal area, however, the septum becomes thicker and more vascular. Incision of the septum should be carried until normal myometrial tissue is identified, generally by its increased vascularity. However, because the liquid distension medium is being injected under pressure, the vascularity of the tissue may not be immediately apparent. It is wise to periodically reduce the distension pressure, observing for bleeding of the incised tissue. Once the incised tissue is noted to be relatively well vascularized, division is discontinued because the likelihood of uterine perforation increases.

If a laparoscope is in place, the intensity of the laparoscopic illumination is occasionally reduced throughout the procedure, allowing the observer to judge the thickness of the uterine fundus as a function of the amount of light transmitted through the hysteroscope. While laparoscopic observation will not guarantee against perforation, it allows early recognition of this complication, reducing the risk of additional injury to surrounding organs. Intraoperative ultrasound monitoring may be used to accurately determine remaining myometrial thickness and in difficult cases may prove to be a useful adjuvant technique.[12]

To maintain a good view of both cornual areas the surgeon must not insert the hysteroscope too far beyond the internal cervical os and should maintain this position relatively fixed, extending only the cutting scissors. Once the septum is divided near the cornu on each side, it is time to stop. Special care must be taken when a broad-based septum is encountered as it is difficult to keep both cornual areas visualized and to maintain proper orientation. Increased bleeding and uterine perforation are more likely to occur in this situation.

If the cervix appears "double" because of the length of the septum (Fig. 30.3), one can cut through the cervical portion of the septum using Metzenbaum scissors. However, there is some concern that this may later lead to an incompetent cervix, and if this division is performed, one should consider placing a cerclage in a subsequent pregnancy. The preferred technique is to insert the operative hysteroscope into one of the uterine cavities, preferably the larger one, cutting a hole through the septum near the level of the internal cervical os (Fig. 30.4). Once this has been accomplished, one can proceed to divide the upper portion of the septum, leaving the lower cervical portion of the septum intact. On occasion, a small opening may be already present in the septum, near the level of the internal os, and division can proceed upward from that point. Alternatively,

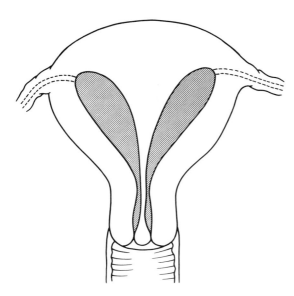

FIGURE 30.3. Complete septate uterus. The septum is thin and extends completely to the external cervical os.

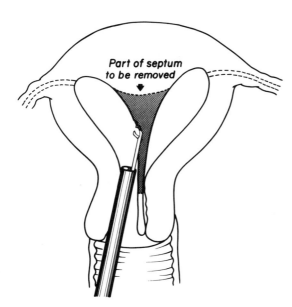

FIGURE 30.4. Hysteroscopic treatment of a complete septate uterus. The septum involves the upper cervix, and the lower margin is difficult to see. However, at laparoscopy both tubes and a normal fundus are visualized. An opening is made in the septum near the level of the cervical internal os and division proceeds as usual.

a no. 8 pediatric Foley catheter may be placed into the cervical canal opposite the hysteroscope to prevent loss of distending medium once the septum has been perforated.[13]

A different situation occurs when the septum is long but does not extend to the external os. With this abnormality, the surgeon may have some difficulty in identifying the lower septum margin and in having enough working room in front of the hysteroscope to allow the use of the scissors. As the lower cervix is often patulous, there may also be difficulty in being able to maintain adequate distension medium pressure. In this situation, Metzenbaum scissors can be used to blindly cut the lower portion of the septum. The hysteroscope is then reinserted and the operation proceeds as usual.

Occasionally a repeat hysteroscopic procedure may need to be performed for incomplete septum resection or because the metroplasty was prematurely terminated as a result of uterine perforation. While this is an inconvenience, it is preferable to incising the septum under unsafe conditions. The surgeon should always incise the septum under good surgical control to avoid serious uterine perforations, particularly in patients with exceedingly wide septa.

Complications

The primary complications of hysteroscopic metroplasty are perforation, bleeding, infection, and those complications related directly to the distending medium employed. The use of large volumes and prolonged operating time are major predisposing factors to the development of complications related to the distension medium.

Uterine perforations generally occur in the fundal area and present little problem with blood loss. In these instances, the procedure should be terminated as continued pressure from distension media may enlarge the perforation. Specific bleeding points at the perforation site can be cauterized with laparoscopic bipolar cautery. An alternate technique is to inject a 5- to 10-ml dilute solution of pitressin (20 mU in 30 ml 0.9% saline) into the uterine fundus, using a long spinal needle placed through the anterior abdominal wall under direct laparoscopic visualization. Hemostasis is usually rapidly apparent, and in general no further therapy is necessary. In fact, observation alone generally suffices for fundal perforations. Alternatively, if the perforation occurs laterally or in the region of the cornua or utero-ovarian ligament, brisk bleeding is likely and laparotomy for repair may be required.

While excessive bleeding from the septum division site is a concern, there is little need for hysteroscopic electrocautery. When excessive bleeding does occur, packing of the uterus or insertion of a balloon catheter to tamponade the uterine cavity is recommended. However, this is rarely necessary. Occasionally, transvaginal injection of pitressin into the myometrium can be used.

The risks of fluid overload and anaphylactic reactions associated with distension media are discussed in Chapter 32. Although these complications are usually related to prolonged operative time or failure to monitor total fluid intake, anomalous uterine vascularity may also play a role in excessive fluid or gas absorption. Fatal air embolism associated with improper use of a Hyskon pump has been reported.[14] Infusion pressures should remain less than 100 mmHg, and pumps should be turned off before changing fluid bottles. Pure gravitational infusion systems or handheld syringe infusion may be the safest alternative for the relatively brief metroplasty procedure. Complete familiarity with all equipment is a mandatory prerequisite for safe hysteroscopic surgery.

Although the operative field is certainly not sterile, infection does not appear to be a major problem with hysteroscopic metroplasties. Nevertheless, few data are available on the use of antibiotic prophylaxis. The authors prefer the administration of a single perioperative dose of a broad-spectrum antibiotic, similar to that employed in a routine vaginal hysterectomy.

Postoperative Care and Follow-up

In general, patients undergoing hysteroscopic metroplasty require little in the way of postoperative care. While the postoperative administration of supplemental estrogen has been mentioned, there are no data to support its use. In fact, a study of 19 patients found no significant synechiae during repeat hysteroscopy at various intervals after septoplasty.[15] If the operation is timed in the early follicular phase of the menstrual cycle, the physiologic preovulatory rise in estrogen levels would make the addition of supplemental estrogen unnecessary. In contrast to the situation noted in Asherman's syndrome (Chapter 27), the endometrial cavity in patients with a septate uterus has abundant healthy endometrium, allowing rapid regeneration.

Some have advocated the placement of an intrauterine device (IUD) or other device to separate the uterine walls following surgery. Again, there is no data to support this maneuver, which in theory could increase the risk of postoperative infection. A prospective study evaluating the use of postoperative estrogen and intrauterine devices (IUD) in 10 patients found this combined therapy to be of no benefit when compared to 10 untreated controls.[16]

It may be advisable to obtain a repeat HSG some 3 months after the procedure to compare to the original radiographs (Fig. 30.5). Frequently the contour of the uterine walls may be less than perfect, which is particularly true when the surgeon has corrected a relatively thick septum or a uterus with a broad fundus. Minor prominences giving the impression of a short septum or an arcuate fundus do not require additional surgical intervention. In fact, in one study residual septa of less than 1 cm were found to be clinically insignificant.[17] If intrauterine adhesions are detected, they are easily eliminated at a repeat hysteroscopy.

As has been previously mentioned, patients can and do become pregnant rather quickly following this operation. There is no need to prevent pregnancy for a period of time as in the case of a Jones or Tompkins abdominal metroplasty, and there is no need for a subsequent cesarean section. However, additional counseling must be undertaken if uterine perforation has occurred. Recently, several cases of poor obstetric outcome associated with spontaneous uterine rupture have been reported in patients with a history of uterine perforation during prior hysteroscopic

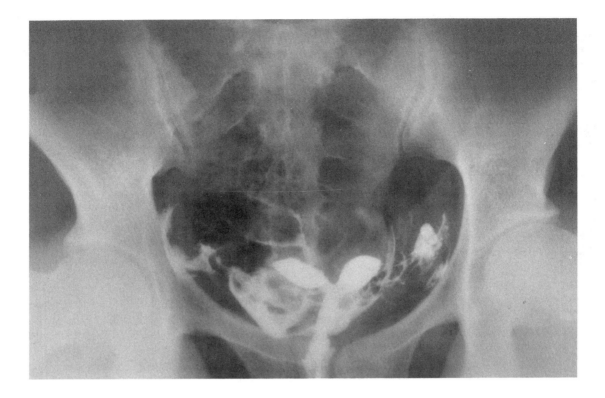

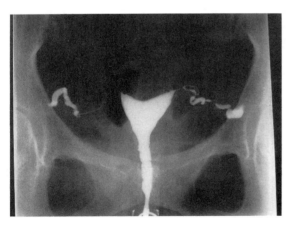

FIGURE 30.5. Preoperative (*top*) and postoperative (*bottom*) HSGs of patient with recurrent abortions and a septate uterus treated by hysteroscopic metroplasty.

procedures.[18] These cases highlight the need to lower the risk of perforation with concomitant laparoscopy or ultrasound monitoring and by maintaining good cervical traction. Although not reported in the literature, laparoscopic suturing of the puncture site using extracorporeal technique may theoretically reduce the risk of subsequent uterine rupture. Finally, given current data on preconceptual folic acid supplementation and the prevention of neural tube defects, we prescribe prenatal vitamins to our patients if they are actively attempting pregnancy.

Results

Several authors have reviewed the literature concerning transcervical division of the uterine septum.[19,20] It is apparent that the results of hysteroscopic metroplasty are excellent, either equal or superior to those obtained by transabdominal approaches. In patients complaining of recurrent fetal wastage and desiring a child, more than 85% have become pregnant, with 75% resulting in full-term live births. Alternatively, when patients have associated primary infertility the results are not nearly as good as only one-third of patients subsequently became pregnant, although almost two-thirds of these deliver a full-term liveborn. Generally, a residual septum of less than 1 cm is not considered to be clinically relevant.

Fewer than 5% of patients in the collected series required a repeat hysteroscopic procedure because of incomplete removal of the septum (residual septum generally greater than 1 cm). Of those patients experiencing an incompetent cervix, more than half had a preoperative history compatible with this disorder, which usually leads to the placement of a prophylactic cerclage in following pregnancies. Overall, replacement of abdominal metroplasty with the outpatient hysteroscopic technique represents a significant advance in the surgical treatment of uterine septae, one that has resulted in greatly improved patient outcome and reduced morbidity.

References

1. Ashton D, Amin HK, Richart RM, Neuwirth RS. The incidence of asymptomatic uterine anomalies in women undergoing transcervical tubal sterilization. *Obstet Gynecol.* 1988;72:28.
2. Rock JA, Jones HW Jr. The clinical management of the double uterus. *Fertil Steril.* 1977;28:798–806.
3. Rock JA, Sclaff WD. The obstetrical consequences of uterovaginal anomalies. *Fertil Steril.* 1985;43:681–692.
4. The American Fertility Society. American Fertility Society classification of Müllerian anomalies. *Fertil Steril.* 1988;49:952.
5. Daly DC, Maier D, Sotos-Albors C. Hysteroscopic metroplasty: six years experience. *Obstet Gynecol.* 1989;73:201–205.
6. Fedele L, Arcaini L, Parazzini F, Vercellini P, Di Nola G. Reproductive prognosis after hysteroscopic metroplasty in 102 women: a life table analysis. *Fertil Steril.* 1993;59:768–772.
7. Nagel TC, Malo JW. Hysteroscopic metroplasty in the DES exposed uterus and similar nonfusion anomalies: effects on subsequent reproductive performance; a preliminary report. *Fertil Steril.* 1993;59:502–506.
8. Hucke J, DeBruyne F, Campo RL, Freikha AA. Hysteroscopic treatment of congenital uterine malformations causing hematometria: a report of three cases. *Fertil Steril.* 1992;58:823–825.
9. Doyle MB. Magnetic resonance imaging in mullerian fusion defects. *J Reprod Med.* 1992;37:33–38.
10. Randolph J, Ying Y, Maier D, et al. Comparison of real-time ultrasonography, hysterosalpingography, and laparoscopy/hysteroscopy in the evaluation of uterine anomalies and tubal patency. *Fertil Steril.* 1986;46:828.
11. Perino A, Chianchiano N, Petronio M, Cittadini E. Role of leuprolide acetate depot in hysteroscopic surgery: a controlled study. *Fertil Steril.* 1993;59:507–510.
12. Querleu D, Brasme TL, Parmentier D. Ultrasound guided transcervical metroplasty. *Fertil Steril.* 1990;54:995–998.
13. Rock JA, Murphy A, Cooper W. Resectoscopic techniques of lysis of a class V complete uterine septum. *Fertil Steril.* 1987;48:495–496.
14. Nachum Z, Kol S, Adir Y, Melamed Y. Massive air embolism—a possible cause of death after operative hysteroscopy using a 32% dextran 70 pump. *Fertil Steril.* 1992;58:836–838.
15. Candiani GB, Vercellini P, Fedele L, Carinelli SG, Merlo D, Arcaini L. Repair of the uterine cavity after hysteroscopic septal incision. *Fertil Steril.* 1990;54:991–994.
16. Vercellini P, Vendola N, Colombo A, Passadore C, Trespidi L, Fedele L. Hysteroscopic metroplasty with resectoscope or microscissors for the correction of septate uterus. *Surg Gynecol Obstet.* 1993;176:439–442.
17. Fedele L, Bianchi S, Marchini M, Mezzopane R, Di Nola G, Tozzi L. Residual uterine septum of less than 1 cm after hysteroscopic metroplasty does not impair reproductive outcome. *Hum Repro.* 1996;11(4):727–729.
18. Howe RS. Third trimester uterine rupture following hysteroscopic uterine perforation. *Obstet Gynecol.* 1993;81(5, part 2):827–829.
19. Hassiakos DK, Zourlas PA. Transcervical division of uterine septa. *Obstet Gynecol Surv.* 1990;45:165–173.
20. Elchalal U, Schenker JG. Hysteroscopic resection of uterus septus versus abdominal metroplasty. *J Am Coll Surg.* 1994;178:637–644.

31

Transcervical Tubal Cannulation, Tuboplasty, and Falloposcopy

Eugene Katz

Etiology and Diagnosis of Proximal Tubal Occlusion

Etiology of Proximal Tubal Occlusion

Tubal disease is the cause of 25% to 30% of female infertility, of which approximately 20% is caused by occlusions located at the uterotubal junction.[1,2] Moreover, until recently one-fifth of laparotomies performed for tubal occlusion were done in connection with such occlusions.

The sequelae of salpingitis and salpingitis isthmic nodosa (SIN) appear to be responsible for the majority of proximal tubal occlusions. For instance, chronic salpingitis can be found in 40% to 60% of tubes being repaired for proximal occlusions.[3] More recently, chronic inflammation or its fibrotic sequelae were described in 60% of excised occluded proximal tubes.[4] SIN is present in 20% to 70% of such tubes,[5] and intramural endometriosis appears to play a role in proximal obstructions in 14% of cases.[4] In fact, remissions of proximal obstructions have been reported following dana-zol therapy.[6] Crystallized tubal secretions can also lead to proximal obstruction.[7] This finding may explain the high false-positive occlusion rate for hysterosalpingograms (HSGs) and provides the rationale for attempting to dislodge such plugs mechanically by cannulating the tubal lumen.

Diagnosis of Proximal Tubal Obstruction

The initial diagnosis of tubal obstructions is commonly made by HSG. Unfortunately, HSGs carry a false-positive rate of 15% to 40%.[8] It is therefore important to complement the HSG with chromotubation during laparoscopy. In fact, it is not uncommon to find a normal proximal tube at the time of surgery despite prior diagnosis of proximal tubal occlusion with both HSG and laparoscopy.[9–11] Several pharmacologic agents have been used to assist the passage of contrast media through the presumable spasmodic uterotubal junction during laparoscopy or HSG. Unfortunately, the administration of terbutaline[12], glucagon,[13] and isoxuprine[14] have not been clearly shown to be effective in alleviating such spasms.[15]

Transuterine Tubal Cannulation and Tuboplasty

Interest in transcervical/transuterine tubal sterilization stimulated research in direct cannulation of the fallopian tube. Interestingly, Smith had attempted in 1849 to pass whalebone sounds into the oviducts to treat infertility, the same year that other researchers reported a method of sterilization by applying silver nitrate to the cornual regions. More recently, Corfman and Taylor[16] described a balloon-tipped metal cannula to directly inject fluid into the tubes. The catheter was introduced into the uterine cavity and aimed at the uterine cornua before injection. Later, catheterization of the tubal ostia under hysteroscopic visualization was accomplished in an effort to occlude the fallopian tubes for contraception,[17] and Platia and Krudy reported the use of fluoroscopically guided wires to recannulize proximal obstructed tubes.[18] The idea was further developed by Thurmond et al.[19] and by Confino et al.[20]; the latter introduced the idea of the balloon dilatation technique, much like angioplasties for coronary artery disease. Tubal cannulation can be performed under fluoroscopy, under sonography, or via hysteroscopy.

Fluoroscopically Guided Tubal Cannulation

All forms of fluoroscopically guided procedures require an undistorted uterine cavity so as to reach the cornual portion of the tubes with the catheters.

Wire Catheterization System

Instruments and Technique

The wire catheterization system as described by Thurmond et al.[21] includes a "hysterocath," three coaxial catheters, three guidewires, and a Tuhoy–Borst adapter (Cook Ob/Gyn, Bloom-

ington, IN). The hysterocath consists of a central 25-cm-long, soft plastic shaft with a central conduit that is 5 mm wide and tapers to 2.5 mm at its acorn-shaped tip (Fig. 31.1). This plastic tube traverses a 2.5-cm-long, semiopaque soft plastic cup. When the sliding shaft is placed into the external os, the cup is slid over the cervix. Cups are available in 3 sizes (25, 30, and 35 mm) and include a side plastic conduit that attaches to a hand vacuum pump to keep the hysterocath in place.[22]

The procedure is performed under IV sedation and paracervical block. An HSG is initially performed through the hysterocath to confirm the diagnosis of proximal tubal obstruction. A 32-cm, 9-Fr. Teflon catheter is introduced though the hysterocath shaft and is placed under fluoroscopic control within the lower third of the uterine cavity. A 50-cm-long, 5.5-Fr. polyethylene catheter with a 3-cm tip curved to a 45° angle is introduced next. A 0.035-in.-diameter curved safe-T-J guidewire is placed inside the 5-Fr. catheter before insertion, and both catheter and guidewire are introduced through the 9-Fr. catheter and directed toward the uterine cornua. Before final

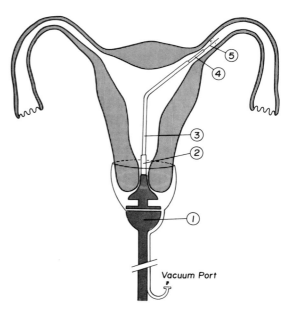

FIGURE 31.1.   Wire catheterization system in place. *1*, Hysterocath; *2*, 9-Fr. catheter; *3*, 5.5-Fr. catheter; *4*, 3-Fr. catheter; *5*, guidewire.

wedging of the catheter against the cornua, the curved wire is replaced by a 0.035-in. straight guidewire. The wire is then removed and a "selective HSG" is performed by injecting contrast medium directly into the tubal cornua.

If the obstruction persists, a 3-Fr. Teflon catheter with a 0.015-in.-diameter cope-mandril guidewire with platinum tip is advanced through the 5.5-Fr. catheter into the fallopian tube (Fig. 31.1). The tube is then probed with back-and-forth movements of the guidewire. When the obstruction is successfully negotiated, the wire is removed and contrast medium is injected through the 3-Fr. catheter. Additional cannulation equipment that can be used if a second distal isthmic obstruction is encountered consists of an even smaller catheter tapering from 3 Fr. to 2.2 Fr. with a guidewire also tapering from 0.016 to 0.013 in. This equipment is used in a fashion similar to the 3-Fr. catheter and wire described. A similar system, consisting of a curved introducing catheter to fit the tubal ostium, a 3-Fr. catheter tapered to 2.4 Fr. distally, and a metal position-ing mandrel, is available as separate compo-nents (Conceptus San Carlos, CA).

Results

Thurmond reported 100 consecutive patients with uni- or bilateral proximal tubal obstruc-tion diagnosed by a single HSG. In this study, the procedure succeeded in opening at least one tube in 86% of the patients, with a 5% inci-dence of uncomplicated tubal perforations. Only 20 patients presented with bilateral proxi-mal obstruction and no other known con-tributing factors to their infertility. In 19 (95%) of these patients, wire catheterization suc-ceeded in opening at least 1 tube; 24 of 39 (89%) tubes were opened, and 9 pregnancies (45%) occurred within 6 months. Only 8 non-pregnant patients returned for a 2- to 8-month follow-up HSG. Reocclusion had occurred bi-laterally in 4 patients (50%) and unilaterally in 2 patients (25%).

Using a similar system, Thompson et al. re-ported the recanalization of 9 of 29 (31%) of proximally obstructed tubes in 28 patients. Eight tubes were found to be obstructed dis-tally as well. Of 8 patients undergoing an HSG 6 to 9 months post surgery, 4 had patent tubes. There were four intrauterine pregnancies in the group.[23]

Transcervical Balloon Tuboplasty

Instruments and Technique

The transcervical balloon tuboplasty (TBT) system (Bard Reproductive Systems, Billerica, MA) consists of an HSG or introducing catheter, an angle guiding or "selective salpin-gography" catheter with a radiopaque tip, a balloon tuboplasty catheter, a wireguide, an in-flation device, and a Tuhoy–Borst adapter (Fig. 31.2). The HSG introducing catheter has a central lumen with a side lumen that allows the injection of contrast media. In addition, two in-flation cuffs are connected to balloons proxi-mal and distal to the cervical os (Fig. 31.2).

The procedure can be done under IV seda-tion or under general anesthesia with the pa-tient in lithotomy position. After cleansing of the cervix with Betadine, the anterior lip of the cervix is grasped with a single-toothed tenacu-lum. The HSG catheter is then introduced into the lower uterine segment and the distal bal-loon inflated with 5 ml of normal saline. The distal balloon is wedged against the internal os and the proximal balloon is then inflated; this stabilizes the catheter and seals the cavity. The presence of a proximal tubal obstruction is confirmed by injecting contrast medium through the central lumen of the HSG catheter. A 2.5-mm guiding catheter is then in-troduced through the central lumen of the HSG catheter and directed toward the tubal os-tium. This catheter has a preshaped curve that allows the operator to position it at the cornua with little difficulty. A "selective HSG" is per-formed by injecting contrast medium directly into the tube through the guiding catheter. If the obstruction is confirmed, a balloon tubo-plasty is performed.

The balloon tuboplasty catheter has a 1-mm-thick shaft with a central lumen. A second lu-men is connected to a small balloon that sur-rounds the distal portion of the catheter. The balloon is available in different diameters (2 and 3 mm) and in different lengths (Fig. 31.3). The longer, but thinner, variety is used in early

FIGURE 31.2. Components of the balloon tuboplasty system. *Left to right:* introducing catheter, guiding catheter, guidewire, and balloon tuboplasty catheter. (*Not shown:* inflation device and Tuhoy–Borst Y-connector.)

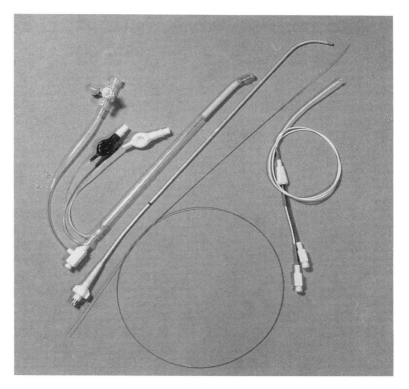

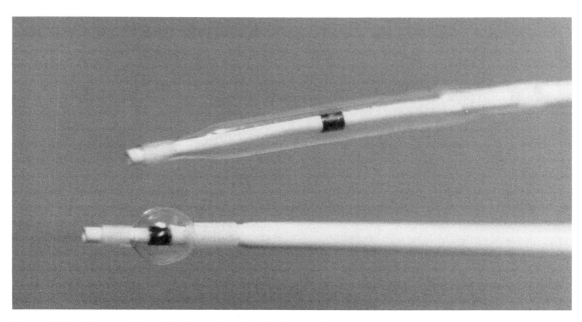

FIGURE 31.3. Two varieties of balloon-tipped tuboplasty catheters.

isthmic segments, while the larger and shorter versions are recommended for obstructions of the cornual portions of the tube. Proximally, the second lumen is connected to an inflation device with a manometer to avoid overinflation and rupture of the balloon (Fig. 31.4). Contrast medium and a 0.6-mm wireguide are introduced through the central lumen of the balloon tuboplasty catheter. Proximally, the guidewire is introduced through the straight lumen of a Tuhoy–Borst Y-connector, the side lumen of which is used for injecting contrast media.

Before insertion, the balloon is purged of air and primed gently with either saline or contrast medium. The balloon is then connected to the manometer and vacuum is applied. A syringe with contrast medium is attached to the side arm of the Tuhoy–Borst Y connector, and a soft-tipped guidewire loaded through the central lumen of the balloon catheter until the wireguide tip extends 1 to 2 mm beyond the balloon. The wireguide is then locked into position by securing the Tuhoy–Borst connector. The entire assembly is then introduced through the guiding catheter already in the cornual portion of the uterus (Fig. 31.4). The

balloon catheter is advanced to the obstructed area. Often, the catheter negotiates the tubal lumen without difficulty. If an obstruction is encountered, the balloon catheter is inflated to 4 to 5 atmospheres. Medium is then injected through the straight arm of the Y-connector. When the obstruction is in the tubal isthmus, the wireguide can be advanced into the strictured area, the TBT catheter tracked over the guidewire, and the balloon inflated. Advancement and ballooning can be repeated until recanalization is achieved.

Results

Among all the fluoroscopically and hysteroscopically guided tubal cannulation procedures, the TBT has been the most systematically studied. In a multicenter evaluation of the TBT system, 77 women underwent this procedure.[24] All had been previously diagnosed with bilateral tubal occlusion by both an HSG and laparoscopic chromotubation. In 92% of the patients, at least one tube was recannulized. Among 64 patients with no other factors for infertility, a 34% pregnancy rate was reported after a median follow-up of 12 months. This represents a 38% pregnancy rate for those subjects whose tubes were successfully recannulized. Although one ectopic pregnancy occurred, it was located distal to the site of the initial obstruction. Unfortunately, despite the fact that this system underwent the most rigorous scientific evaluation of all the cannulation procedures available, it is no longer manufactured in the United States.

Sonographically Directed Tubal Cannulation

In an attempt to avoid the potential risk of radiation, particularly on the ovaries, associated with fluoroscopy, color Doppler has been used to guide the cannulation of proximally obstructed tubes. Using a coaxial catheter containing a 0.016-in. flexible wire, Bustillo et al.,[25] successfully negotiated the obstruction in 24 of 25 tubes (96%) of 13 women with bilateral proximal tubal obstruction. Five women (38%) achieved pregnancies within 1 year after the procedure.

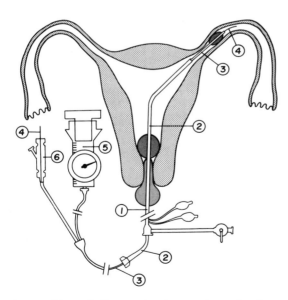

FIGURE 31.4. Balloon tuboplasty catheter in place. 1, Introducing catheter; 2, guiding catheter; 3, balloon tuboplasty catheter; 4, guidewire; 5, inflation device; 6, Tuhoy–Borst Y-connector.

Hysteroscopically Guided Tubal Cannulation

Instruments and Technique

The procedure described by Novy uses CO_2 as the distending media for the rigid hysteroscope and concomitant laparoscopy. A 30-cm-long, 5.5-Fr. clear Teflon catheter with a metal obturator is introduced into the uterine cavity through the operating channel of the hysteroscope (Cook Ob/Gyn, Bloomington, IN). A Y-adaptor ending in Luer-lock hubs is attached to its proximal end. The straight arm is used to inject dye or irrigation fluid, and is sealed with a screw cap when not in use. The other arm has an adjustable O-ring through which a 3-Fr. catheter will be introduced (Fig. 31.5). This 3-Fr. catheter is tapered to 2.5 Fr. at its distal 3 cm.

A Teflon-coated stainless steel guidewire, 0.018 in. in diameter with a flexible blunt tip, is placed into the lumen of the 3-Fr. catheter. The 5.5-Fr. catheter is placed at the tubal ostium under hysteroscopic visualization. The 3-Fr. catheter and guidewire are introduced next, with the wire protruding slightly from the catheter tip. If resistance is met, the catheter is advanced over the guidewire, the wire is removed, and dye (methylene blue or indigo carmine) is injected. Visualization of dye or the catheter tip through the fimbriated end of the tube by laparoscopy signals a successful cannulation. The procedure can also be performed using a flexible hysteroscope.

Results

Novy et al. reported the successful cannulation of 11 of 12 tubes in 10 patients.[26] Five subjects presented with bilateral proximal occlusion, and 3 had a unilateral obstruction with an absent contralateral tube. The pregnancy rate in patients with bilateral proximal obstruction has not been reported to date.

Conclusions

Multiple studies have demonstrated that traditional tubal surgery for proximal tubal obstruction carries a pregnancy rate that at best does not exceed 40%. In addition, such surgery requires a lengthier hospitalization and recuperative time. It is therefore anticipated that some of these proximal tubal surgeries will soon be replaced by transcervical tubal cannulation.

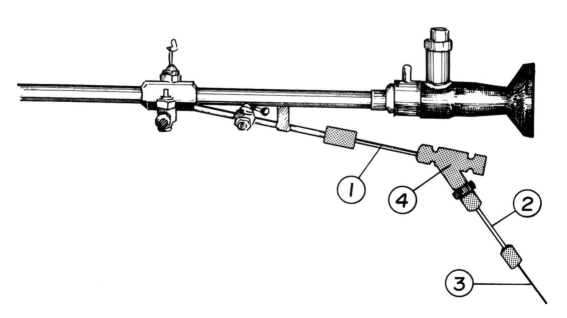

FIGURE 31.5. Wire catheterization system introduced through an operating hysteroscope. *1*, 5.5-Fr. catheter; *2*, 3-Fr. catheter; *3*, guidewire; *4*, Y-connector.

Transcervical tubal cannulation should be offered to patients with proximal tubal obstruction before attempting laparotomy repair or in vitro fertilization.

Falloposcopy

New instrumentation is currently being developed to visually explore the lumen of the fallopian tubes. The system as described by Kerin et al.[27] consists of a 30-cm-long operating hysteroscopy with an outside diameter (OD) of 3.3 mm and an accessory operating channel (1.8 mm in internal diameter). The proximal 25 cm of the hysteroscope is semirigid and the distal 5 cm is flexible and steerable (Olympus Corp., Lake Success, NY). The falloposcope is a miniature fiberoptic endoscope with an OD of 0.5 mm that is guided into the lumen of the fallopian tube through the operating channel of the flexible hysteroscope.

The flexible hysteroscope is introduced into the uterine cavity and directed toward the tubal ostia. A Teflon-coated, floppy, stainless steel, platinum-tipped, tapered guidewire (similar to that described for hysteroscopic cannulation) is introduced through the operating channel of the hysteroscope into the fallopian tube for about 15 cm or until resistance is met. A 1.2- to 1.3-mm-OD Teflon catheter is then introduced over the entirety of the guidewire and the wire subsequently removed. A Tuhoy–Borst Y connector is placed at the proximal end of the catheter, and the falloscope is introduced through one arm of the connector into the catheter. The other arm of the connector is used to irrigate and minimally distend the tube, thus facilitating visualization. Cannulation is not always possible because of the tortuosity of some otherwise normal tubal lumens.

In-office falloposcopies can be well tolerated by patients.[28] A hands-free cannulation technique without the need for a hysteroscopy is also possible.[29] The procedure is diagnostic in that it provides information about the tubal lumen and is possibly therapeutic if debris or intraluminal adhesions are mechanically disrupted.[30] Nevertheless, falloposcopy is not yet widely used. Large studies in fertile women have yet to be conducted to better assess the significance of the findings described in infertile patients, and its definitive diagnostic value remains to be defined.

References

1. Musich JR, Behrman SJ. Surgical management of tubal obstruction of the uterotubal junction. *Fertil Steril.* 1983;40:423–441.
2. Holst N, Abyholm T, Borgerson A. Hysterosalpingography in the evaluation of infertility. *Acta Radiol.* 1983;24:253–257.
3. Grant A. Infertility surgery of the oviduct. *Fertil Steril.* 1971;22:496–503.
4. Fortier KJ, Haney AF. The pathologic spectrum of utero-tubal junction obstruction. *Obstet Gynecol.* 1985;65:93–98.
5. Hellman LM. Tubal plastic operations. *J Obstet Gynaecol Br Commonw.* 1956;68:852–860.
6. Ayers JW. Hormonal therapy for tubal occlusion: Danazol and tubal endometriosis. *Fertil Steril.* 1982;38:748–750.
7. Sulak PJ, Letterie GS, Coddington CC, et al. Histology of proximal tubal occlusion. *Fertil Steril.* 1987;48:437–440.
8. World Health Organization. Comparative trial of tubal insufflation, hysterosalpingogram and laparoscopy with dye hydrotubation for assessment of tubal patency. *Fertil Steril.* 1986;46:1101–1102.
9. Musich JR, Behrman SJ. Infertility laparoscopy in perspective: review of 500 cases. *J Obstet Gynaecol.* 1982;143:293–303.
10. Hutchins CJ. Laparoscopy and hysterosalpingography in the assessment of tubal patency. *Obstet Gynecol.* 1977;49:327–328.
11. Okonofua FE, Essen UI, Nimalaraj T. Hysterosalpingography versus laparoscopy and tubal infertility: comparison based on findings at laparotomy. *Int J Gynecol Obstet.* 1989;28:143–147.
12. Thurmond AS, Novy, Rosch J. Terbutaline in diagnosis of interstitial fallopian tubal obstruction. *Invest Radiol.* 1988;23:209–210.
13. Winfield AC, Pittaway D, Maxson W, Daniel G, et al. Apparent cornual occlusion by hysterosalpingography: reversal by glucagon. *AJR* 1982;139:525–527.
14. Page EP. Use of isoxuprine in uterosalpingography and uterotubal insufflation. *Am J Obstet Gynecol.* 1968;101:358–364.
15. Cooper JM, Rigberg HS, Houck R, et al. Incidence, significance and remission of tubal

spasm during attempted hysteroscopic tubal sterilization. *J Reprod Med.* 1985;30:9–13.

16. Corfman PA, Taylor HC. An instrument for transcervical treatment of the oviducts and uterine cornua. *Obstet Gynecol.* 1966;27: 880–884.

17. Siegler AM, Haulka J, Peretz A. Reversibility of female sterilization. *Fertil Steril.* 1985;43: 499–510.

18. Platia MP, Krudy AG. Transvaginal laparoscopic recanalization of approximately occluded oviduct. *Fertil Steril.* 1985;44:704–706.

19. Thurmond AS, Novy M, Uchida BT, et al. Fallopian tube obstruction: selective salpingography and recanalization. *Radiology.* 1987;163: 511–514.

20. Confino E, Friberg I, Gleicher N. Transcervical balloon tuboplasty. *Fertil Steril.* 1986;46: 963–966.

21. Thurmond AS, Rosch J. Nonsurgical tube recanalization for treatment of infertility. *Radiology* 1990;174:371–374.

22. Thurmond AS, Uchida BT, Rosch J. Device for hysterosalpingography for fallopian tube catheterization. *Radiology* 1990;174:571–572.

23. Thompson KA, Kiltz RJ, Koci T, Cabus ET, Kletzky OA. Transcervical fallopian tube catheterization and recanalization for tubal obstruction. *Fertil Steril.* 1994;61:243–247.

24. Confino E, Tur-Kaspa I, DeCherney A, et al. Transcervical balloon tuboplasty. A multicenter study. *JAMA.* 1990;264:2079–2082.

25. Bustillo M, Coulam CB. Colour Doppler ultrasound guidance for wire tuboplasty. *Hum Reprod.* 1993;8:1715–1718.

26. Novy ML, Thurmond AS, Patton P, et al. Diagnosis of cornual obstruction by transcervical fallopian tube cannulation. *Fertil Steril.* 1988;50: 434–440.

27. Kerin J, Daykhovsky L, Segalowitz J, et al. Falloscopy: a microendoscopic technique for visual exploration of the human fallopian tube from the uterotubal ostium to the fimbria using a transvaginal approach. *Fertil Steril.* 1990;54: 390–400.

28. Ingleson B, Hartman D, Dodd C. A comparison of pain experienced during hysterosalpingography and in-office falloposcopy. *Fertil Steril.* 1994; 62:67–70.

29. Pennehouat G, Risquez F, Naouri M, Thebault Y, Gugliemina JN, Deval B, Moya B, Madelenat P. Transcervical falloposcopy; preliminary experience. *Hum Reprod.* 1993;8:445–489.

30. Kerin JF, Williams DB, San Roman GA, Pearlstone AC, Grundfest WS, Surrey ES. Falloscopic classification and treatment of fallopian tube lumen disease. *Fertil Steril.* 1992;57: 731–741.

32

Minimizing, Recognizing, and Managing Hysteroscopic Complications

Samuel Smith

Although hysteroscopic complications are uncommon, they are potentially severe. This chapter focuses on the prevention, recognition, and management of the most common complications associated with hysteroscopy. For a more detailed discussion, see Corfman et al.[1]

Complications of Operative Hysteroscopy

The American Association of Gynecologic Laparoscopists (AAGL) 1991 membership survey on operative hysteroscopy had a 15% response rate (Table 32.1).[2] The complication most commonly reported was uterine perforation not requiring blood transfusion (11.1 per 1000 procedures). The overall major complication rate, excluding benign uterine perforations, was 13.7 per 1000 procedures.[2] Compared to the 1988 AAGL survey, laparotomies to manage hemorrhage and bowel and urinary tract injuries, as well as CO_2 embolism and procedure-related deaths, were more common.[3] Although simple perforation, water intoxication, and pulmonary edema were less common, more serious complications such as bowel and urinary tract injury, CO_2 embolism, and death were reported with disturbing frequency in 1991.

Performing the procedure in a patient who has an undiagnosed pregnancy is a possible adverse occurrence during hysteroscopy. This complication is best avoided by scheduling procedures before ovulation and asking the patient to practice barrier contraception. Thermal injury to the intestinal tract without uterine perforation can also occur during operative hysteroscopy. Peritonitis developing postoperatively as a result of this type of injury is managed by laparotomy and bowel resection.[4]

Complications Related to Distension Media

The distension media most widely used for hysteroscopy are carbon dioxide (CO_2), 32% dextran-70 (Hyskon), 5% dextrose in water, and other nonelectrolyte solutions such as glycine or sorbitol. Any of the aforementioned

TABLE 32.1 Complications of operative hysteroscopy: data from the 1988 and 1991 AAGL surveys.

	Rate/1000 procedures		
Complication	1988	1991	Change, 1988 to 1991
Uterine perforation not requiring transfusion	13.0	11.1	−0.9-fold
Water intoxication or pulmonary edema	3.4	1.4	−0.4-fold
Hospital readmission	1.5	0.9	−0.6-fold
Hemorrhage requiring transfusion	1.0	0.3	−0.3-fold
Laparotomy to manage hemorrhage	0.5	1.4	1.4-fold
Nerve injuries	0.5	0.1	−0.2-fold
Laparotomy to manage bowel or urinary tract injury	0	0.3	
CO_2 embolism	0	0.1	
Death	0	0.1	

Adapted from Peterson HB, Hulka JF, Phillips JM. American Association of Gynecologic Laparoscopists 1988 membership survey on operative hysteroscopy. *J Reprod Med.* 1990:35;590–591; and Hulka JF, Peterson HB, Phillips JM, Surrey MW. Operative hysteroscopy: American Association of Gynecologic Laparoscopists 1991 membership survey. *J Reprod Med.* 1993;38:572–573

liquid media may be used for operative hysteroscopy because visualization is satisfactory and they do not conduct electrical current.

Intravascular intravasation of Hyskon, a high-viscosity liquid, has been associated with anaphylaxis, disseminated intravascular coagulation, adult respiratory distress syndrome, and noncardiogenic pulmonary edema.[5-10] Risks of pulmonary edema are increased when a hysteroscopic procedure lasts more than 45 mins, large areas of endometrium are traumatized, more than 500 ml of Hyskon is infused, or infusion pressures exceed 150 mmHg.[9] Hyskon is a plasma expander, and when it enters the vascular system it draws more than sixfold its volume of extracellular fluid into the patient's vascular space, thus predisposing her to hyperoncotic pulmonary edema.[9,10] Limiting Hyskon infusions to less than 300 ml and infusion pressure to less than 100 mmHg reduces the risks of pulmonary edema, adult respiratory distress syndrome (ARDS), and disseminated intravascular coagulation (DIC) by reducing the amount of Hyskon absorbed into the patient's bloodstream.[5-10] At present, it is unclear whether ARDS and DIC are idiosyncratic reactions to Hyskon or are related to fluid overload.[8-10]

Treatment of pulmonary edema is symptomatic with oxygen, diuresis, and other supportive measures. Treatment may be protracted because of the long half-life of Hyskon.[8,9] In very severe cases with renal failure, plasmapheresis may be necessary to remove Hyskon from the circulation.[7] ARDS is treated similarly, but ventilation support may be necessary.[8,9] DIC is managed with replacement of coagulation factors.

Anaphylaxis can occur regardless of the volume of Hyskon used. When an anaphylactic reaction is diagnosed, Hyskon infusion should be discontinued immediately and treatment with epinephrine (intratracheal and intravenous), hydrocortisone, or antihistamines initiated.[8] The risk of anaphylaxis can be reduced by the intravenous administration of dextran-1 (Promit, Medisan Pharmaceuticals, Inc., Parsippany, NJ) before surgery.

Low-viscosity liquids such as glycine, sorbitol, dextrose, saline, and Ringer's lactate have largely replaced Hyskon for operative hysteroscopy procedures and are used in continuous-flow systems. Electrosurgical instruments, such as the resectoscope, cannot be used with saline or lactated Ringer's because their electrolytes will conduct the electrical current and dissipate it throughout the uterine cavity. Current can also be carried into the peritoneal cavity.[8,9]

Solutions of 1.5% glycine and 3% sorbitol have become the mainstay of operative hysteroscopy procedures. Absorption of large volumes of these liquids into the circulation can cause significant morbidity. Originally called the "post-transurethral resection of prostate (TURP) syndrome" by urologists, hyper-volemia, dilutional hyponatremia, and decreased serum osmolarity associated with excessive absorption of these fluids induces bradycardia and hypertension with subsequent hypotension, pulmonary edema, and cerebral edema. Symptoms consist of nausea, vomiting, headache, respiratory distress, visual disturbances, agitation, cognitive dysfunction, lethargy, and seizures.[8,9] Coma, cardiovascular collapse, and death have occurred in severe cases.

The basic underlying feature is water intoxication, and treatment involves diuresis of excess fluid and correction of the hyponatremia (Fig. 32.1). Asymptomatic patients may be treated with water restriction until spontaneous diuresis occurs, but this is risky because seizures and respiratory arrest can occur abruptly without warning.[8,11,12] Even though it is now agreed that therapy should be initiated promptly, there are only general treatment guidelines available. Serum sodium should be raised slowly over several hours, at 1 to 2 mEq/liter per hour and generally not more than 12 mEq/liter in a 24-hr period. Intravenous administration of normal or hypertonic saline solution is used in combination with diuretics such as furosemide or mannitol. Urine output is monitored with a Foley catheter, which helps to guide the rate of infusion of saline solution.[8]

The length of the hysteroscopic procedure, as well as the amount of raw uterine surface created, are important factors predisposing to dilutional hyponatremia.[13] Infusion of chilled distension medium, which promotes vasoconstriction, under low pressure through a cervix that is slightly overdilated to facilitate egress of the medium are safety measures that may reduce the risk of dilutional hyponatremia. Fluid intake and output through the continuous-flow hysteroscope need to be monitored frequently

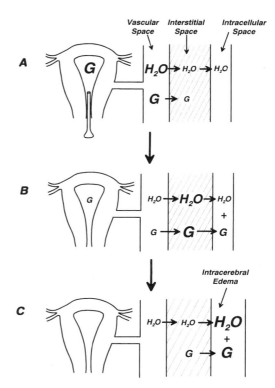

FIGURE 32.1. Development of cerebral edema after absorption of glycine irrigation fluid. **A:** Glycine is absorbed into the intravascular space, moves into the interstitial space, and finally passes into cells. **B:** Intravascular osmolarity decreases, and as a result water moves preferentially into the interstitial and intracellular spaces. **C:** Intravascular hypoosmolarity promotes the movement of water across the blood–brain barrier into the intracerebral space causing cerebral edema. (Modified from Witz CA, Silverberg KM, Burns WN, Schenken RS, Olive DL. Complications associated with the absorption of hysteroscopic fluid media. *Fertil Steril* 1993;60: 745–56. Reproduced with permission of the publisher, the American Society for Reproductive Medicine [Formerly the American Fertility Society].)

during the procedure, and furosemide (Lasix) is given intraoperatively if an excess of distension medium is absorbed into the circulation. In general, 10 mg of furosemide is given when urologic fluid intake exceeds output by 1000 ml. Electrolytes should be checked in the recovery room after the procedure.

In addition to morbidity associated with hyponatremia and hypoosmolarity, ammonia toxicity may occur with the use of glycine solutions. Some patients metabolize glycine rapidly and produce ammonia, which can cause central nervous system (CNS) symptoms.[8] Glycine can also act as an inhibitory neurotransmitter to interfere with retinal function and cause transient visual impairments.[8]

Carbon dioxide (CO_2) is generally a safe distension medium for diagnostic hysteroscopy. However, if excessive CO_2 insufflation rates are used, fatal cardiac irregularity and cardiac arrest, can occur. Hysteroscopic insufflators should not exceed 100 ml CO_2/min for this reason.[9] Fatal gas embolism has also been reported in association with the use of CO_2 as the distension medium for hysteroscopic laser procedures[4,14]; the Food and Drug Administration now discourages the use of CO_2 for uterine distension during hysteroscopic laser procedures.

Air Embolism

Air embolism is an infrequent but life-threatening complication of operative hysteroscopy. In a recently published series of five patients, four died and the fifth sustained permanent brain damage.[15] During operative hysteroscopic procedures, uterine venous channels are opened. Room air can enter these vessels through the vagina and cervix via the speculum and possibly the uterine manipulators. The clinical presentation is variable and will depend on the amount of air, the position of the patient, and the size of the air bubbles.[16] Gas embolism should be suspected if there is sudden development of acute cardiovascular/respiratory symptoms such as marked bradycardia, marked hypotension, significant decrease in oxygen saturation, cyanosis, or asystole. With a slight or steep Trendelenburg position, gas accumulates in the heart and pulmonary tree; pressure in the right side of the heart increases and cardiac output from the left side of the heart decreases. Cardiac auscultation typically reveals a "millwheel" murmur caused by the mixing of gas with blood, and frothy blood can be aspirated from the heart.

Gas bubbles trapped in the microcirculation may cause late manifestations such as DIC. The brain is the main target for gas emboli when the head is higher than the heart. Neurologic symptoms such as seizures, loss of consciousness, paralysis, visual symptoms, and altered sensorium can occur. The earliest clinical sign of gas embolism is a precipitous decrease in end-tidal CO_2 as blood flow to the lungs decreases. If CO_2 or air embolism is suspected, the insufflator should be turned off, intrauterine instruments removed, and the open cervix and vagina occluded with packing. The patient should be placed in the Trendelenburg position to protect the brain. Emergency resuscitative measures include 100% oxygen and IV fluids until the patient can be transferred to a hyperbaric treatment facility. Prompt recognition, diagnosis, and treatment may be life saving.[15,16]

Complications Related to the Surgical Procedure

Cervical dilatation can be complicated by formation of false passages and tenaculum tears. Uterine perforation can occur during cervical dilatation, during the insertion of the hysteroscope, or during the operative portion of the procedure. If not immediately recognized, uterine perforation should be suspected if large volumes of media fail to distend the uterus. Perforations may be managed expectantly, although laparoscopic assessment is indicated if intraabdominal or broad ligament bleeding or intestinal damage is suspected. The management of uterine perforations is outlined next.

Trauma to intraabdominal organs can occur even in the absence of uterine perforation. For example, the Nd:YAG laser has caused thermal intestinal injury during the course of endometrial ablation procedures.[17] Laser energy can be transmitted through an intact uterine wall to adjacent loops of intestine or bladder.

Finally, acute pelvic infection may occur after operative hysteroscopy. This is a very uncommon occurrence unless the procedure is performed in a patient who has an unrecognized infection. If a patient develops peritonitis following a procedure in which thermal or laser energy was used, the surgeon should also consider the possibility of intestinal damage.

Uterine Perforations

Uterine perforation may complicate any endoscopic surgery and can occur during the insertion of uterine manipulators, uterine manipulation per se, or hysteroscopic surgery. If a uterine perforation is suspected, the procedure should be discontinued. Using electrosurgery or the Nd:YAG laser inside the uterus after a perforation has occurred will increase the risk for adjacent bowel, bladder, or vascular injury (Fig. 32.2).[18,19] If there is a possibility of bowel or other organ damage, a laparoscopy should be performed. Alternatively, it may be elected to observe the patient. Damage to the integrity of the uterine cavity generally prevents continuation of the hysteroscopic procedure because of leakage of gas or dextran. If the intrauterine procedure must be continued, as in the case of incomplete removal of products of conception, a concomitant laparoscopy is performed.

Anterior and posterior wall and fundal perforations do not usually bleed much, and bipolar electrocoagulation of the bleeding site generally achieves hemostasis. In contrast, perforations in the cornual region tend to bleed more vigorously. Electrocoagulation can usually obtain hemostasis, but extensive tubal destruction can result. Microfibrillar collagen (Aviten) may also be used to secure hemostasis in this area. If this fails, and the patient desires preservation of fertility, suturing of the injured site laparoscopically or by laparotomy is indicated. Perforations of the lateral uterine wall are usually concealed between the layers of the broad ligament and may become evident only when a hematoma distends the ligament. If a broad ligament hematoma is observed, a laparotomy should be performed, the area carefully dissected, and the ureter identified before ligation of the uterine artery.[20] Bowel, bladder, and vascular injuries are repaired as described in Chapter 24.

Uterine perforations are best avoided by gentle insertion of the hysteroscope under direct vision. If laparoscopy is to be performed concomitantly, abdominal access should be established first. Laparoscopy during difficult hysteroscopic procedures decreases the incidence of uterine perforations and prevents additional damage should this occur. Fortunately, perforation sites are usually small and heal without remote adverse consequences. How-

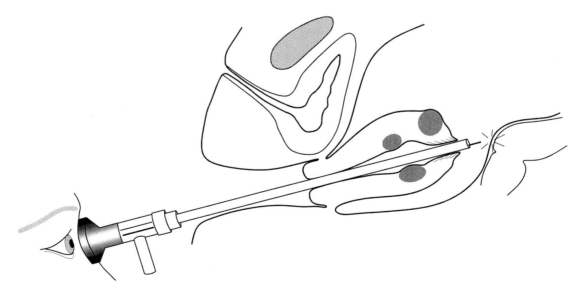

FIGURE 32.2.   Uterine perforation occurring during an operative procedure to resect submucous uterine fibroids. The Nd:YAG laser can damage the bowel even though the fiber does not directly contact the intestines.

ever, catastrophic uterine rupture during pregnancy has occurred after uterine perforation at operative hysteroscopy.[21] Women suffering seemingly innocuous uterine perforations during hysteroscopy procedures should be advised of this rare complication.[21]

Conclusions

Hysteroscopic complications are infrequent but potentially severe. Most complications associated with the uterine distension media are avoidable, although idiosyncratic reactions may occur. The surgeon must be able to recognize and manage complications associated with the distension media as well as procedurally related complication. Laparoscopy and laparotomy may occasionally be required to evaluate and manage intraperitoneal complications, and the surgeon should not hesitate to use them to evaluate suspected injury.

References

1. Corfman RS, Diamond MP, DeCherney A, eds. *Complications of Laparoscopy and Hysteroscopy.* Cambridge: Blackwell Scientific Publishers; 1993.

2. Hulka JF, Peterson HB, Phillips JM, Surrey MW. Operative hysteroscopy: American Association of Gynecologic Laparoscopists 1991 membership survey. *J Reprod Med.* 1993;38:572–573.

3. Peterson HB, Hulka JF, Phillips JM. American Association of Gynecologic Laparoscopists' 1988 membership survey on operative hysteroscopy. *J Reprod Med.* 1990;35:590–591.

4. Siegler AM, Valle RF. Therapeutic hysteroscopic procedures. *Fertil Steril.* 1988;50:685–701.

5. Jedeikin R, Olsfanger D, Kessler I. Disseminated intravascular coagulopathy and adult respiratory distress syndrome: life-threatening complications of hysteroscopy. *Am J Obstet Gynecol.* 1990;162:44–45.

6. Leake JF, Murphy AA, Zacur HA. Noncardiogenic pulmonary edema: a complication of operative hysteroscopy. *Fertil Steril.* 1987;48:497–499.

7. McLucas B. Hyskon complications in hysteroscopic surgery. *Obstet Gynecol Rev.* 1991;46:196–200.

8. Witz CA, Silverberg KM, Burns WN, Schenken RS, Olive DL. Complications associated with the absorption of hysteroscopic fluid media. *Fertil Steril.* 1993;60:745–756.

9. Loffler FD. Complications from uterine distention during hysteroscopy. In: Corfman RS, Diamond MP, DeCherney A, eds. *Complications of Laparoscopy and Hysteroscopy.* Cambridge: Blackwell Scientific Publishers; 1993:177–186.

10. Managar D, Gerson JI, Constantine RM, Lenzi V. Pulmonary edema and coagulopathy due to Hyskon (32% dextran 70) administration. *Anesth Analg.* 1989;68:686–687.

11. Arieff AE. Hyponatremia, convulsions, respiratory arrest, and permanent brain damage after elective surgery in healthy women. *N Engl J Med.* 1986;314:1529–1535.

12. Carson SA, Hubert GD, Schriock ED, Buster JE. Hyperglycemia and hyponatremia during operative hysteroscopy with 5% dextrose in water distention. *Fertil Steril.* 1989;51:341–343.

13. Istre O, Skajaa K, Schjoensby AP, Forman A. Changes in serum electrolytes after transcervical resection of endometrium and submucous fibroids with use of glycine 1.5% for uterine irrigation. *Obstet Gynecol.* 1992;80:218–222.

14. Brundin J, Thomasson K. Cardiac gas embolism during carbon dioxide hysteroscopy: risk and management. *Eur J Obstet Gynecol Reprod Biol.* 1989;33:241–245.

15. Corson SL, Brooks PG, Soderstrom RM. Gynecologic endoscopic gas embolism. *Fertil Steril.* 1996;65:529–533.

16. Weissman A, Kol S, Peretz BA. Gas embolism in obstetrics and gynecology: a review. *J Reprod Med.* 1996;41:103–111.

17. Perry CP, Daniell JF, Gimpelson RJ. Bowel injury from Nd:YAG endometrial ablation. *J Gynecol Surg.* 1990;6:199–203.

18. Sullivan B, Kenney P, Seibel M. Hysteroscopic resection of fibroid with thermal injury to sigmoid. *Obstet Gynecol.* 1992;80:546–547.

19. March CM. Hysteroscopy. *J Reprod Med.* 1992;37:293–312.

20. Borten M. *Laparoscopic Complications: Prevention and Management.* Philadelphia: BC Decker; 1980.

21. Howe RS. Third-trimester uterine rupture following hysteroscopic uterine perforation. *Obstet Gynecol.* 1993;81:827–829.

Index